WS 115 WAT

(23).

50·00

MMB

45·00

20/11/92

D1643447

Protein-energy malnutrition

John C Waterlow, CMG, MD, ScD, FRCP (London), FRS
Emeritus Professor of Human Nutrition, London School of Hygiene and Tropical Medicine, University of London

with contributions by
Andrew M Tomkins MB, FRCP (London)
Professor of International Child Health,
Institute of Child Health, University of London
and
Sally M Grantham-McGregor MD, DPH
Professor of Child Health, Tropical Metabolism Research Unit,
University of the West Indies, Kingston, Jamaica

Edward Arnold
A division of Hodder & Stoughton
LONDON MELBOURNE AUCKLAND

© 1992 J C Waterlow

First published in Great Britain 1992

British Library Cataloguing in Publication Data
Waterlow, J. C.
  Protein-energy malnutrition.—2nd ed.
  I. Title   II. McGregor, Sally
  III. Tomkins, Andrew
  616.3009172

ISBN 0-340-50127-8

Whilst the advice and information in this book is believed to be
true and accurate at the date of going to press, neither the author
nor the publisher can accept any legal responsibility or liability for
any errors or omissions that may be made.

Typeset in 10/11pt Linotron Times Roman by
Rowland Phototypesetting Limited, Bury St Edmunds, Suffolk
Printed and bound in Great Britain for Edward Arnold,
a division of Hodder and Stoughton Limited, Mill Road, Dunton Green,
Sevenoaks, Kent TN13 2YA by St Edmundsbury Press Limited,
Bury St Edmunds, Suffolk and Hartnoll Limited, Bodmin, Cornwall

Contents

Foreword   vii

1 Protein-energy malnutrition:general introduction   1
   A note on history   1
   Nomenclature   3
   Classification   5
   Multiplicity of causes   9

2 Some general questions   14
   What is meant by deficiency?   14
   Bases of reference   15
   Adaptation   21
   Analysis of associations   22

3 Body composition and body water   26
   Changes in organ pattern   26
   Changes in chemical composition   28
   Clinical implications of changes in body water   35

4 Electrolytes and major minerals   40
   Introduction   40
   Potassium   41
   Sodium   44
   Calcium   45
   Magnesium   48
   Phosphorus   49

5 Effects of PEM on structure and function of organs   54
   Cardiac function   54

Anaemia   58
Liver   61
Pancreas   65
Gastrointestinal tract   66
Kidney   69
Skin and hair   71
The nervous system   74

6 Metabolic changes   83
Energy metabolism   83
Nitrogen metabolism   89
Albumin metabolism   97

7 Biochemical measurements for the assessment of PEM   104
Introduction   104
Early detection of PEM and the search for 'sensitive' tests   104
Measures of severity and prognosis   106
Biochemical distinction between kwashiorkor and marasmus   107
Estimates of protein intake from the partition of urinary nitrogen 108

8 Endocrine changes in severe PEM   112
Introduction   112
Insulin and blood sugar   113
Glucocorticoids   115
Growth hormone   116
Somatomedins   117
Thyroid hormones   121

9 Trace elements   126
Introduction   126
Zinc   127
Copper   130
Selenium   131
Conclusion   132

10 Cell membranes and free radicals   136
Changes in cell membranes   136
Free radicals in the pathogenesis of kwashiorkor   138

11 Causes of oedema and its relation to kwashiorkor 146
Causes of oedema 146
Aetiology of kwashiorkor 154

12 Treatment of severe PEM 164
Where should children be treated? 164
Treatment 167
Phase 1: treatment of acute complications 168
Phase 2: initiation of cure 172
Phase 3: rehabilitation 177

13 Nutrition and growth 187
Introduction 187
Classification of growth deficits 188
Growth standards and references 191
Natural history of stunting 195
Causes of retardation of linear growth 200
Functional consequences and associations of stunting 202
The question of adaptation 203

14 Assessment of nutritional state in the community 212
Introduction 212
Measurements, indices and indicators 212
Analysis and presentation of data 216
Applications of anthropometric data 220

15 Energy and protein requirements of infants and young children 222
Energy requirements 222
Protein requirements 241
Energy and protein requirements for catch-up growth 251

16 Breast feeding and weaning 260
Introduction 260
Volume of breast milk 261
Energy and protein content of breast milk 265
Factors affecting the volume and composition of breast milk 267
Protective factors in breast milk 270
Protective effect of breast feeding—the epidemiological evidence 272

Adequacy of exclusive breast feeding 273
Supplementary feeding 275
Duration of partial breast feeding 279
Diet at and after weaning 281

17 Nutrition and infection (in collaboration with A M Tomkins) 290

Outline of the problem 290
General mechanisms of response to infection and their effect
on nutritional state 292
Effects of specific infections and pathological states 296
Specific nutrient deficiencies and the development and
course of infections 309
Nutritional state and morbidity 311
Long-term effects of infection on growth 313

18 Malnutrition and mortality 325

Introduction 325
Patterns of infant mortality 328
Patterns of child mortality 331
Effect of low birth weight on mortality 331
Contribution of PEM to mortality 333
Anthropometric assessment of the risk of death 336

19 The effect of malnutrition on mental development (by S M Grantham-McGregor) 344

Introduction 344
Effect of undernutrition on behaviour 344
Studies of severely malnourished children 348
Studies of mild to moderate malnutrition 354

20 Prevention of protein-energy malnutrition 361

Introduction 361
The political and economic background 362
The contribution of developed countries 364
Strategies for prevention 365
Primary health care and community participation 381
Conclusion 386

Index 393

Foreword

This is the third book on protein-energy malnutrition that has been published by Edward Arnold. The first was the classic *Kwashiorkor* by Trowell, Davies and Dean, published in 1954 and reproduced by the Nutrition Foundation of America in 1982. This book, although it was centred on the authors' observations in Uganda, provided for the first time a wide survey of the world literature on malnutrition in children. In the second book, published in 1977, there were six co-authors from the two Medical Research Council Units in Uganda and Jamaica (Alleyne *et al.*, 1977). This work differed from the earlier one in two ways: in the 1960s and 70s a great deal of new information had been produced in many parts of the world on the biochemical and endocrine changes in PEM, which needed to be summarized, because earlier fairly extensive reviews (Waterlow *et al.*, 1960; Waterlow and Alleyne, 1971) were already out of date. Secondly, the Uganda group had given much attention to PEM in the community—how and why it developed and how it should be treated and prevented. It was important to describe current thinking and experience on those topics.

When about four years ago I was invited to produce a new book, I had many doubts. Factors in favour were that the earlier volumes were out of print and hard to obtain; that there were a number of new ideas about the pathophysiology of PEM; above all, that the time was ripe for a more extensive review of the public health and community aspects of PEM. Although subjects such as protein and energy requirements, the assessment of nutritional state and the interactions of nutrition and infection had been well documented in many specialized reviews and books, they had never been brought together in one volume. Moreover, it might be useful to give some account of the heated debates in the last two decades on strategy and tactics for the prevention of PEM. On the opposing side was the difficulty of undertaking such a formidable task, particularly since my own experience has for the most part been of the clinical and biomedical aspects of PEM and it could be argued nowadays that these are largely irrelevant.

However, I decided to have a go and to try to produce a book that might be interesting and useful to physicians and public health workers, especially in Third World countries, even if it did no more than act as a source of references. That in itself presents a difficulty; it is impossible to be comprehensive over such a wide field, and the choice of papers that are quoted inevitably reflects my own contacts and my own bias. To those authors whom I have neglected I can but extend my apologies. Some readers may feel that it is unnecessary to recall once again older work that has been discussed in previous books and reviews, but I think that it is impossible to do justice to any topic without some reference to the historical background. The pioneers should not be forgotten, particularly since they were often working under very difficult conditions. I have also not hesitated to express my own views on subjects that are controversial. The important point is not that the reader should agree with those views, but rather that he or she should realize that differences of opinions exist, and perhaps be stimulated to undertake studies that might resolve those differences.

Professor Andrew Tomkins made a major contribution to the chapter on nutrition and infection (Chapter 17) and Professor Sally Grantham-McGregor has been entirely responsible for the chapter on the effects of malnutrition on mental development (Chapter 19). These are subjects on which I have little first-hand knowledge, but they are essential for the balance of the book. For the rest I must take full responsibility, but I should like to record my gratitude to my colleagues, too numerous to mention individually, in the Tropical Metabolism Research Unit, Jamaica, and the Department of Human Nutrition, London School of Hygiene and Tropical Medicine, whose research and ideas have been a continuing stimulus over more than forty years.

References

Alleyne, G. A. O., Hay, R. W. *et al.* (1977). *Protein-energy malnutrition*. Edward Arnold, London.

Trowell, H. C., Davies, J. N. P., Dean, R. F. A. (1954). *Kwashiorkor*. Edward Arnold, London. Reprinted 1982 by Academic Press, New York.

Waterlow, J. C., Alleyne, G. A. O. (1971). Protein malnutrition: advances in knowledge in the last ten years. *Advances in Protein Chemistry* **25**: 117–241.

Waterlow, J. C., Cravioto, J., Stephen, J. M. L. (1960). Protein malnutrition in man. *Advances in Protein Chemistry* **15**: 131–238.

1
Protein-energy malnutrition: general introduction

A note on history

We use the term 'severe protein-energy malnutrition' (PEM) to cover a spectrum of clinical pictures, ranging from frank kwashiorkor to severe marasmus. The description of kwashiorkor (Table 1.1) given by Williams in her first published article (1933) is as vivid and accurate today as it was more than 50 years ago, although she did not introduce the name kwashiorkor until her second paper in 1935.

The earliest account of the syndrome that we have been able to trace was published by Hinajosa in Mexico in 1865. After that there seems to be a gap, because the older literature in Latin America is not readily accessible and has not been seriously researched.

The book *Kwashiorkor* published in 1954 by Trowell, a physician, Davies, a pathologist and Dean, a paediatrician, is one of the classics of our subject. Trowell gives a very full account of the early history of kwashiorkor and of the controversies surrounding it, with a list of papers published up to that time. A short account that brings us closer to the present time is included in a recent history of paediatrics (Waterlow, 1991). The highlights in the development of knowledge and ideas about kwashiorkor are summarized in Table 1.2.

Table 1.1 Characteristics of children with kwashiorkor as described by Williams, 1933

Age   1–4 years
History of an 'abnormal' diet; breast-feeding by an old or pregnant woman with supplementary feeds of maize paps
Oedema
Wasting
Diarrhoea
Sores of mucous membranes
Desquamation of skin on legs and forearms
'Diffluent' fatty liver
Uniformly fatal unless treated

Table 1.2 Highlights in the history of kwashiorkor

1865	Hinajosa's first description (Mexico).
1890–1910	Nutritional oedema in infants described in Germany, France and England.
1920s–1930s	Many descriptions of kwashiorkor and childhood oedema from Latin America, Central Africa and China.
1933	Williams' first paper from the Gold Coast.
1935	Williams introduces the name 'Kwashiorkor'.
1940s	'Infantile pellagra' (Uganda) and 'Fatty liver disease' (West Indies) recognized as kwashiorkor. Kwashiorkor and nutritional oedema in infants described in several countries of Europe after World War II.
1950s	First descriptions of kwashiorkor from India. Surveys by FAO/WHO in Africa, Central America and Brazil.
1954	Publication of *Kwashiorkor* by Trowell, Davies and Dean (Uganda).
1959	Introduction of term 'Protein-calorie malnutrition' (Jelliffe).
1950s–1960s	Peak period of *clinical* research: in Uganda, Belgian Congo, Cairo, Cape Town, Hyderabad, Calcutta, Thailand, Mexico, Guatemala, Jamaica, Chile. General acceptance of theory of protein deficiency.
1960s	Development of high protein weaning foods promoted by UN Agencies.
1968	Gopalan questions protein deficiency theory.
1970	Wellcome classification introduced.
1973	Publication of FAO/WHO report on energy and protein requirements. Protein deficiency begins to seem irrelevant. Increasing attention to energy deficiency.
1970s	Increasing interest in community assessment, anthropometry and the effect of infections (Scrimshaw).
1980s	Concentration on community nutrition and primary health care.
Late 1980s:	Development of free radical theory of kwashiorkor (Golden).

Williams' two papers were not the first description of the kwashiorkor syndrome in this century. As Trowell's list shows, in the 1920s and 1930s there were many accounts of what was later recognized to be kwashiorkor from Latin America and Africa, particularly the then Belgian Congo. In the early 1950s it was described from India (Achar, 1950; Gopalan and Patwardhan, 1951). The United Nations Organizations were quick off the mark and organized surveys in Africa (Brock and Autret, 1952), Central America (Autret and Behar, 1955) and Brazil (Waterlow and Vergara, 1956).

It was soon recognized that kwashiorkor was worldwide, nor was it confined to countries that may be described as tropical. It occurred in Italy, Greece and Hungary in the near-famine conditions of the last war; and it was reported from Egypt, Turkey and countries of the Middle East, although not as commonly as marasmus. Since oedema is such an important feature of kwashiorkor, the parallel was drawn with the nutritional oedema of infants described by paediatricians in Germany, France and England in the early years of the century, and to which Czerny and Keller (1925) gave the name 'flour-feeding injury'. Thus it would seem that not only is kwashiorkor ubiquitous but that it has probably always been with us, appearing wherever and whenever there is poverty, deprivation and inadequate infant feeding.

We are inclined, following Williams, to think of the kwashiorkor syndrome as occurring mainly in young children. However, it is very clear from earlier accounts that the condition was often seen in older children also, and Trowell *et al.* (1954) devoted a whole chapter to protein-energy malnutrition in adults. There are many reports from India (e.g. Gopalan *et al.*, 1952) of nutritional oedema in adults, which do not seem to differ in any important way from kwashiorkor in young children. This is a controversial subject. McCance

(1951), in his exhaustive discussion of famine oedema in adults, claimed that it was not the same as kwashiorkor. He laid particular emphasis on energy deficit as the main cause (see Chapter 11). However, the Indian workers reported that there were 'important differences between the conditions [in adults] observed here and in [post-war] Europe, probably arising from the fact that the subjects here have suffered from a more prolonged and severe dietary restriction' (Srikantia *et al.*, 1953).

Nomenclature

Names are important and the history of their use is illuminating. Asher (1986) has justly said that a disease does not exist until it has a name. Broadly, names are of two kinds, descriptive and causal, and medical science aims to move from one to the other. For names used as code names to conjure up a syndrome or clinical picture the original meaning of the word is not important. We recognize cirrhosis of the liver without having to know that in Greek it means tawny, and we can recognize kwashiorkor without having to know that in the Ga language of West Africa it could be translated as 'the disease of the deposed child' (Williams, 1935).

Trowell *et al.* (1954) listed some 70 names that have been applied in different parts of the world to the condition that we now call kwashiorkor. Why, then, out of all these choices did the obscure dialect name proposed by Williams in her second paper (1935) gain such wide acceptance? And why is it still used today?

The general acceptance probably depended on two factors: first, the description was in English, and most anglophone workers did not read or did not have access to the papers published in French or Spanish. As recently as 1979 Fondu *et al.*, working in Zaïre, remarked: 'We sometimes feel that papers of non-English speaking people are systematically ignored by some authors.' A second reason for the widespread acceptance of 'kwashiorkor' was perhaps that it first appeared in a paper published in the *Lancet*, an international journal of general medicine (Williams, 1935). Virtually all the previous accounts had been either in local journals or in journals devoted to tropical medicine. Thus to Asher's dictum that before a disease can exist it must have a name we might add that the name must also be published in a widely read journal.

The next stage is the transition from descriptive to causal names. The early Latin American workers generally regarded what we call kwashiorkor as a multiple deficiency state (distrofia pluricarencial or polycarencial). In the scientific climate of the 1930s, when the attention of nutritional scientists was largely concentrated on the vitamins, it was natural to suppose that the oedema might be a manifestation of beri-beri and the skin lesions of pellagra. As early as 1926 Normet, working in Indo-China, proposed that the oedema of children, described as 'la bouffissure d'Annam' was a result of protein deficiency. He cited as evidence the fact that they had a decreased urinary urea excretion—perhaps the first application of biochemistry to the study of kwashiorkor. Williams' work implicitly supported the theory of protein deficiency, with her description of kwashiorkor developing in children fed starchy paps after being deposed from the breast, and being cured by milk. She quite clearly regarded this as the most likely cause. In 1963 she said explicitly: 'kwashiorkor is a disease primarily due to protein deficiency' (Williams, 1963). Although there were for a time dissenting voices, as evidenced, for example, by the controversy over infantile pellagra (Trowell, 1941), by the 1950s the concept of protein deficiency became fully established as the cause of kwashiorkor in tropical countries, even if it was not clear what role it played in hunger oedema of adults.

Thus the causal name 'protein malnutrition' was born (e.g. Jamaica Conference, 1955) and seemed ready to supersede the name kwashiorkor which Williams herself described as 'cacophonous'.

It did not, however, hold the field for very long. Marasmus has been recognized for centuries (Gürson and Saner, 1982), and although it is less spectacular than kwashiorkor, it is probably far commoner in many parts of the world. If marasmus is in fact semi-starvation, marasmic children must be deficient in protein as well as energy. Moreover, dietary studies began to show that children who developed kwashiorkor had inadequate intakes of energy as well as of protein. This led to the concept of a spectrum of combined deficiency, with protein being most limiting at the kwashiorkor end and energy at the marasmus end. The natural consequence was that 'protein malnutrition' was modified to protein-calorie malnutrition (PCM) or protein-energy malnutrition (PEM) to cover the whole range of malnutrition, other than states caused primarily by deficiencies of specific nutrients (Jelliffe, 1959). Recently there has been a move to supersede PEM with the term 'energy-nutrient malnutrition' (ENM), which gives pride of place to energy deficiency and subsumes protein among all other nutrients. The wheel has turned full circle, back to the 'multiple deficiency syndrome' of the early Latin American workers.

Here we are not concerned with whether the changing views on causality implied by these names are correct: that question will be dealt with later (Chapter 11). We are concerned only with their general implication. Blanket names such as PEM and ENM have advantages and disadvantages. The disadvantage is that they ignore real differences. To the clinician kwashiorkor and marasmus are different, and names are needed to describe them and to stimulate us to find out why they are different. For this reason we still talk of kwashiorkor even after more than 50 years.

The strength of the general names is that they relate to causes, and not to clinical pictures. Thus it is possible to think about subclinical or early deficiency states and to accept that fully developed clinical malnutrition is only the tip of the iceberg. One can talk of subclinical ascorbic acid deficiency, but not of subclinical scurvy. The general names, by avoiding specificity, carry the implication that particular types and causes of malnutrition are of little importance compared with the general causes—poverty and deprivation. These blanket names therefore have moved us inexorably from the clinical to the public health approach and the history of names mirrors the history of ideas in this field.

Classification

For practical purposes the two approaches, clinical and public health, require different types of classification. The distinction between kwashiorkor and marasmus is essentially qualitative; the assessment of 'subclinical' PEM in the community must be quantitative and is based on weight and height. That subject is discussed in a later chapter (Chapter 14). Here we are concerned with severe PEM. An early attempt at classification is shown in Table 1.3.

Table 1.3 An early attempt to distinguish systematically between kwashiorkor and marasmus

	Fatty liver disease	Undernourished without liver damage
Number of children	15	21
Number with BSP retention[a]	14	0
Number with:		
palpable liver	14	5
oedema	11	1
glossitis	11	5
angular stomatitis	7	1
cheilosis	8	2
'mosaic' skin	6	3
raised serum bilirubin	8	1
Mean weight, % of standard	68	50
Mean haemoglobin, % of Haldane standard	56	60
Mean serum total protein, g/dl	4.5	5.7
Mean serum alkaline phosphatase, KA units	19.7	19.4
Liver fat, % of wet weight	40.2	4.6
	(4 cases)	(6 cases)

From Waterlow (1948)
[a] Bromsulphthalein

In the decades after the war, when paediatricians all over the world were describing slightly different pictures of childhood malnutrition as they saw it in hospitals, the question naturally arose: what exactly are the criteria for the diagnosis of kwashiorkor and its distinction from marasmus? Many children present features of both; many cases of kwashiorkor have some but not all the characteristics listed in Table 1.1. Different workers put emphasis on different factors: Trowell (1941), impressed by the skin lesions, suggested the causal name 'infantile pellagra'. Waterlow (1948) described cases seen in the Caribbean as 'fatty liver disease'. Brock and Autret (1952) insisted that the *sine qua non* for the diagnosis of kwashiorkor was discoloured, reddish hair. McLaren *et al.* (1967) proposed a scoring system by which points were given for different clinical features, including low serum albumin, so that marasmus had a low score and kwashiorkor a high score. The situation could only be described as chaotic. The Wellcome Trust came to the rescue by promoting a symposium in Jamaica in 1969 to reach an agreed definition of these forms of severe PEM.

It turned out that there was only one characteristic other than weight deficit which all participants agreed must be present for the diagnosis of kwashiorkor, namely oedema. It was accepted that marasmus simply represents a severe loss of body weight; the cut-off point was taken at 60 per cent of the expected weight for age by the Harvard standard. These two characteristics led to the two-way classification that has been called the Wellcome classification (Table 1.4) (Wellcome Trust Working Party, 1970). On this system one could logically abandon the name kwashiorkor and substitute 'oedematous malnutrition'.

Table 1.4 The Wellcome Classification of severe protein-energy malnutrition

Weight for age (% of expected[a])	Oedema	
	Present	Absent
80–60	Kwashiorkor	Undernutrition
< 60	Marasmic kwashiorkor	Marasmus

[a] Expected weight for age by Harvard standards

The basic premise of this classification is that the presence or absence of oedema has some interest and importance. If oedema is not important, the classification is pointless. Because of its simplicity it inevitably has some disadvantages. Obviously weight is distorted by the presence of oedema, although this can be allowed for by using the minimum weight after oedema is lost. More serious is that the classification takes no account of length or height. A child may be 60 per cent of expected or normal weight for age either because it is very wasted or because it is very small—the so-called 'nutritional dwarf'. The two conditions are quite different (Chapter 14), and this ambiguity about the definition of marasmus has led to much confusion. Bhattacharyya (1981, 1986) attempted to get round the problem of including both qualitative and quantitative characteristics with a classification containing 16 cells, which is rather too complicated for general use. However, it has the important merit of drawing attention to chronicity and recurrence. In Calcutta Bhattacharyya probably sees a wider spectrum of PEM than in most other places nowadays. McLaren (1984) has given an excellent general account of the problems of classification and aetiology, based on his experience in Lebanon.

The fact that clinical signs other than oedema, such as fatty liver and dermatosis, are ignored in the Wellcome classification is less serious. Although these characteristics are not always present, in Jamaica a statistically significant association was found of fatty liver with oedema (Waterlow et al., 1957), and it is clear from the data of McLaren et al. (1967) in the Lebanon that there was a strong association of dermatosis with oedema. This association was reported also by Golden et al. (1985) in Jamaica and by Coulter et al. (1988) in the Sudan. Bhattacharyya (1972) said that the dermatosis of kwashiorkor was never seen in the absence of oedema, although oedema may occur without dermatosis. He suggested that 'the presence of a considerable amount of subcutaneous fat seemed to be essential for the development of dermatosis'.

Crude though the Wellcome classification is, it has valuable uses. It has directed attention to the prevalence of marasmus, which tended to be ignored because kwashiorkor is so much more dramatic. It can be used to compare the relative prevalences of marasmus, marasmic kwashiorkor and kwashiorkor in different places; a few examples are shown in Table 1.5. Certainly these figures, taken from hospital admissions, are subject to selection bias, but nevertheless they have a certain interest. The classification can be used to tabulate and compare systematically the characteristics of the different types of PEM as they present at hospital or clinic. As one example, the age on admission is of obvious interest in relation to natural history and cause. In India a substantial number of cases of kwashiorkor and marasmic kwashiorkor were more than three years old (Bhattacharyya, 1986). Of 43 cases, mostly of marasmic kwashiorkor, reported by Vis *et al.* (1965) in Zaïre, more than half were over three years old, with many up to six or eight years, whereas in Jamaica the average age of admission is around one year. By contrast, in Chile kwashiorkor has virtually disappeared; PEM presents only as marasmus, and almost always below one year (Mönckeberg, 1988). Marasmus usually, but not always, presents at a younger age than kwashiorkor (Table 1.6).

Table 1.5 Relative prevalence (%) of marasmus, marasmic kwashiorkor and kwashiorkor in some hospital series

Country	Marasmus	Marasmic kwashiorkor	Kwashiorkor	Reference
India	35	21	43	Chaudhuri *et al.* (1961)
India	18	31	51	Bhattachariyya (1986)
Jamaica	40	24	35	Garrow (1966)
Uganda	12	16	72	Wharton (1973)
Turkey	84	11	5	Gürson *et al.* (1975)
Lesotho	37	14	49	Tolboom *et al.* (1986)
Sudan	38	27	35	Coulter *et al.* (1988)

Table 1.6 Age of children on admission to hospital

Country and reference	Mean age (months)		
	Marasmus	Marasmic kwashiorkor	Kwashiorkor
Jamaica (Garrow, 1966)	11.7	–	12.5
Jamaica (Waterlow and Rutishauser, 1974)	11.4	12.8	12.7
Jordan (McLaren, 1966)	7.7	20.7	rare
Baghdad (Shakir *et al.*, 1972)	16.9	21.8	21.0
India (Chaudhuri *et al.*, 1961)[a]	25.5	22.0	21.6
Lesotho (Tolboom *et al.*, 1986)	12.3	17.5	20.2

[a] Estimated; cases below 3 years only.

Another difference of interest is that the deficit in linear growth tends to be greater in marasmus than in kwashiorkor (Waterlow and Rutishauser, 1974) (Table 1.7). Considerations of this kind have led us to suggest a differ-

Table 1.7   Length for age in children with PEM in Jamaica and Baghdad

| | Length for age (% of standard[a]) | |
	Jamaica	Baghdad[b]
Marasmus	86	83.5
Marasmic kwashiorkor	84.5	79.5
Kwashiorkor	92	87

Mean age was about 9 months greater in Baghdad than in Jamaica.
[a] 50th centile Harvard standard
[b] From Shakir *et al.* (1972)

ence in the natural history of these two forms of PEM, depicted schematically in Fig. 1.1. According to this scheme, in marasmus the onset of malnutrition would be earlier and the duration longer, perhaps as a result of repeated and long-lasting episodes of gastroenteritis in addition to inadequate food, whereas kwashiorkor is typically precipitated by an acute infection such as measles. The Wellcome classification could be used, but seldom has been, to examine environmental and social differences between the two conditions, and perhaps give some insight into the contentious question of the cause of kwashiorkor. Fondu *et al.* (1979) have stressed that 'PEM is not a single disease but a group of disorders with different signs from one region to another. Any speculation about the results obtained in another region may be misleading.' This is wise advice, but it is precisely these regional comparisons which may be illuminating, providing always that they are made in a systematic and comparable way.

The earlier authors who described what they saw as a multiple deficiency

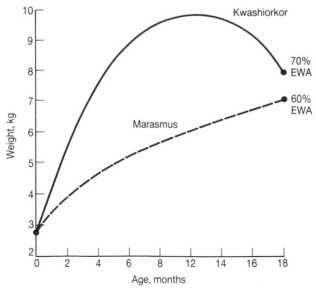

Fig. 1.1   Hypothetical diagram of body weight in the first 18 months of life in children who develop kwashiorkor or marasmus. EWA, expected weight for age. After Garrow (1966).

state were undoubtedly right. In a child with PEM, whatever the type, the tissues are wasted and therefore depleted of the minerals and micronutrients which, together with energy and protein, are essential for life. It is food that is eaten, not nutrients, and a diet that is inadequate in one way is likely to be inadequate in other ways also. Thus in PEM specific deficiencies are often superimposed on or underlie the more obvious changes. This is one source of the variation between regions mentioned by Fondu *et al.* (1979). The common and most serious deficiency that may accompany PEM is that of vitamin A. In other cases specific deficiencies only become apparent when other factors that were limiting have been restored. This sequence has been recorded for rickets and folic acid deficiency.

It is therefore probably wise to regard severe PEM as a multiple deficiency state—an approach that has obvious implications for treatment. In spite of all the research that has been done in the last 50 years the mortality, even in hospitals, is still deplorably high. The basic challenge remains: to prevent children from becoming severely malnourished, and for that to be achieved it is necessary to understand the causes.

Multiplicity of causes

There is a hierarchy of causes of PEM. Almost everyone who has written on the subject has produced a chart, model or diagram, of which Fig. 1.2 is a simple example. Causes operate at different levels and those at a higher level in a sense override those lower down. There is nothing to be gained by argument about whether one level is more important than another. The prevention or elimination of PEM requires the collaboration of people in many different disciplines, from politics to biochemistry. We return to this subject in the last chapter of the book.

At every level there are multiple causes. Social scientists, for example, have shown that famine is not simply the result of a bad harvest, for which in turn there are many causes as well as adverse climatic changes. This book is concerned with the factors operating at the level of the individual child, which can be grouped under three headings: lack of food, infection and psychosocial deprivation, the last two perhaps acting through the final common pathway of anorexia.

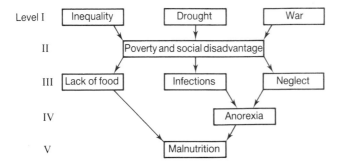

Fig. 1.2 Hierarchical model of the causes of protein-energy malnutrition.

A treatise with the title 'protein-energy malnutrition' naturally concentrates on the factor food, and in Chapter 11 I have set out my ideas about the relative importance of deficiencies of energy and protein in producing the classical syndromes of PEM. The impact of infections is discussed in Chapter 17. Something remains to be said about psychosocial deprivation, which is difficult to quantify but may be a contributing factor in many cases of PEM.

Stimulation and bonding to the mother in the first weeks of life make an essential contribution to the health and growth of the child. Maternal deprivation as a cause of growth failure is well recognized in affluent societies and has been vividly described by MacCarthy (1974). (For a useful review of the literature, see Frank and Zeisel, 1988.) These deprived children are apathetic, with a pale skin and cold extremities, as in anorexia nervosa. Sometimes there is even oedema. MacCarthy considered the rather contradictory evidence for impairment of growth hormone secretion by the pituitary, presumably as a result of hypothalamic dysfunction, but concluded that the basic cause of the stunting in growth was a reduced food intake. Often this resulted from maternal neglect, but anorexia undoubtedly plays an important role: the child rejects food in response to rejection by its mother. In Jamaica, where marasmic children usually have a voracious appetite, we have seen stubborn refusal of food by children who had been transferred to the ward from an orphanage, refusal that was overcome by attention and mothering. Widdowson's account (1951) is well known, of the effect of an uncongenial matron on the growth of children in an orphanage.

As mentioned earlier, Williams (1935) translated the Ga name kwashiorkor to mean the disease of the displaced child—displaced by the next baby. Goodall (1979) began a superb account of psychological deprivation in kwashiorkor by recording how 'Frederick II in the thirteenth century is said to have tried to bring up a group of newborn babies in absolute silence in an attempt to discover the natural evolution of language. The children all failed to thrive to the point of death, history relating that they could not live without the petting . . . and loving words of their foster-mothers.'

What is the background to this maternal deprivation? In Uganda Goodall compared the family situation of a group of children with kwashiorkor to that of healthy children and showed that a significant proportion of those with kwashiorkor had been separated from their mothers—she called them 'exiled weanlings'—or belonged to families in which the parents were not living together. Dixon et al. (1982) reported on a tribe in Kenya where the nutritional situation was relatively good. The few cases of severe PEM that were seen were the children of mothers who were alcoholics or were unmarried or divorced; these are conditions frowned upon in that society, so that other relatives did not rally round to help.

Maternal competence or ignorance are factors that are often invoked. In a Mexican village where socioeconomic conditions were rather uniform some children became malnourished while others did not. The factor most strongly correlated with the development of malnutrition was the extent to which the mother listened to the radio and used the national rather than the local language (Cravioto et al., 1967).

The marasmic children of rich parents and the well-nourished children of very poor ones are just as interesting as those who fit the model, but they are seldom shown in it. The healthy children of the poor, sometimes referred to as 'positive deviants', have only recently attracted the attention of research workers (Zeitlin and Ghassemi, 1986).

Such social and psychological factors may go a long way to explaining why, in an apparently homogeneous community, only some children develop malnutrition. Clearly, food alone will not solve such problems.

References

Achar, S. T. (1950). Nutritional dystrophy among children in Madras. *British Medical Journal* 1: 701–703.

Asher, R. (1986). In Avery Jones Sir Francis (ed) *Talking sense.* Churchill Livingstone, London.

Autret, M., Behar, M. (1955). Le syndrome de polycarence en Amerique Centrale (Kwashiorkor). FAO Nutritional Studies No. 13. FAO, Rome.

Bhattacharyya, A. K. (1972). Concomitants of kwashiorkor dermatosis. *Bulletin of the Calcutta School of Tropical Medicine* 20: 46–48.

Bhattacharyya, A. K. (1981). Kwashiorkor-marasmus syndrome (KMS): a suggested nomenclature for protein-energy malnutrition (PEM) and a composite (clinical and anthropometric) classification. *Bulletin of the Calcutta School of Tropical Medicine* 29: 125–130.

Bhattacharyya, A. K. (1986). Protein-energy malnutrition (kwashiorkor-marasmus syndrome): terminology, classification and evolution. *World Review of Nutrition and Dietetics* 47: 80–133.

Brock, J. F., Autret, M. (1952). *Kwashiorkor in Africa.* WHO Monograph Series No. 8. World Health Organization, Geneva.

Chaudhuri, R. N., Bhattacharyya, A. K., Basu, A. K. (1961). Kwashiorkor and marasmus in Calcutta. *Journal of the Indian Medical Association* 36: 557–565.

Coulter, J. B. S., Suliman, G. I. *et al.* (1988). Protein-energy malnutrition in Northern Sudan: clinical studies. *European Journal of Clinical Nutrition* 42: 787–796.

Cravioto, J., Birch, H. G. *et al.* (1967). The ecology of infant weight gain in a pre-industrial society. *Acta Paediatrica Scandinavica* 56: 71–84.

Czerny, A., Keller, A. (1925–28). *Des kindes Ernährung, Ernährungs Störungen u. Ernährungs Therapie,* 2nd edn. Franz Deutiche, Leipzig u. Wien.

Dixon, S. D., Levine, R. A., Brazelton, T. B. (1982). Malnutrition: a closer look at the problem in an East African village. *Developmental Medicine and Child Neurology* 24: 670–685.

Fondu, P., Mandelbaum, J. M., Vis, H. L. (1979). The erythrocyte membrane in protein-energy malnutrition. *American Journal of Clinical Nutrition* 31: 717–719.

Frank, D. A., Zeisel, S. H. (1988). Failure to thrive. *Pediatric Clinics of North America* 35: 1187–1206.

Garrow, J. S. (1966). "Kwashiorkor" and "Marasmus" in Jamaican infants. *Archivos Latinoamericanos de Nutricion* 16: 145–154.

Golden, M. H. N., Golden, B. E., Bennett, F. I. (1985). Relationship of trace element deficiencies to malnutrition. In Chandra, R. K. (ed) *Trace elements in nutrition of children.* Nestlé Nutrition, Vevey/Raven Press, New York, pp. 185–204.

Goodall, J. (1979). Malnutrition and the family: deprivation in kwashiorkor. *Proceedings of the Nutrition Society* 38: 17–28.

Gopalan, C. (1970). Some recent studies in the Nutrition Research Laboratories, Hyderabad. *American Journal of Clinical Nutrition* 23: 35–51.

Gopalan, C., Patwardhan, V. N. (1951) Some observations on the "nutritional oedema syndrome". *Indian Journal of Medical Sciences* 5: 312–317.

Gopalan, C., Venkatachalam, P. S. *et al.* (1952). Studies on nutritional oedema. *Indian Journal of Medical Sciences* 6: 277–295.

Gürson, C. T., Saner, G., Yüksel, T. (1975). Some etiological aspects of protein-calorie malnutrition in the Marmara region of Turkey. *Environmental Child Health* **21**: 311–314.

Gürson, C. T., Saner, G. (1982). Historical introduction. In McLaren, D. S., Burman, D. (eds) *Textbook of paediatric nutrition*, 2nd edn. Churchill-Livingstone, Edinburgh, pp. 3–17.

Hinojosa, F. (1865). Apuntes sobre una enfermedad del pueblo de la Magdalena. *Gaceta Médica de Mexico* **1**: 137–139.

Jamaica Conference (1955). Waterlow, J. C. (ed) *Protein malnutrition*. Proceedings of a Conference held in Jamaica 1953. FAO/WHO/Josiah Macy Jr Foundation, Cambridge University Press.

Jelliffe, D. B. (1959). Protein-calorie malnutrition in tropical pre-school children. *Journal of Pediatrics* **54**: 227–256.

MacCarthy, D. (1974). Effects of emotional disturbance and deprivation (maternal rejection) in somatic growth. In Davis, J. A., Dobbing, J. (eds) *Scientific foundations of paediatrics*. Heinemann Medical, London, pp. 56–67.

McCance, R. A. (1951). The history, significance and aetiology of hunger oedema. In *Studies of undernutrition, Wuppertal, 1946–9*. Medical Research Council Special Report Series No. 275. HM Stationery Office, London.

McLaren, D. S. (1966). A fresh look at protein-calorie malnutrition. *Lancet* **2**: 485–488.

McLaren, D. S. (1984). Forms and degrees of protein-energy deficits. In Brozek, J., Schürch, B. (eds) *Malnutrition and behaviour: critical assessment of key issues*. Nestlé Foundation, Lausanne, pp. 42–50.

McLaren, D. S., Pellett, P. L., Read, W. W. C. (1967). A simple scoring system for classifying the severe forms of protein-calorie malnutrition of early childhood. *Lancet* **1**: 533–535.

Mönckeberg, F. (ed) (1988). *Desnutricion infantil*. Impresora Creces, Santiago, Chile.

Normet, L. (1926). La "boufissure d'Annam". *Bulletin de la Societé de Social Pathologie Exotique* **19**: 207–213.

Shakir, A., Demarchi, M., El-Milli, N. (1972). Pattern of protein-calorie malnutrition in young children attending an outpatient clinic in Baghdad. *Lancet* **2**: 143–146.

Srikantia, S. G., Venkatachalam, P. S., Gopalan, C. (1953). Electrolyte studies in nutritional edema. *Metabolism* **2**: 521–528.

Tolboom, J. J. M., Ralitapole-Maruping, A. P. *et al.* (1986). Severe protein-energy malnutrition in Lesotho, death and survival in hospital, clinical findings. *Tropical Geographical Medicine* **38**: 351–358.

Trowell, H. C. (1941). Infantile pellagra. *Transactions of the Royal Society of Tropical Medicine and Hygiene* **33**: 389–404.

Trowell, H. C., Davies, J. N. P., Dean, R. F. A. (1954). *Kwashiorkor: Part I Reports of kwashiorkor in children and a discussion of terminology. Part II The history of kwashiorkor*. Edward Arnold, London. Reprinted in 1982 by the Nutrition Foundations, Academic Press, New York and London.

Vis, H., Dubois, R. *et al.* (1965). Etude des troubles electrolytiques accompagnant le kwashiorkor marastique. *Revues Français d'Études Biologie Clinique* **10**: 729–741.

Waterlow, J. C. (1948). *Fatty liver disease in infants in the British West Indies*. Medical Research Council Special Report Series No. 263. HM Stationery Office, London.

Waterlow, J. C. (1991). History of kwashiorkor. In Nichols, B. L., Guesry, P. (eds) *History of pediatrics. 1850–1950*. Nestlé Nutrition Workshop No. 22. Raven Press, New York, pp. 233–247.

Waterlow, J., Vergara, A. (1956). *Protein malnutrition in Brazil*. FAO Nutritional Studies No. 14. FAO, Rome.

Waterlow, J. C., Rutishauser, I. H. E. (1974). Malnutrition in man. In Cravioto, J.,

Hambraeus, L., Vahlquist, B. (eds) *Early malnutrition and mental development.* The Swedish Nutrition Foundation, Uppsala, pp. 13–26.

Waterlow, J. C., Bras, G.,De Pass, E. (1957). Further observations on the liver, pancreas and kidney in malnourished infants and children. II. The gross composition of the liver. *Journal of Tropical Pediatrics* **2**: 189–198.

Wellcome Trust Working Party (1970). Classification of infantile malnutrition. *Lancet* **2**: 302–303.

Wharton, B. (1973). Metabolic effects of malnutrition in childhood. *Journal of the Royal College of Physicians, London* **7**: 259–270.

Widdowson, E. M. (1951). Mental contentment and physical growth. *Lancet* **1**: 1316–1318.

Williams, C. D. (1933). A nutritional disease of childhood associated with a maize diet. *Archives of Disease in Childhood.* **8**: 423–433.

Williams, C. D. (1935). Kwashiorkor: a nutritional disease of children associated with a maize diet. *Lancet* **2**: 1151–1152.

Williams, C. D. (1963). The story of kwashiorkor. *Courrier* **13**: 361–369. Reprinted in *Nutrition Reviews* (1973) **31**: 334–340.

Zeitlin, M. F., Ghassemi, H. (1986). Positive deviance in nutrition: adequate child growth in poor households: a workshop report. In Taylor, T. G., Jenkins, N. K. (eds) *Proceedings of the XIIIth International Congress of Nutrition.* John Libbey, London, pp. 158–161.

Additional references for general reading

Alleyne, G. A. O., Hay, R. W. *et al.* (1977). *Protein-energy malnutrition.* Edward Arnold, London.

Golden, M. H. N. (1985). The consequences of protein deficiency in man and its relationship to the features of kwashiorkor. In Blaxter, K. L., Waterlow, J. C. (eds) *Nutritional adaptation in man.* John Libbey, London, pp. 169–188.

Jackson, A. A. (1990). The aetiology of kwashiorkor. In Harrison, G. A., Waterlow, J. C. (eds) *Diet and disease in traditional and developing societies.* Cambridge University Press, pp. 76–113.

Somerswara Rao, K., Swaminathan, M. C. *et al.* (1959). Protein malnutrition in South India. *Bulletin of the World Health Organization* **20**: 603–639.

Viteri, F., Béhar, M. *et al.* (1964). Clinical aspects of protein malnutrition. In Munro, H. N., Allison, J. B. (eds) *Mammalian protein metabolism* **2**: chapter 22, Academic Press, New York and London.

Waterlow, J. C., Alleyne, G. A. O. (1971). Protein malnutrition in children: advances in knowledge in the last ten years. *Advances in Protein Chemistry* **25**: 117–241.

Waterlow, J. C., Cravioto, J., Stephen, J. M. L. (1960). Protein malnutrition in man. *Advances in Protein Chemistry* **15**: 131–238.

Williams, C. D., Jelliffe, D. B. *et al.* (1985). *Mother and child health: delivering the services.* Oxford University Press.

2

Some general questions

The purpose of this chapter is to clear the way for the description of PEM and discussion of its causes. In the author's experience it is very easy to get tangled up with words whose meaning at first sight seems perfectly obvious.

What is meant by deficiency?

The words 'diet' and 'deficiency' are cases where confusion may occur. To a dietitian prescribing a diet means specifying both amount and composition. In other contexts 'diet' means simply a particular mixture of foods, with the composition or quality specified, but not the quantity. The word will be used here in the first sense.

A deficient diet is one that leads to a state of deficiency in the person or animal living on it. This statement is not a tautology; it makes the point that the adequacy of a diet, the extent to which it meets requirements, can only be defined in terms of functions of the consumer—growth, health, activity, etc. Moreover, dietary deficiency and adequacy are relative: the quality of a diet may be deficient for growth in children but adequate for maintenance in adults. Therefore the adequacy of a diet has to be defined in terms of a particular situation and a particular function.

States of deficiency in the consumer are of two kinds, specific and general, which may or may not co-exist. Specific deficiencies, such as the classical avitaminoses, lead to defined clinical outcomes, often described by code-names (Chapter 1) such as scurvy, beri-beri or rickets. Very often there are biochemical changes which accompany or precede the clinical signs and which make possible the early diagnosis of subclinical or impending deficiency. In many specific deficiencies there is a decreased concentration of the particular nutrient in blood or tissues. The problem of biochemical diagnosis then becomes one of drawing dividing lines between normal and deficient or at risk. The history of attempts to establish requirements for vitamins and some other nutrients shows how difficult this is.

A general deficiency is reflected by failure to grow or by loss of weight, usually without specific clinical or biochemical changes. It results from a quantitatively inadequate intake, which in turn may be caused by lack of a specific nutrient. An example is the profound anorexia when the intake of all nutrients is reduced; this characteristically occurs with diets low in zinc.

It is self-evident that new tissue cannot be deposited in a growing organism unless all the components of cytoplasm—protein, minerals, essential fatty acids, etc.—are available together. Conversely, when lean body tissue is lost all the components are lost, because for most of them there are no body stores. Iron is an outstanding exception to this generalization. If one component is missing the others cannot be utilized, even if available in excess. Hence arises the concept of a limiting factor. Zinc again is an example of being a limiting factor for growth on an otherwise adequate diet (Chapter 9).

Protein provides a good illustration of the difficulty of defining deficiency. A young animal on a low protein diet does not grow, but the protein concentration in the tissues is normal. When it was supposed that kwashiorkor was a result of protein deficiency, the question arose: how can a state of protein deficiency be diagnosed if tissue composition is normal? This question led to the idea of 'depletion', representing a quantitative rather than a qualitative deficiency (Waterlow, 1955). The only way of diagnosing depletion is by relating the amount of a component such as nitrogen to the DNA content of the tissue. Each diploid cell contains a fixed amount of DNA, which is not altered by malnutrition, so that in the depleted state the cytoplasm shrinks round the nucleus and the cell is like a half-empty bag. Animal studies and measurements on human tissues have indeed shown a reduction in the ratio N/DNA in malnutrition (Kosterlitz, 1947; Waterlow and Weisz, 1956).

This approach provides no distinction between kwashiorkor and marasmus. If it is supposed that kwashiorkor results from protein deficiency, the only way of demonstrating it is by identifying a specific effect, over and above the general depletion of protein. That is why so much importance attaches to the cause and significance of hypoalbuminaemia, as discussed in Chapters 6 and 11.

Alleyne (1970) extended the concepts of deficiency and depletion to potassium. A child with a low total body K, expressed as mmol/kg, may either have a reduced active tissue mass (depletion), which Alleyne called a reduction in K capacity, or a low K concentration in the tissues (specific deficiency), or both. The K concentration is rapidly restored when potassium is given, but the reduction in capacity takes longer to make good, and of course requires other nutrients.

The distinction was further extended by Golden (1988), who classified reduced concentration and reduced capacity as 'type I' and 'type II' deficiencies, as shown in Table 2.1. This is a useful contribution, because Golden's system covers a wide range of nutrients and emphasizes the important point that PEM is a multiple deficiency state.

Bases of reference

Garrow and co-workers (1968), in their book on electrolytes in malnutrition, raised the fundamental question: what is the appropriate control for a malnourished child? Should it be a normal child of the same age, the same weight or the same height? It is impossible to have a control that combines all three.

Table 2.1   Tentative classification of nutrients into type I and type II

Type I Initial normal growth Reduced tissue concentration Specific signs	Type II Primary growth failure Normal tissue concentration No specific signs
IA *No identified stores* Selenium	IIA *No identified stores* Nitrogen Essential amino acids Zinc Potassium Sodium Phosphorus
IB *Stored* Iodine Iron Copper Calcium Thiamin Riboflavin Ascorbic acid Retinol Tocopherol Cobalamin	IIB *Stored* Energy
IC Defect in longitudinal growth with specific signs Manganese deficiency Vitamin D deficiency	IIC No specific signs

From Golden (1988)

As these authors showed, the answer can be very different according to the type of control that is used. There is no general solution; the choice depends on the particular question being asked.

There are three kinds of comparisons.

Absolute comparisons of body size

The anthropometric diagnosis of malnutrition is based on absolute comparisons of body size (Chapter 14). One of the three variables has to be fixed, usually age but sometimes height. This gives us comparisons of weight or height at the same age, or of weight at the same height.

Size-independent comparisons

Measures of development, such as bone age or mental development, can be used for comparison and are independent of body size. Here age has to be fixed, because the question being asked is whether the child's progress over time is normal. Body size in itself is irrelevant, but height may be used as an index of biological age, i.e. the age of a normal child of the same height. This refinement is quite important, because a stunted child has a bone age that is retarded compared with a normal child of the same age, but advanced compared with a normal child of the same height (Chapter 13). What this means is that two aspects of development, growth in length and maturation of ossification centres, are no longer synchronized in the normal way. Whether the same applies to mental development has not been investigated. For practical purposes the relationship to age is the most important, since children go to school at a certain age and not at a certain height.

Comparisons based on a relation to body size

Weight, some power of weight, height or surface area are the factors most often used for comparison. In the analysis that follows the basal metabolic rate (BMR) will be used as an example, because physiologists and paediatricians have devoted a great deal of attention to finding the best way of expressing it so that comparisons between normal and malnourished children may be meaningful. The term BMR is used here, although it cannot be guaranteed that in all cases the metabolic rate was measured under the strict conditions defined as 'basal', particularly in young children.

A tissue composed of cells may be regarded as having an *intrinsic* rate of oxygen uptake, and the more cells the greater the uptake. Other things being equal, the BMR/kg should express the intrinsic metabolic rate and should be constant. However, other things are never equal. Figure 2.1 shows how in normal children the BMR/kg varies with age from birth to five years. The factors that affect the BMR/kg are body composition, maturity (i.e. age), shape (as expressed by height or surface area) and weight itself.

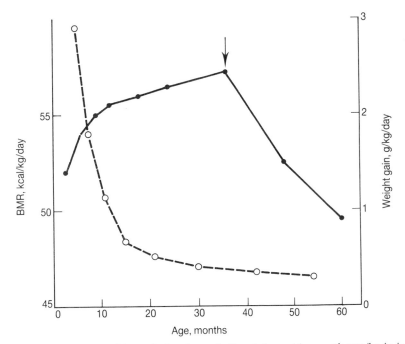

Fig. 2.1   Changes with age in basal metabolic rate/kg and in growth rate/kg in infants and pre-school children (boys). Calculated from the equations of Schofield *et al.* (1985) for BMR and from the WHO reference median weights:
0 – 3 years: BMR = 60.9W − 54 kcal/day
3 – 10 years: BMR: 22.7W + 495 kcal/day
     Note the discontinuity in the BMR curve at 3 years (arrow).This reflects partly but not entirely the change from the first to the second equation. Note also the lack of correspondence between growth rate and BMR.

Body composition

It may be supposed that the BMR/kg increases during the first year of life because the baby is losing fat and gaining lean. However, the fact that BMR/kg at maturity is only half that at three years cannot be explained by changes in body composition alone.

Maturity

Intrinsic metabolism is undoubtedly faster in young than in mature animals. This can be shown *in vitro*; for example, the rates of protein synthesis in muscle and to a lesser extent in liver are greater in the young than in the mature rat (Millward, 1978; Waterlow, 1988). In general rates of protein turnover parallel rates of oxygen uptake; the rate of whole-body protein turnover per kg in young children is about twice that of adults (Waterlow, 1984).

Shape: height and surface area

In young children in particular height or length has an important effect on BMR, independent of weight. At the same weight a tall child will have a higher BMR than a short one. The classical explanation of this phenomenon is that the tall child has a greater ratio of surface to volume and hence a higher rate of heat loss. This concept dominated the physiology of energy metabolism for a long time and there is a very large literature about it. It was customary, particularly in children, to relate BMR to surface area (e.g. Talbot, 1921), although intuitively the idea that heat production should be determined by heat loss seems to be putting the cart before the horse. Nevertheless, there may be a physiological basis for surface area as a basis of reference, since many functions, such as absorption of nutrients in the gut and exchange of gases in the lungs are dependent on area. In fact, Coulson (1986) has argued that oxygen uptake depends on the perfusion of tissues by the blood, and this in turn depends on the cross-sectional area of the capillary bed, which is a function of surface rather than mass.

Weight

In inter-species comparisons the BMR/kg is inversely related to body weight or size, both *in vivo* and *in vitro* (Davies, 1961). The classical work of Kleiber (1961) showed that in mature animals, with body weights ranging over five orders of magnitude (0.01 to 1000 kg) the BMR could be expressed by a power function of weight: $M = CW^b$, where C is a constant. By regression analysis Kleiber obtained a value of 0.73 for the exponent b. This gave rise to the concept of 'metabolic mass', represented by $W^{0.73}$, or more simply, by $W^{3/4}$. Heuser (1984) has argued on physical grounds that Kleiber's value of 0.73 for the exponent is a statistical artefact and that the correct value should be 2/3, which has the dimensions of surface area.

Young children appear to be an exception to this general relationship. The observed relationship of BMR to body weight in infants has an exponent that is closer to 1 than to either 3/4 or 2/3. Karlberg (1952) made a detailed analysis of the older literature. He showed that in four studies from different countries, over a weight range of 1 to about 10 kg, the value of the exponent ranged from 0.91 to 1.11, and was never as low as 3/4. Hill and Rahimtulla (1965) obtained an exponent of approximately 1 up to the age of 18 months.

A value of 1 would mean that BMR was a direct linear function of body weight. Figure 2.2 shows the relationship of BMR to weight calculated from the data summarized by Schofield *et al.* (1985). In this log-log plot, the slope gives the value of the exponent b. From birth to 15 kg in weight, corresponding to about three years in age, the slope is 1.19. Thereafter the slope changes; it seems clear that even in a logarithmic plot the relationship between MR and W must be curvilinear. When the exponent is less than 1, as it is in older children and adults, it means that weight has an independent effect, such that the BMR/kg decreases as weight increases. The reason for such a relationship is not clear, but one possibility is that it results from changes in body composition as size increases. Quite apart from a tendency to increased amounts of fat in heavier people, a small animal has a larger ratio of visceral tissues to muscle than a large one, and a child has a larger ratio than an adult. Since visceral tissues metabolize more rapidly than muscle, the result will be a higher overall metabolic rate. An exponent greater than 1, as shown in Fig. 2.2, could represent a decrease in body fat with increasing age, as mentioned earlier.

Whatever the reason, it is clear that except in young children weight has an effect on BMR that is independent of its action as a scaling factor. A good example is a study by Walker *et al.* (1990), in which it was shown that the BMR/kg lean body mass was greater in stunted than in normal children, being inversely related to height. It was suggested in correspondence about this paper that the difference between the BMRs of stunted and normal children could be eliminated by covariance analysis. This would remove from consideration an effect of physiological interest—i.e. the inverse relationship between BMR/kg and body size. On the other hand, it would make it possible to find out whether the BMR was determined by any factor other than size, such as age or maturity.

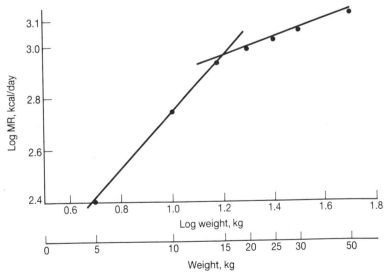

Fig. 2.2 Log-plot of basal metabolic rate *versus* body weight in infants and children. Constructed from the equations of Schofield *et al.* (1985) as in Fig. 2.1.

This case is cited as an example of how difficult it is to find a basis of reference that reveals rather than obscures functional differences. The problem was discussed but not solved many years ago by Tanner (1949).

Equations for predicting metabolic rate

Schofield *et al.* (1985) analysed the world literature and produced a series of linear equations for predicting BMR from weight, with or without height, over different age ranges (Chapter 6). These equations have the form MR = A + B.W. They do not represent physiological relationships, but are simply arithmetical compilations of the available data. Taking account of weight only, at zero body weight MR would have a finite value A, which is impossible. In reality the equations represent linear segments of a curve, but that does not reduce their value for prediction, provided that they are only used over the ranges of age and weight from which they were derived.

When height is included in the Schofield equations it makes little difference to the prediction of group average BMRs, but it can play a dominant role in predicting the BMR of an individual. There is little difference in BMR predicted from weight alone, or from weight and height, when the values are those of an average child with a normal ratio of weight to height, but at the extremes there is a substantial difference, at constant weight, between a tall and a short child. The equations of Karlberg (1952) also show the same difference between tall and short children of equal weight.

None of these equations includes a separate factor for age, independent of weight and height. Butte (1990) has produced such as equation, but it only covers the very restricted age-range of one to four months.

Assessment of metabolic rate in PEM

It is apparent that the determinants of BMR in children are both complex and interrelated. In PEM what we are really interested in is to find out whether there is any alteration or abnormality in what I have called the intrinsic metabolism of the tissues of the body, taken as an aggregate. Over the important age range of one to three years it is reasonable to ignore the age-factor, since the BMR/kg is fairly constant (Fig. 2.1). It is impossible, virtually by definition, for any normal child to be both the same weight and the same height as a malnourished child. They could, however, have the same surface area (SA). Since SA depends on weight and height, at equal SA the normal child would be shorter but heavier than the malnourished child. This does not seem a very satisfactory basis for comparison. Moreover, measuring the SA is very difficult. Boyd *et al.* (1929) showed that in young children the measured SA varied as the 2/3 power of the weight, but we do not know whether this or any other equation for SA derived from normal children can be applied to malnourished children with a greatly distorted ratio of weight to height. Boyd and Scammon (1929) measured the SA of children by enclosing them in plaster except for the nose and determining the area of the cast made from the mould, but this is hardly a method than can be applied to sick children.

We are left, then, with weight, i.e. BMR/kg, as the only practical and theoretically reasonable basis of comparison. It is fortunate that in normal children over the crucial age-range of one to three years the BMR/kg is rather constant (Fig. 2.1). In the logarithmic equation calculated from the data of Schofield *et al.* (1985), the exponent over this very restricted range is 1.09, which may not be significantly different from unity. It is true that any difference in BMR between normal and malnourished will be increased by using $W^{2/3}$ rather than weight as a basis of reference, but that is no justification for using an approach that is theoretically unsatisfactory. It would certainly be desirable, if it were possible, to take some account of height as well as weight, but in practice differences in body composition between normal and malnourished children are likely to be far more important than differences in height. That aspect of the problem is discussed in Chapter 6.

A final question is whether this reasoning can be applied to functions other than metabolic rate. It is traditional, for example, to relate cardiac output and renal clearances to SA rather than weight. The basic concern is whether such a method of expression is physiologically reasonable for those particular functions. For comparisons in adults it may well be empirically better because it will reduce the effects of differences in body composition, of oedema, etc. For malnourished children, the same arguments against the use of surface area apply as in the case of metabolic rate.

Adaptation

The concept of adaptation comes up in a number of contexts, such as conservation of energy and nitrogen (Chapter 6) and reduction in growth (Chapter 13). It has been invoked to differentiate marasmus from kwashiorkor (Chapter 11). It is difficult to define adaptation in a useful way and to distinguish it from related concepts such as homoeostasis. (For more detailed discussion see Waterlow, 1985 and 1990*a*, *b*).

From a general biological point of view, every organism that survives and reproduces is by definition adapted to its environment. It follows that an adapted state must be sustainable, although sometimes it is the species that is sustained at the expense of the individual.

Whenever someone is described as adapted to a particular situation or stress, there are four questions that it is interesting and useful to ask.

1. What are the limits of this adaptation? At what point does it break down? For example, in adults the simplest way of adapting to a low energy intake is to reduce body weight, which leads to a fall in BMR and in the energy cost of many activities. However, there is obviously a limit below which weight loss becomes excessive, morbidity increases and work output falls. It has been tentatively suggested that in terms of body mass index (BMI, weight/height squared, kg/m^2), this limit or cut-off point might be set at 17, which is about 20 per cent below the average BMI of normal adults in less developed countries (James *et al.*, 1988).
2. What are the costs of the adaptation? Almost by definition adaptation confers benefits compared with the unadapted state, but it also usually involves costs. For example, to walk a given distance slowly economizes energy but it uses up time—what the economists call opportunity costs (Waterlow, 1990*a*).

3. What kind of relationship does the adapting organism's response have to the stress imposed (Waterlow, 1990*b*)? In some cases it is more or less linear; when energy is limiting, a small deficit leads to a small weight loss, a larger deficit to a larger loss. In other cases there is a threshold; for example, human beings can adapt to a low nitrogen intake by economizing nitrogen losses without drawing to any significant extent on body protein stores. However, there is a threshold below which the mechanisms of economy break down and body protein will be lost. The shape of such relationships is very important. Children who are stunted in linear growth often show some degree of retardation in mental development (Chapter 19). Does any degree of growth deficit carry some risk? or is there a threshold, above which function is unimpaired, and if so, where is it?

4. The final question about any adaptation is: what are the mechanisms? In the context of PEM they may be behavioural, physiological, metabolic, etc. A better understanding of mechanisms will help to answer the preceding questions.

It must also be remembered that adaptation is relative; 'adapted' and 'normal' are two sides of the same coin. Thus the dweller at high altitude may regard those of us who live at sea level as having achieved a remarkable degree of adaptation to high oxygen pressure. Since oxygen can be toxic, e.g. in relation to free radical production (Chapter 10), it is possible that this adaptation has been achieved at a cost which so far has not been appreciated.

It may be useful to reflect on these points in order to counteract a tendency to regard 'adapted' as a synonym for 'satisfactory'. As discussed in Chapter 13, in relation to stunting of growth, an adaptation may be the best that can be achieved under the circumstances: this need not deter us from trying to eliminate those circumstances that make the adaptation necessary.

Analysis of associations

The concept of cause (Chapter 1) is full of pitfalls. As everyone recognizes, all that can usually be shown is an association between two events or situations, A and B, without proof of cause or indication of its direction. However, in ordinary life it is justifiable to postulate cause and effect if a reasonable hypothesis can be developed for a mechanism linking A to B. Understanding the mechanisms of linkage is necessary as a basis for any intervention that might prevent B from happening. Interventions are also tests of a causal hypothesis—perhaps indeed the final arbiter. The therapeutic test has played a very important part in the history of nutrition.

In a system in which the outcome depends on many factors, the question of which are the most important is usually tackled by multiple regression analysis. The purpose of what follows is to emphasize that just as a statistician ought to be involved in the planning of a study, so should the investigator be intimately involved in the analysis of it. Computers make it possible to handle large numbers of subjects and also large numbers of input variables. Such an analysis is not simply a statistical exercise. First, a decision has to be made about the variables to be included in what has come to be called the 'model'. This decision depends on experience, common sense and preconceived ideas about possible causal relationships. Secondly, a choice has to be made about the order in which the variables are put into the equation. If there are N variables, there are N! possible orders. The choice of order will depend on the investigator's particular interest. The factors that are put in first will generally make the largest contribution to the variance of the outcome. The effect of this is that, referring to Fig. 1.2, if a 'higher level' variable is put in first, it will tend to obscure relationships at a 'lower' level. A simple example might be a supposed relationship between vitamin A deficiency and morbidity from respiratory infections. On biological grounds such a relationship would be plausible because of the known effects of vitamin A on epithelia. Analysis of a model which included these two variables only, one dependent, one independent, might show a strong association, supporting the hypothesis. Suppose that the investigator is now told he must take account of 'confounding' factors such as poverty. Suppose further that all vitamin A deficient subjects are poor. If some measure of poverty is put first into the equation, it will make a major contribution to the variance of the outcome, morbidity and vitamin A deficiency coming second will add nothing more. Thus the introduction of poverty into the analysis could obscure a real biological relationship. On the other hand, if vitamin A deficiency is put in first, poverty will make no further contribution, unless it is a proxy for another independent causal factor.

In general, higher level variables are harder to define. If one is interested in causes, there could well be a case for working *up* the chain of causation rather than down, i.e. to adjust for the most specific variables first. Suppose that instead of poverty the other factor to be considered is, more specifically, the number of people in a room, since overcrowding will increase the risk of transmission of infection. Some people are vitamin A deficient but not overcrowded; others are overcrowded but not vitamin A deficient. The order in which these two variables, which are at the same level, are put into the equation only matters if they overlap substantially in their explanatory power. If the interpretation of the orderings is important, the results for both orderings should be given. The final choice depends on the question being asked. Thus in practice it may be easier to prevent vitamin A deficiency than to reorganize housing. Putting the deficiency second into the equation will show whether it has a large enough independent effect, after adjusting for overcrowding, to support a policy of prophylactic intervention.

The point of this foray into the philosophy of statistical analysis is that the way in which an analysis is made depends very much on the questions being asked by the investigator. A social scientist may be more interested in housing, a nutritionist in vitamin deficiency. Too often published accounts concentrate on the details of statistical analysis and give little or no information on the choices on which the model was based and how the analysis was organized. A second point is that analysis of a complex multifactorial system may obscure rather than illuminate important biological relationships, particularly when the model includes factors that operate at different levels.

I am grateful to Dr, T. J. Cole for constructive advice on this section.

References

Alleyne, G. A. O. (1970). Studies on total body potassium in malnourished infants: factors affecting potassium repletion. *British Journal of Nutrition* **24**: 205–212.

Boyd, E., Scammon, R. E. (1929). Measurements of surface area in children. *Proceedings of the Society of Experimental Biology and Medicine* **27**: 449–453.

Boyd, E., Scammon, R. E., Donovan, L. (1929). The determination of surface area of living children. *Proceedings of the Society of Experimental Biology and Medicine* **27**: 445–449.

Butte, N. F. (1990). Basal metabolism of infants. In Schürch, B., Scrimshaw, N. S. (eds) *Activity, energy expenditure and energy requirements of infants and children*. Nestlé Foundation, Lausanne.

Coulson, R. A. (1986). Metabolic rate and the flow theory: a study in chemical engineering. *Comparative Biochemistry and Physiology* **84A**: 217–229.

Davies, M. (1961). On body size and tissue respiration. *Journal of Cellular Comparative Physiology* **57**: 135–147.

Garrow, J. S., Smith, R., Ward, E. E. (1968). *Electrolyte metabolism in severe infantile malnutrition*. Pergamon Press, London.

Golden, M. H. N. (1988). The role of individual nutrient deficiencies in growth retardation of children as exemplified by zinc and protein. In Waterlow, J. C. (ed) *Linear growth retardation in less developed countries*. Nestlé, Vevey/Raven Press, New York, pp. 143–163.

Heusner, A. A. (1984). Biological similitude: statistical and functional relationships in comparative physiology. *American Journal of Physiology* **246** (*Regulatory Integrative Comparative Physiology* **15**): R 839–R 845.

Hill, J. R., Rahimtulla, K. A. (1965). Heat balance and the metabolic rate of new-born babies in relation to environmental temperature; and the effect of age and of weight on basal metabolic rate. *Journal of Physiology* **180**: 239–265.

James, W. P. T., Ferro-Luzzi, A., Waterlow, J. C. (1988). Definition of chronic energy deficiency in adults. *European Journal of Clinical Nutrition* **42**: 969–981.

Karlberg, P. (1952). Determination of standard energy metabolism (basal metabolism) in normal infants. *Acta Paediatrica Scandinavica* **41**, Suppl. 89: 79–123.

Kleiber, M. (1961). *The fire of life*. Wiley, New York.

Kosterlitz, H. W. (1947). The effects of changes in dietary protein on the composition and structure of the liver cell. *Journal of Physiology* **106**: 194–210.

Millward, D. J. (1978). The regulation of muscle-protein turnover in growth and development. *Biochemical Society Transactions* **6**: 494–499.

Schofield, W. N., Schofield, C., James, W. P. T. (1985). Basal metabolic rate—review and prediction, together with an annotated bibliography of source material. *Human Nutrition: Clinical Nutrition* **39C**: Suppl. 1, 1–96.

Talbot, F. B. (1921). Severe infantile malnutrition: the energy metabolism with the report of a new series of cases. *American Journal of Diseases of Children* **22**: 358–370.

Tanner, J. M. (1949). Fallacy of per-weight and per-surface area standards and their relation to spurious correlation. *Journal of Applied Physiology* **2**: 1–15.

Walker, J. M., Bond, S. A. et al. (1990). Treatment of short normal children with growth hormone—a cautionary tale? *Lancet* **336**: 1331–1334.

Waterlow, J. C. (ed) (1955). *Protein malnutrition*. FAO/WHO/Josiah Macy Jr Foundation, Cambridge University Press.

Waterlow, J. C. (1984). Protein turnover with special reference to man. *Quarterly Journal of Experimental Physiology* **69**: 409–438.

Waterlow, J. C. (1985). What do we mean by adaptation? In Blaxter, K. L., Waterlow, J. C. (eds) *Nutritional adaptation in man*. John Libbey, London, pp. 1–12 and 233–236.

Waterlow, J. C. (1988). The variability of energy metabolism in man. In Blaxter, K. L., Macdonald, I. (eds) *Comparative nutrition*. John Libbey, London, pp. 133–140.

Waterlow, J. C. (1990*a*). Mechanisms of adaptation to low energy intakes. In Harrison, G. A., Waterlow, J. C. (eds) *Diet and disease in traditional and developing societies*. Cambridge University Press, pp. 5–23.

Waterlow, J. C. (1990*b*). Nutritional adaptation in man: general introduction and concepts. *American Journal of Clinical Nutrition* **51**: 259–263.

Waterlow, J. C., Weisz, T. (1956). The fat, protein and nucleic acid content of the liver in malnourished human infants. *Journal of Clinical Investigation* **35**: 346–354.

3

Body composition and body water

A severely malnourished underweight child is not just a scaled-down version of a normal child. It differs in two ways: in the relative proportions of the various organs and tissues—what may be called the organ pattern—and in the chemical composition of the body. These differences make comparisons between malnourished and normal children very difficult to interpret.

Changes in organ pattern

It is illuminating to concentrate on two organs or tissues which show a clear contrast and which both contribute substantially to the weight of the whole body—brain and muscle. Other organs commonly weighed by pathologists, such as kidneys and heart, only make a small contribution. With liver the picture is often complicated by excess fat. The skin is indeed a major component but it is very unusual for any quantitative measurements to be made of it.

Brain weight

Kerpel-Fronius and Frank (1949) were perhaps the first to record that even in children dying of malnutrition the weight of the brain, compared with that of other organs, was relatively well preserved (Fig. 3.1). It is true that brain weight and DNA content are less than would be expected in a child of the same age (Garrow et al., 1965; Winick et al., 1970) and these findings at autopsy have been confirmed in vivo by computerized tomography (Househam and de Villiers, 1987). However, this deficit, like stunting in height, should probably be regarded as a result of retarded development rather than as an actual loss.

In the normal child at one year the brain accounts for about 9 per cent of body weight (Coppoletta and Wolbach, 1933), compared with up to 20 per cent in severe PEM (Alleyne et al., 1969). This increase in brain weight as a

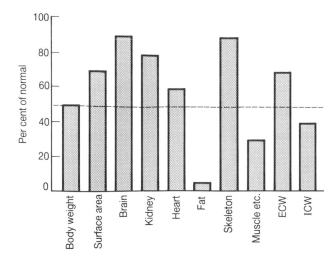

Fig. 3.1 Weights of organs at death in atrophic children as percentages of normal age-controls. Horizontal line shows total body weight. From Kerpel-Fronius and Frank (1949).

proportion of body weight has important consequences for measurements made on the whole body. Normally at one year the brain would contain about 20 per cent of total body potassium (TBK) and its metabolism would account for about 50 per cent of the basal metabolic rate (BMR) (Holliday *et al.*, 1967). Therefore, if the proportion of brain is doubled in malnutrition, it should follow that TBK and BMR per kg body weight would be actually increased, unless there are specific deficits. We shall return to these questions later.

Muscle mass

The contrasting tissue is muscle. Figure 3.1 shows that in marasmic infants muscle mass was 30 per cent of normal (although no information is given about how muscle mass was measured), while the body weight was 50 per cent of normal. It is evident that muscle bore the lion's share of tissue loss. This conclusion has been amply confirmed by indirect measurements on children with PEM in Jamaica. Montgomery (1962) and Hansen-Smith *et al.* (1979) demonstrated gross wasting of muscle fibres microscopically. Standard *et al.* (1959) found that in severe PEM 24-hour creatinine excretion, which is often used as a measure of muscle mass, was 37 per cent of normal. The conversion of creatinine excretion to muscle mass depends on the assumption that an output of 50 mg creatinine in 24 hours corresponds to 1 kg of muscle (Cheek *et al.*, 1970). If this factor can be applied to both normal and malnourished children, the creatinine outputs recorded by Standard would correspond to a muscle mass of 27 per cent of body weight in the normal and 10 per cent in the malnourished infant. The value of the factor depends on the creatine concentration in muscle. Reeds and co-workers (1978) examined this question in studies with ^{15}N-labelled creatine. In children with PEM the muscle mass was on average 10 per cent of body weight and after recovery 22 per cent. The value in PEM may actually be an overestimate, because the creatine concentration in muscle was higher than after recovery, while the creatine turnover rate was unchanged.

Another way of estimating muscle wasting, which nowadays would not be regarded as ethically acceptable, is by measurements of the protein/DNA ratio in muscle biopsies (see Chapter 2). In malnutrition this ratio was reduced (Waterlow, 1956; Cheek *et al.*, 1970; Reeds *et al.*, 1978).

In experimental animals on a low protein diet the skin lost even more protein than muscle (Waterlow and Stephen, 1966), but we have little information for children. Halliday (1967) found that in two malnourished children who died, the skin accounted for 15 per cent and 17 per cent of body weight, but loss of protein from the skin may be masked by an increase in water content (Frenk *et al.*, 1957). No values have been found for total skin weight in normal children.

We can conclude that in PEM there is a preferential loss of muscle and probably of skin, tissues which in the resting state have a low metabolic activity, while essential organs with high rates of activity are relatively well preserved. This would seem to be a mechanism for survival.

Changes in chemical composition

There are two ways of looking at body composition. One is in terms of compartments: fat tissue and lean tissue, the latter in turn being divided into extra- and intra-cellular compartments. The other is in terms of chemical components: water, protein, fat and minerals.

Methods

The subject of body composition is one where methods are all-important. Direct analysis of the bodies of children who died (Garrow *et al.*, 1965; Picou *et al.*, 1966; Halliday, 1967) has given baseline information of great importance and there is probably little need for further studies along these lines. Certainly none have been made. Advances in instrumentation involving very high technology, such as neutron activation analysis (NAA), magnetic resonance imaging and computerized tomography make it possible to obtain a great deal of information *in vivo* and have given a tremendous impetus to studies of body composition (for reviews see Burkinshaw, 1985; Forbes, 1987; Coward *et al.*, 1988; Fuller *et al.*, 1990). With NAA it is possible to measure the amounts of a range of elements in the body: C, N, H and O. The other two methods provide images of organs and enable fat to be distinguished from lean. So far, however, these new instruments have not been applied in any systematic way to the study of malnourished children.

Measurements of body water and its compartments and of total body potassium (TBK) have been of fundamental importance for understanding the changes in body composition that are found in PEM. Measurement of TBK requires a sensitive and well-shielded whole-body counter, which again is an expensive and 'high-tech' instrument, to which only two groups have had access in regions where PEM occurs, in Jamaica and South Africa. Determination of total body water (TBW) therefore remains the most important and widely used tool, as it was in the 1960s and 1970s.

The 'gold-standard' for measurement of TBW is the use of stable isotopes of water, ^2H_2O or $H_2^{18}O$. The method is non-invasive, since the isotope can be given by mouth and the measurements made on urine, saliva or expired air (Schoeller *et al.*, 1980). The determination of stable isotope concentration is admittedly not simple, but at least the samples can be sent to a laboratory equipped to do it, an exercise that depends on but also promotes international collaboration.

Two new relatively simple instruments have come into use, which have great potential for clinical purposes. Both are based on the principle that the impedance, resistance and electrical conductivity of a body of fluid depend on its volume and electrolyte content. One instrument, called the TOBEC (total body electrical conductivity), is a large coil in which an oscillating electromagnetic field is generated. The subject is placed inside the coil and the water content calculated from the change in signal, which is a function of the conductivity (Cochran *et al.*, 1986; Fiorotto *et al.*, 1987*a,b*). In the second method, bioelectric impedance (BEI), an alternating current is applied through electrodes attached to the dorsal surface of one hand and foot. The voltage drop is measured through two other electrodes placed close to those that induced the current.

The strength of the signal depends not only on the volume but also on the shape of the body, so that length has to be taken into account in interpreting the readings obtained. Both instruments have been calibrated against independent measurements of body water by $H_2^{18}O$ (Cochran *et al.*, 1989; Fjeld *et al.*, 1990; Gregory *et al.*, 1991). Fjeld *et al.* (1990) summarized the results obtained in different laboratories by the BEI method; they seem to be quite consistent, the calibration equation being of the form:

TBW = A + [B.L^2/R] where A and B are constants, L is length/height in cm and R impedance in ohms. The constant A is small, so that the calibration line goes almost through the origin, which is satisfactory (Chapter 2).

With both instruments the signal strength is determined not only by size and shape but also by the concentrations of electrolytes in body fluids. Preliminary studies with the TOBEC instrument indicate that changes in the proportion of extracellular fluid do not introduce errors in the prediction of TBW (Fiorotto *et al.*, 1987*b*; Cochran *et al.*, 1989). However, since different ions have different activities, it is not yet clear what may be the effects of distortions in electrolyte pattern, such as the potassium deficiency and hyponatraemia that may be found in severe PEM (Chapter 4). If this problem can be solved, it may be expected that both instruments will be of great value in the clinical management of PEM.

Method of expressing TBW

The expression of TBW presents a difficult problem, for which there is no satisfactory solution (Garrow *et al.*, 1968). TBW is usually expressed as a percentage or fraction of body weight or lean body mass. This is not very satisfactory, for two reasons. First, the percentage of weight accounted for as water will be affected by changes in components other than water. For example, Hansen *et al.* (1965) showed a linear relationship between percentage of body water and degree of weight deficit (Fig. 3.2). This could result

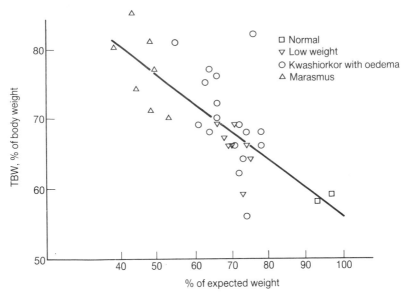

Fig. 3.2   Relationship between total body water (% of body weight) and weight deficit (% expected weight for age) in normal and malnourished children. Reproduced by permission from Hansen *et al.* (1965).

simply from the fact that the greater the weight deficit, the smaller the proportion of fat in the body, so that increases in TBW in marasmus may be apparent rather than real.

The second difficulty is that water appears in both the numerator and the denominator of the fraction (Garrow *et al.*, 1968). Thus for purely arithmetical reasons the usual method of relating TBW to body weight will, other things being equal, underestimate the size of any changes, whether increases or decreases (Table 3.1). In clinical practice it is changes in the course of treatment that are the main concern, and for this purpose absolute values are the most appropriate. Another way of representing excess or deficit of water would be to relate measured TBW to the amount expected in a normal child of the same length and hence biological age, using as standards the values of Fomon *et al.* (1982) (Fig. 3.3). This will take account of the normal decrease in percentage body water that occurs in the first few months after birth.

Table 3.1   Comparison of three methods of expressing changes in total body water (TBW)

	'True' body weight	Observed body weight	
		Oedematous	Dehydrated
Weight, kg	10.0	12.0	9.0
TBW, kg	6.5	8.5	5.5
TBW, % of observed weight	65	71	61
Absolute Δ TBW, kg	–	+2.0	−1.0
Δ TBW, % of true body weight	–	+20	−10
Δ TBW, % of true TBW	–	+31	−15

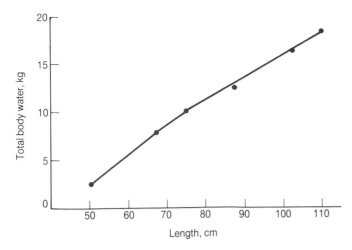

Fig. 3.3 Relationship between total body water (kg) and length (cm) in normal children (boys). Calculated from data of Fomon *et al.* (1982).

Changes in body water in PEM

Some of the results of measurements of TBW in malnourished children found in the literature are summarized in Table 3.2. Considering differences in method and the likelihood of differences in fatness, the results in control or fully recovered children are reasonably consistent, but this cannot be said for the findings in PEM.

Hansen *et al.* (1965) emphasized the relationship of excess water to deficit in body weight (Fig. 3.2). They attributed their low results in kwashiorkor to the fact that their cases were less underweight than those of other authors. They say 'oedema *per se* does not seem to be related to TBW'. Their results would imply that as far as body water is concerned there is no distinction

Table 3.2 Total body water (TBW) as a percentage of body weight in normal and malnourished children

	TBW, % of body weight		
	Controls or fully recovered	Malnourished	
Reference		With oedema	No oedema
Fomon *et al.* (1982)			
1–2 years: M	62–63		
F	60–62		
Schneider *et al.* (1958)	64.5	80.5	–
Smith (1960)	62.6	84.5	–
Hansen *et al.* (1965)	59	70	77
Alleyne (1968)	57.4	66.5 (mixed cases)	
Reeds *et al.* (1978)[a]	63	63	64

[a] Cases studied within 3 days of admission: four described as kwashiorkor or marasmic kwashiorkor, three as marasmus or undernutrition

between kwashiorkor and marasmus. Alleyne (1968) did not report separately on cases with and without oedema. It would clearly be useful to have more studies of body water, particularly in marasmic children.

Distribution of body water

On the basis of the earlier work it was generally accepted that in oedematous PEM, as in famine oedema of adults, the greater part of the excess fluid was extracellular (ECW) (Waterlow *et al.*, 1960). However, there is very little hard evidence for this. The results of three series are shown in Table 3.3. There is a major problem of methodology; the markers used for measuring ECW are supposed not to enter cells, but they may do so in the malnourished state if cell membranes are damaged, as suggested by the work of Patrick and Golden discussed in Chapter 10. The effect would be to overestimate the ECW. The values of Fomon *et al.* (1982) for normal children were obtained indirectly from measurements of TBW and TBK and the concentrations of K in extra- and intra-cellular water. This approach avoids the problem of membrane permeability. It is therefore remarkable that Fomon's estimates of ECW as a percentage of TBW should be higher than those found by Friis-Hansen (1954) in normal children using classical methods. One point, however, which does emerge from these studies is a significant inverse relationship between ECW and body weight (Alleyne, 1968). Hansen *et al.* (1965) suggested that the relative increase in ECW in malnutrition represented a reversion to an earlier stage of development.

Table 3.3   Extracellular water (ECW) as a percentage of total body water

| | ECW, % of TBW | | |
| | Controls or fully recovered | Malnourished | |
Reference		With oedema	No oedema
Fomon *et al.* (1982)	51–54		
Hansen *et al.* (1965)	42	47	44
Brinkman *et al.* (1965)	38	47	
Alleyne (1968)	47	59	

   The results of both Hansen *et al.* and Alleyne show an absolute increase in intracellular water during recovery, although this calculation, being by difference (TBW − ECW), is always precarious. It is not possible to tell whether it resulted from an absolute increase of cell mass, as seems likely, or from intracellular dilution. Patrick *et al.* (1978) re-analysed the earlier Jamaican data of Smith (1960) and Alleyne (1968), together with some new information of Reeds *et al.* (1978), in relation to diet and reported that when children were put on to a high energy diet after the loss of oedema, there was a substantial increase in TBW from about 63 to 71 per cent of body weight. They suggested that this increase was intracellular. Part of it could be accounted for by water associated with newly deposited glycogen, since muscle glycogen had been shown to increase ten-fold in the early stages of treatment, from 2 mg/g to 20 mg/g (Alleyne and Scullard, 1969), and 3–4 ml water are retained per g glycogen stored (Olsson and Saltin, 1970; Chan *et al.*, 1982). In addition Patrick *et al.* invoked potassium repletion and altered membrane transport to explain an increase in intracellular water, since the time interval would have been too short for a significant increase in cellular protein.

The question of intracellular dilution is very important (Chapter 11). Another approach to it is by measurements on tissues. Samples taken at autopsy, unless it is immediate, are not satisfactory for this purpose, because there is a rapid redistribution of water and sodium post-mortem. The results of measurements on muscle biopsies were summarized by Garrow *et al.* (1968). Calculations of the distribution of water between intra- and extracellular compartments were based on the assumption that all chloride is extracellular. This may not be true if cell membranes are damaged. The values obtained from muscle biopsies were very variable and do not give any clear indication of whether or not in PEM intracellular water is increased in relation to tissue solids.

Lean body mass and body fat

The difference between body weight and body water represents body solids. As soon as measurements of TBW began to be made in children with PEM, it was clear that, however they were expressed, total solids were greatly reduced. The problem is to separate the fat from the lean.

The classical methods used in adults for measuring body fat cannot readily be applied to children who are ill. Skinfold measurements are of no value in the presence of oedema, and in any case equations for relating skinfold thicknesses to body fat content, of the kind that have been developed for adults (Durnin and Womersley, 1974), do not exist for preschool children. Attempts to measure body volume, and hence density and fat, by helium dilution (Siri, 1961) were not successful because gas in the infants' gastrointestinal tracts introduced unacceptably large errors (Halliday, 1971).

Another approach that has been widely used in work on body composition is to determine lean body mass (LBM) from TBW on the assumption that water represents 73 per cent of lean tissue. However, if the amount and distribution of body water are abnormal this assumption does not hold. Estimates of LBM derived from total body potassium (TBK) run into similar difficulties. It is necessary to assume a constant factor for the average K concentration in the lean tissue of the normal body. The factor will not be correct if there is specific K depletion (Chapter 4), and the normal value will not be appropriate when there is an alteration in the proportions of the different tissues, as discussed above. Nevertheless, TBK probably gives the best available estimate of *cell* mass.

In the context of PEM, lean body mass is not of prime interest. Its main value is to give an estimate of fat mass by difference from body weight. Lean tissue has two components, structural and cellular, and it is the latter that is important. Picou *et al.* (1966) measured the collagen and non-collagen nitrogen in the whole bodies of children who died. In two children considered to be well-nourished collagen accounted for 27 per cent of total body protein and in eight malnourished children it accounted for 36–48 per cent. These authors concluded that even in severe PEM the collagen framework of the body is maintained more or less intact while the active cell mass shrinks round it. In a study on adults, total body nitrogen was measured by neutron activation analysis and cellular N estimated from TBK (James *et al.*, 1984). The difference represents structural or extracellular N, most of which is collagen. This fraction accounted for 35 per cent of whole body N in normal subjects and much more in those who were wasted, confirming the trend found in the children.

Table 3.4 shows computations of body protein in malnourished and recovered children, derived (A) from TBK, which provides an estimate of cellular protein; and (B) from TBW, which, after correction for ECW, gives a value for whole body protein on the assumption of constant hydration of the lean body mass. The proportion of the total that is structural protein is given by $(B-A)/B$. Although the proportions are lower than in the examples quoted above, the trend is the same: the proportion of structural protein is twice as great in the malnourished state as after recovery. The table also shows a significant decrease in cellular protein, expressed as a percentage of body weight.

Table 3.4 Distribution of body protein in eight children with PEM, when malnourished and after recovery (median interval 50 days); SDs in parentheses

	Malnourished	Recovered
Body weight, kg	5.73 (1.53)	7.41 (1.35)
A. Cellular protein, % of body weight	11.45 (1.67)	14.55* (1.10)
B. Total protein, % of body weight	15.8 (3.6)	16.85* (1.50)
Structural protein, % of total protein $(B-A)/B$	27.5 (9.6)	13.4 (6.2)

Summarized from Waterlow and Alleyne (1971) Table VII.
* Difference from malnourished $P < 0.01$.
Cellular protein calculated from TBK; total body protein from TBW and ECW.

In Fig. 3.4 an attempt is made to give an overall picture of the body composition of a child with severe PEM compared with a normal child of the same height. The decrease in the absolute amount of cellular protein is a measure of the extent to which the child is depleted. It is remarkable that a child can survive such a tremendous loss. It can only do so because muscle and perhaps skin protect the more essential organs. It is logical, therefore, to use muscle mass, represented by the creatinine/height index (Viteri and Alvarado, 1970), as a measure of the degree of depletion. A timed urine collection, even over a period of six hours, would be useful for this purpose, since the excretion of creatinine appears to be regular provided that there is an adequate urine flow. However, the variability increases with shorter collection periods (Viteri *et al.*, 1971).

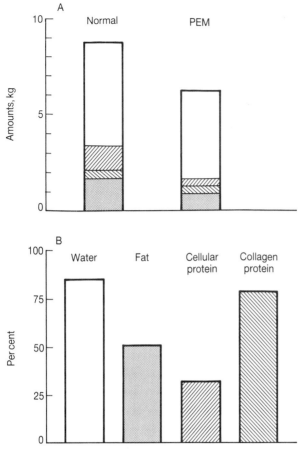

Fig. 3.4   Changes in body composition in severe PEM.
A. Absolute amounts compared with a normal child of the same height (70 cm).
B. Amounts of body components in PEM as a percentage of amounts in a normal child.
▢, water; ▨, fat; ▨, cellular protein; ▧, structural protein.
Derived from data of Picou *et al.* (1966).

Clinical implications of changes in body water

The characteristics of oedema in PEM have been described so often that only a brief summary is needed. Some authors have stated that oedema first appears in the buccal pads—hence the term 'moonface'. Sometimes, even when there is no obvious pitting, the subcutaneous tissues have a characteristic spongy feel, which has been regarded as 'pre-oedema' (Waterlow, 1948). Pitting oedema first appears on the feet and lower legs and then may become generalized. Almost all authors agree that ascites is never found. If it is present, particularly if abdominal veins are enlarged, the most likely cause is toxic liver damage, such as the 'veno-occlusive disease' caused by Senecio poisoning, which used to be observed quite commonly in Jamaica (Chapter 6).

There seem to be two somewhat different presentations of oedema in PEM. In frank kwashiorkor the child, in spite of generalized oedema, still retains considerable amounts of subcutaneous fat. This is the picture that Platt called 'sugar baby'. The history usually suggests that the onset has been quite recent, often following an infection. The other picture is seen in many cases of marasmic kwashiorkor: pitting oedema is confined to the feet and legs, while the subcutaneous tissues of the thorax and arms show reduced turgor and eyes and fontanelle are sunken. This combination of overhydration of the tissues in one part of the body and underhydration in another has often been described. Many authors agree that the prognosis is worse in marasmic kwashiorkor than in the other types of PEM (Chapter 12).

If these clinical impressions are correct, they lead to the possibility that oedematous PEM is not a clinical entity, varying only in the degree of wasting that accompanies the oedema, as would be suggested by the Wellcome classification (Chapter 1). It may be that the different presentations reflect a different balance of factors causing fluid retention. We return to the question of the cause of oedema in Chapter 11.

It is consistent with this hypothesis of multiple causation that, as Gürson *et al.* (1976) have emphasized, the degree and severity of oedema do not affect the prognosis. However, from the point of view of clinical management the increase in body water presents a problem. When a child fails to gain weight for two or three weeks, it is difficult to know whether is it genuinely making no progress, perhaps because of an undetected infection, or whether loss of excess water is masking an increase in body solids (Fig. 3.5).

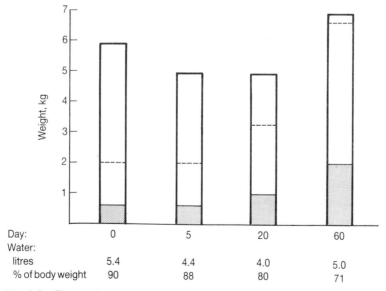

Day:	0	5	20	60
Water:				
litres	5.4	4.4	4.0	5.0
% of body weight	90	88	80	71

Fig. 3.5 Changes in body water and body solids during treatment in one child with kwashiorkor. Solids = body weight − body water. ☐ , water; ▨ , solids; ---- indicates the amount of water that would be expected from the measured amount of solids if body composition were normal. Data from Smith (1960).

The clinician dealing with PEM has to consider under- as well as over-hydration. Garrow *et al.* (1968) stressed that it is unrealistic to describe infantile malnutrition without also considering the changes due to gastroenteritis, since the two conditions so often occur together. In such cases there is a deficit rather than an excess of body water. The classical signs of dehydration are subjective and difficult to quantify (Chapter 12). Objective estimates of the degree of dehydration have been retrospective, based on the change in body weight after rehydration. It is very important not to overhydrate malnourished children; therefore the new instruments for determining body water by electrical conductivity or resistance, which are quick, non-invasive and can be used in the ward, will hopefully make an important contribution to the management of dehydrated malnourished children.

The measurement of body water is fundamental to understanding the changes in body composition that occur in the different forms of PEM. The research work described in this chapter, most of which was done a generation ago, has provided some insight into these changes and, as a result, a sounder basis for treatment. However, inconsistencies between different studies remain a cause for concern and more work on this subject could usefully be done. Moreover, we are still a long way from a clear and agreed understanding of the mechanisms of fluid retention in PEM. This subject is taken up again in Chapter 11.

References

Alleyne, G. A. O. (1968). Studies on total body potassium in infantile malnutrition: the relation of body fluid spaces and urinary creatinine. *Clinical Science* **34**: 199–209.

Alleyne, G. A. O., Scullard, G. M. (1969). Alterations in carbohydrate metabolism in Jamaican children with severe malnutrition. *Clinical Science* **37**: 631–642.

Alleyne, G. A. O., Halliday, D., Waterlow, J. C. (1969). Chemical composition of organs of children who died of malnutrition. *British Journal of Nutrition* **23**: 783–790.

Brinkman, G. L., Bowie, M. D. *et al.* (1965). Body water composition in kwashiorkor before and after loss of edema. *Pediatrics* **36**: 94–103.

Burkinshaw, L. (1985). Measurement of human body composition in vivo. *Progress in Medical Radiation Physics* **2**: 113–137.

Chan, S. T. F., Johnson, A. W. *et al.* (1982). Early weight gain and glycogen-obligated water during nutritional rehabilitation. *Human Nutrition: Clinical Nutrition* **36C**: 223–232.

Cheek, D. B., Hill, D. E. *et al.* (1970). Malnutrition in infancy: changes in muscle and adipose tissue before and after rehabilitation. *Pediatric Research* **4**: 135–144.

Cochran, W. J., Klish, W. J. *et al.* (1986). Total body electrical conductivity used to determine body composition in infants. *Pediatric Research* **20**: 561–564.

Cochran, W. J., Fiorotto, M. L. *et al.* (1989). Reliability of fat-free mass estimates derived from total body electrical conductivity measurements as influenced by changes in extra-cellular fluid volume. *American Journal of Clinical Nutrition* **49**: 29–32.

Coppoletta, J. M., Wolbach, S. B. (1933). Body length and organ weights of infants and children. *American Journal of Pathology* **9**: 55–70.

Coward, W. A., Parkinson, S. A., Murgatroyd, P. R. (1988). Body composition measurements for nutrition research. *Nutrition Research Reviews* **1**: 115–124.

Durnin, J. V. G. A., Womersley, J. (1974). Body fat assessed from total body density and its estimation from skinfold thickness: measurements on 481 men and women aged from 16–72 years. *British Journal of Nutrition* **32:** 77–97.

Fiorotto, M. L., Cochran, W. J., Klish, W. J. (1987*a*). Fat-free mass and total body water of infants estimated from total body electrical conductivity measurements. *Pediatric Research* **22:** 417–421.

Fiorotto, M. L., Cochran, W. J. *et al.* (1987*b*). Total body electrical conductivity measurements: effects of body composition and geometry. *American Journal of Physiology* **252:** (*Regulatory Integrative Comparative Physiology* 21) R794–800.

Fjeld, C. R., Freundt-Thurne, J., Schoeller, D. A. (1990). Total body water measured by ^{18}O dilution and bioelectrical impedance in well and malnourished children. *Pediatric Research* **27:** 98–102.

Fomon, S. J., Haschke, F. *et al.* (1982). Body composition of reference children from birth to age 10 years. *American Journal of Clinical Nutrition* **35:** 1169–1175.

Forbes, G. B. (1987). *Human body composition: growth, aging, nutrition and activity.* Springer-Verlag, New York and London.

Frenk, S., Metcoff, J. *et al.* (1957). Intracellular composition and homeostatic mechanisms in severe chronic infantile malnutrition. II. Composition of tissues. *Pediatrics* **20:** 105–120.

Friis-Hansen, B. (1954). The extracellular fluid volume in infants and children. *Acta Paediatrica Scandinavica* **43:** 444–458.

Fuller, M. F., Fowler, P. A. *et al.* (1990). Body composition: the precision and accuracy of new methods and their suitability for longitudinal studies. *Proceedings of the Nutrition Society* **49:** 423–436.

Garrow, J. S., Fletcher, K., Halliday, D. (1965). Body composition in severe infantile malnutrition. *Journal of Clinical Investigation* **44:** 417–425.

Garrow, J. S., Smith, R., Ward, E. E. (1968). *Electrolyte metabolism in severe infantile malnutrition.* Pergamon Press, London.

Gregory, J. W., Greene, S. A. *et al.* (1991). Body water measurement in growth disorders: a comparison of bioelectric impedance and skinfold techniques with isotope dilution. *Archives of Disease in Childhood* **66:** 220–222.

Gürson, C. T., Yüksel, T., Saner, G. (1976). The short-term prognosis of protein-calorie malnutrition in Marmara region of Turkey. *Journal of Tropical Pediatrics* **22:** 59–62.

Halliday, D. (1967). Chemical composition of the whole body and individual tissues of two Jamaican children whose death resulted primarily from malnutrition. *Clinical Science* **33:** 365–370.

Halliday, D. (1971). An attempt to estimate total body fat and protein in malnourished children. *British Journal of Nutrition* **26:** 147–153.

Hansen, J. D. L., Brinkman, G. L., Bowie, M. D. (1965). Body composition in protein-calorie malnutrition. *South African Medical Journal* **39:** 491–495.

Hansen-Smith, F. M., Picou, D., Golden, M. H. (1979). Growth of muscle fibres during recovery from severe malnutrition in Jamaican infants. *British Journal of Nutrition* **41:** 275–282.

Holliday, M. A., Potter, D. *et al.* (1967). The relation of metabolic rate to body weight and organ size. *Pediatric Research* **1:** 185–195.

Househam, K. C., de Villiers, J. F. F. (1987). Computed tomography in severe PEM. *Archives of Disease in Childhood* **62:** 589–592.

James, H. M., Dabek, J. T. *et al.* (1984). Whole body cellular and collagen nitrogen in healthy and wasted men. *Clinical Science* **67:** 73–82.

Kerpel-Fronius, E., Frank, K. (1949). Einige Besonderheiten der Körperzusammensetzung und Wasserverteilung bei der Säuglingsatrophie. *Annals Paediatrica* **173:** 321–330.

Montgomery, R. D. (1962). Muscle morphology in infantile protein malnutrition. *Journal of Clinical Pathology* **15:** 511–521.

Olsson K-E., Saltin, B. (1970). Variation in total body water with muscle glycogen changes in man. *Acta Physiologica Scandinavica* **80:** 11–18.

Patrick, J., Reeds, P. J. *et al.* (1978). Total body water in malnutrition: the possible role of energy intake. *British Journal of Nutrition* **39:** 417–424.

Picou, D., Halliday, D., Garrow, J. S. (1966). Total body protein, collagen and non-collagen protein in infantile protein malnutrition. *Clinical Science* **30:** 345–351.

Reeds, P. J., Jackson, A. A. *et al.* (1978). Muscle mass and composition in malnourished infants and children and changes seen after recovery. *Pediatric Research* **12:** 613–618.

Schneider, H., Hendrickse, R. G., Haigh, C. P. (1958). Studies in water metabolism in clinical and experimental malnutrition. *Transactions of the Royal Society of Tropical Medicine and Hygiene* **52:** 169–175.

Schoeller, D. A., Van Santen, E. *et al.* (1980). Total body water measurements in humans with ^{18}O and ^{2}H labelled water. *American Journal of Clinical Nutrition* **33:** 2686–2693.

Siri, W. S. (1961). Body composition from fluid spaces and density: analysis of methods. In Brozek, J., Henschel, A. (eds) *Techniques for measuring body composition.* National Academy of Sciences, Washington DC, pp. 223–244.

Smith, R. (1960). Total body water in malnourished infants. *Clinical Science* **19:** 275–285.

Standard, K. L., Wills, V. G., Waterlow, J. C. (1959). Indirect indicators of muscle mass in malnourished infants. *American Journal of Clinical Nutrition* **7:** 271–279.

Viteri, F., Alvarado, J. (1970). The creatinine height index: its use in the estimation of the degree of protein depletion and repletion in protein-calorie malnourished children. *Pediatrics* **46:** 696–706.

Viteri, F. E., Alvarado, J., Alleyne, G. A. O. (1971). Reply to Drs Mendez and Buskirk. *American Journal of Clinical Nutrition* **24:** 386–387.

Waterlow, J. C. (1948). *Fatty liver disease in infants in the British West Indies.* Medical Research Council Special Report Series No. 263. HM Stationery Office, London.

Waterlow, J. C. (1956). The protein content of liver and muscle as a measure of protein deficiency in human subjects. *West Indian Medical Journal* **5:** 167–174.

Waterlow, J. C., Alleyne, G. A. O. (1971). Protein malnutrition in children: advances in knowledge in the last ten years. *Advances in Protein Chemistry* **25:** 117–241.

Waterlow, J. C., Stephen, J. M. L. (1966). Adaptation of the rat to a low protein diet: the effect of a reduced protein intake on the pattern of incorporation of L-^{14}C-lysine. *British Journal of Nutrition* **20:** 461–484.

Waterlow, J. C., Cravioto, J., Stephen, J. M. L. (1960). Protein malnutrition in man. *Advances in Protein Chemistry* **15:** 131–238.

Winick, M., Rosso, P., Waterlow, J. C. (1970). Cellular growth of cerebrum, cerebellum and brain stem in normal and marasmic children. *Experimental Neurology* **26:** 393–400.

4

Electrolytes and major minerals

Introduction

There is no clear dividing line between the elements traditionally referred to as electrolytes (K, Na) and those described as major minerals (Ca, Mg, P), since the latter also have important functions as ions in aqueous solution.* The difference is that the greater part of the body's calcium, a substantial part of the phosphorus and about two-thirds of the magnesium are located in bone. Even this difference is not absolute, since bone has the highest sodium content of any tissue (Forbes, 1987).

The amounts of these elements in the newborn and the adult are shown in Table 4.1. From the point of view of quantity, iron and zinc occupy an intermediate position between what may be called the macro-elements and the trace elements. Iron enters the PEM story in two ways; iron deficiency is considered in the section on anaemia (Chapter 5) and iron excess in the

Table 4.1 Amounts of selected elements in the whole body in order of decreasing quantity

| | Newborn (3.4 kg) | | Child 4½ years (14 kg) | |
	(g)	(mmol)	(g)	(mmol)
Nitrogen	66	2360	535	19000
Calcium	28	700	295	7400
Phosphorus	16	520	147	4700
Sodium	10.4	240	–	
Magnesium	0.76	32	5	208
Iron	0.32	5.7	0.9	16
Zinc	0.053	0.8	0.31	4.7
Copper	0.014	0.2	0.046	0.7

From Forbes (1987), Table 4.3.

* In this and the succeeding chapter the elements are written with superscripts, e.g. K^+, Ca^{++}, only when reference is being made specifically to their actions as ions.

chapter on free radicals (Chapter 10). We treat zinc in the traditional way as one of the trace elements (Chapter 9).

The foundations of our knowledge of electrolyte changes in PEM were laid before 1970 by studies in Mexico, Chile, Jamaica, South Africa and the Congo, and little new work on the subject has been done since then, except for the studies of Patrick and co-workers on electrolyte transport in leucocytes (Chapter 10). The earlier investigations were described in detail in the books by Garrow *et al.* (1968) and Alleyne *et al.* (1977) and an excellent review by Patrick (1978) provides a valuable discussion of the physiology of electrolytes in PEM. Electrolyte changes are so important that we must recapitulate the results of these older studies, in the context of more recent experimental work, particularly that of Clausen and co-workers (Dørup and Clausen, 1989).

Potassium

Hansen (1956) was the first to document K deficiency in PEM, by balance studies in which he showed that with treatment there was a much greater retention of K compared to N than could be accounted for by their proportions in body tissues.

In the 1960s the Tropical Metabolism Research Unit, Jamaica, obtained a small whole-body counter with which total body potassium (TBK) could be determined from the radiation of the natural isotope ^{40}K. With this instrument serial measurements could be made even in children who were very ill. Results obtained by Alleyne are shown in Fig. 4.1. The normal range is 40–45 mmol/kg. Alleyne *et al.* (1970) emphasized the importance of distinguishing between the reduction in K *capacity* which results from tissue wasting and represents depletion (Chapter 2); and reduction in the *saturation* of that capacity, i.e. in the concentration of K in cells, or the ratio of K to N, which represents true K deficiency (Fig. 4.2).

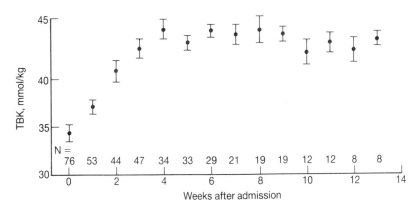

Fig. 4.1   Total body potassium concentration in children as they recovered from severe malnutrition. Vertical bars are standard errors. Reproduced by permission from Alleyne (1970).

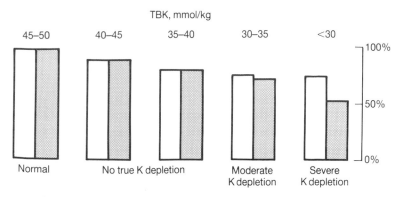

Fig. 4.2   Potassium capacity and potassium content in malnourished children in relation to total body potassium concentration. ⬜, potassium capacity; ▨, potassium content. Reproduced by permission from Alleyne *et al.* (1970).

It could be argued that the initially low values shown in Fig. 4.1 are simply a result of oedema, consisting mainly of extracellular fluid containing very little K. Indeed, it was soon found that oedematous children tended to have particularly low values of TBK/kg (Garrow, 1965; Alleyne, 1968). As might be expected, there was an inverse correlation between TBK and extracellular fluid volume. However, Alleyne (1968) was able to show a significant decrease in the concentration of K in intracellular water, which was linearly correlated with TBK. This finding is the strongest direct evidence for our belief that specific K deficiency is a common and important feature of PEM.

Since body fat also 'dilutes' the cell mass, lean body mass should be a better basis of reference for TBK than body weight. Mann and Hansen (1972) found that in normal infants a more precise prediction of TBK could be obtained if the measurements of ^{40}K were related to skinfold thickness and weight for height, which in effect provide estimates of lean body mass. In this way they were able to diagnose mild degrees of K deficiency in children with gastroenteritis uncomplicated by malnutrition.

Another approach used in the early days for investigating K status was by measurements on muscle biopsies. Muscle K per unit weight or nitrogen was initially low compared with the level on recovery. When muscle K and TBK were measured at the same time, it appeared that values for TBK down to about 35 mmol/kg reflected mainly a decrease in K capacity; below that there was a true deficiency, according to Alleyne's definition (Fig. 4.2) (Nichols *et al.*, 1969; Alleyne *et al.*, 1970).

Although muscle is the main reservoir of K in the body, the brain comes next; the K content of the brain has been found to be reduced at autopsy (Alleyne *et al.*, 1969), although not to the same extent as muscle which bears the brunt of the loss of K. Garrow (1967), by an ingenious adaptation of the whole-body counter, estimated the K content of the head, which effectively represents brain K, in children with PEM. When TBK was less than 35 mmol/kg 'brain' K was only 60 per cent of the level found after recovery. This may well have something to do with the apathy, weakness and hypotonia characteristic of severe PEM.

Consequences of K deficiency

Since the concentration of K in cells affects many biochemical and biophysical processes, it is to be expected that deficiency of K will have serious consequences. Some have been demonstrated in man, others so far only in experimental animals.

There is good evidence that K deficiency promotes retention of water and sodium and therefore may produce oedema, which disappears on administration of K (Black and Milne, 1952; Waterlow and Bunje, 1966). The mechanism is not entirely understood. In PEM potassium supplements were followed by a rapid decrease in extracellular fluid volume (Mann *et al.*, 1975*a*). Krishna *et al.* (1987) showed that even mild K deficiency promotes renal Na retention and decreases excretion of a Na load. In rat muscle K deficiency produces an increase in intracellular Na and a decrease in the number of Na^+–K^+ pumps (Kjeldsen *et al.*, 1984; Clausen, 1986). Reduction in the concentration gradient of Na^+ across the cell membrane lowers the capacity for extruding H^+ ions through the Na^+/H^+ exchange mechanism. This leads to a combination of intracellular acidosis with extracellular alkalosis. It is interesting that Kingston (1973) observed alkalosis in hypokalaemic children when they were treated, even though no bicarbonate or lactate was given. The electrolyte imbalance in muscle cells also impairs the extrusion of calcium (Clausen and Kjeldsen, 1987). Accumulation of Ca^{++} could lead to membrane damage, through stimulation of phospholipases; to mitochondrial swelling and leakiness; to increased protein breakdown through stimulation of calcium-dependent proteases, and to decreased protein synthesis (Dørup and Clausen, 1989). Loss of K^+ with increase in Ca^{++} could reduce the contractile power in the myocardium and thus be a factor in the reduction of cardiac output that is a feature of severe PEM (see Chapter 5). How far these possible effects of K deficiency are translated into reality in PEM we do not know.

Diagnosis of K deficiency

Hypokalaemia is not a constant characteristic of PEM. Kingston (1973) summarized data from 11 countries. In five of them mean serum K was 4.0 mmol/l or above. In his own study in Liberia the mean serum K was 2.2 mmol/l, which is exceptionally low. In Jamaica there was a relationship between TBK and serum K concentration. The symptoms of K deficiency mentioned above are non-specific but if there is hypokalaemia ECG changes and arrhythmias may occur. It is wise to assume that all children with severe PEM are deficient in K; treatment based on this assumption has not led to complications.

Causes of K deficiency

The causes of deficiency are an inadequate intake and excessive losses of K in stools. There is surprisingly little information in the literature on the K content of children's diets in regions where PEM is common. Animal and vegetable foods and unrefined cereals contain 6–9 mmol K/100 g dry weight, giving a ratio of K:N similar to that of human tissues. Refined cereals such as white rice, high extraction corn meal, arrowroot, etc., have a much lower

K content. In cassava it is particularly low. Any diet which is low in protein, like many of the weaning foods commonly used, will be low in K and in other intracellular components such as magnesium, zinc and phosphorus.

Diarrhoea has been recognized since the time of Darrow (1946) as causing an important loss of K in children with gastroenteritis, even when uncompli- cated by malnutrition. Many but not all children with severe PEM have a history of diarrhoea. Alleyne (1970) observed a relationship between TBK on admission and the number of stools passed in the first five days in hospital. The K content of diarrhoeal stools has been given as 20–40 mmol/l stool water. Thus a child weighing 6 kg, with a TBK of 270 mmol, in a severe bout of diarrhoea could easily lose 30 mmol K, or more than 20 per cent of its total body K. Mann *et al.* (1975*b*) report a child in whom an attack of severe diarrhoea reduced TBK from 42 to 35 mmol/kg in five days. The combination of acute loss of K from diarrhoea with an inadequate intake over some time is bound to be serious and may be fatal.

Michaelson and Clausen (1987) have pointed out that many of the staple foodstuffs distributed for emergency relief to populations affected by famine contain inadequate amounts of K and Mg to cover normal requirements and make good losses. This could seriously reduce the effectiveness of the relief programme.

Sodium

If the extracellular fluid volume (ECFV) is increased (Chapter 3) one would expect total body sodium to be increased also, and there is evidence that this is so. In two cadavers analysed by Halliday (1967) the Na content was 104 and 113 mmol/kg, values substantially higher than the 82 mmol/kg found by Widdowson and Spray (1951) in a normal full-term infant. Dubois *et al.* (1968) measured total exchangeable Na before and after treatment in five malnourished children, four of whom had oedema. Exchangeable Na fell from 73 to 61 mmol/kg. The recovery figure is much lower than that of Widdowson, presumably because the proportion of ECFV in the body is much greater at birth than later in childhood. The increase in total body Na was confirmed by balance studies, which showed massive excretion of Na in the early stages of recovery (Hansen, 1956; Vis *et al.*, 1965).

Paradoxically, the increase in total body Na is sometimes accompanied by hyponatraemia. This seems to occur particularly in marasmic kwashiorkor. In the words of Garrow *et al.* (1968), 'there is an excess of Na in an even greater excess of water'. There are two possible explanations for the paradox: Na may be either diluted in the ECF or diverted out of it. In an article with the provocative title 'The charted and uncharted waters of hyponatraemia' Gross *et al.* (1987), discussing particularly cardiac failure, prefer the first possibility and treat the subject almost entirely in terms of increased anti- diuretic hormone (ADH) activity. The evidence for this and for the involve- ment of other hormones that influence water and salt retention is considered in Chapter 8.

The other possible explanation of hyponatraemia is that Na has entered the cells. From the experimental work of Clausen (1986) one would expect this to happen as a consequence of K deficiency. Direct measurements on muscle biopsies in children with PEM were summarized by Garrow *et al.* (1968). The Na content per g fat-free tissue did tend to be high, but it could not be determined with certainty whether or not this simply reflected wasting of muscle fibres and expansion of the muscle's extracellular space. Estimates of this space from measurements of muscle chloride are not entirely reliable because of the possibility that some chloride crosses the cell membrane. Measurements on leucocytes have shown an increased Na content in both kwashiorkor and marasmus, which was attributed to leakiness of their membranes (Patrick and Golden, 1977) (Chapter 10). If Na^+ leaks in, K^+ should leak out, and Flear and Singh (1973) showed a correlation between low serum Na and low TBK. Morgan and Thomas (1979) suggested that, if the membrane is leaky, the cell loses anionic soluble molecules. If the cell volume is to be maintained, the intracellular fluid must become hypotonic; this in turn leads to hypotonicity of the extracellular fluid. A cell in such a state could well be regarded as suffering from what has been called the 'sick cell syndrome'.

Whether or not this explanation of hypotonicity is correct, the fact remains that in PEM hyponatraemia is a very bad prognostic sign (Garrow, 1962). Moreover, in a wide range of conditions—congestive heart disease, pulmonary tuberculosis and trauma—the serum Na level has been shown to be correlated inversely with the severity of clinical state (Tindall and Clark, 1976). It does, therefore, seem to make sense to regard hyponatraemia as evidence of 'sickness' at the cellular level.

Calcium

Calcium has received very little attention in studies on PEM, and is not mentioned even in the indices of the main books on the subject (Olson, 1975; Alleyne *et al.*, 1977). Ninety-eight per cent of the Ca in the body is in bone, so that from the point of view of maintaining the concentration in other tissues, there is a huge reserve. In spite of large differences in intake the concentration of ionized Ca^{++} in plasma and extracellular fluids is regulated within narrow limits by the combined activity of three hormones, parathyroid hormone, calcitonin and the vitamin D metabolite 1,25-dihydroxycholecalciferol (Fraser, 1981; MacIntyre, 1986).

The intracellular concentration of Ca^{++} is 1000 times lower than the extracellular; the constancy of the cytoplasmic Ca^{++} concentration is of great importance, since it plays a fundamental role in the integrated control of membrane permeability, the cellular response to stimulation and intracellular signalling (Matthews, 1986; Campbell, 1990). The very large concentration gradient across the cell membrane is maintained by a 'calcium pump', and it is possible that in the body as a whole this pump is responsible for a larger oxygen uptake than the sodium pump (Clausen *et al.*, 1991). A breakdown of this pump as a result of hypoxia leads to accumulation of intracellular Ca^{++} and serious cell damage (Jackson, 1990). One might speculate that an effect of this kind could be a component of the 'sick cell syndrome' in severe PEM.

Although hypocalcaemia in the newborn, particularly in prematures, is well recognized, by the time that PEM develops the mechanisms that regulate extracellular Ca^{++} concentration appear to be well established. Clinical signs suggestive of tetany may be due to magnesium deficiency or to hypocalcaemia associated with Mg deficiency (Shils, 1969a, b). About half the Ca in serum is bound to albumin so that a low total Ca concentration may result from hypoalbuminaemia. A small but significant fall in ionized Ca^{++} has been reported in marasmus (Nanda *et al.*, 1984).

If there is a deficiency of Ca, its most likely impact is on bone growth. As Fraser (1988) has pointed out, bone growth may be affected in two ways: it may continue but with inadequate mineralization, or it may be held back to a rate at which mineral deposition is normal. According to Fraser the rat appears to adopt the first alternative, except in very severe deficiency, but we have little information on what happens in man. Walker (1972) summarized evidence showing that in Third World children on low Ca intakes cortical bone density was normal. Radiological measurements of bone density are no longer considered to be ethical and we have to wait for results by the non-invasive method of single photon absorptiometry for wider confirmation of this finding. Prentice *et al.* (1990), using this method, have shown that after adjusting for differences in body size the bone mineral content of the radius in Gambian children was 12 per cent lower than that of children in the UK. The Gambian children at two to three years were some 5 cm shorter than their British counterparts, a deficit of more than 1 SD, which represents a decrease in linear growth that is not negligible. How far children adopt the other alternative, of limiting their skeletal growth in response to a low Ca intake, is at present an unsolved question, because Ca in foods is associated with other factors that could be limiting, such as protein or zinc (Chapter 13). Preliminary results from a longitudinal study in Thailand of the development of stunting from birth to two years showed that between one and two years there was a small fall, averaging 0.3 mg/dl, in total serum Ca concentration. The extent of this fall was negatively correlated with growth in height, the children who gained most showing the smallest decrease in Ca (K. Chusilp *et al.*, personal communication).

It seems entirely possible that the Ca intake of the Third World child will become limiting after the first six months of life. The daily increments in body Ca of the reference infant, as calculated by Fomon (1974), are 155 mg/day between birth and four months, and 130 mg/day from four to 12 months. The Ca content of mature human milk from Western mothers is about 300 mg/l (Mellander *et al.*, 1959; Fomon, 1974; Laskey *et al.*, 1990). In The Gambia the content at three months was lower, about 250 mg/l, falling to less than 200 mg/l at nine to 12 months. At four months 800 ml of breast milk will contain about 200 mg Ca. Therefore, in order to provide an increment of 130 mg/day, 65 per cent of the intake would have to be absorbed. Fortunately, the availability of Ca in human milk is very high. At one year, when both intake and Ca concentration of breast milk begin to fall off, it will be difficult for the child's requirement to be met. The only other foods rich in Ca are cow's milk, in which the concentration is four times as high as in human milk, and green leafy vegetables (Sherman, 1947). Moreover, the weaning diet is likely to contain interfering factors, such as phytic acid, which reduce Ca absorption. It is hard to avoid the conclusion that by one year of age skeletal growth could be limited by the supply of calcium.

More than fifty years ago Aykroyd and Krishnan (1937) found that a supplement of skimmed milk stimulated growth in height of school children.

They followed this up with a trial in which calcium lactate was given to pre-school children aged about three years (Aykroyd and Krishnan, 1939). This also produced a significant increase in linear growth. Pettifor and co-workers (1979) in South Africa found that in rural school children, with an estimated Ca intake of only 125 mg/day, 40 per cent had raised serum alkaline phosphatase and 13 per cent had low serum Ca. Bone biopsy in three cases showed the typical histological changes of osteomalacia (Marie *et al.*, 1982). These abnormalities were not observed in urban children with a higher Ca intake.

An interesting possibility has been raised by Clements *et al.* (1987), that a low Ca intake increases the requirement for vitamin D. This might help to explain the high prevalence of rickets in a zone which stretches from North Africa through Egypt and Iran to North India and China. In many parts of the Middle East the staple is unrefined wheat flour, with high concentrations of fibre and phytate, which impair the absorption of Ca. Synthesis of vitamin D in the skin under the influence of ultra-violet radiation is thought to be a more important source of the vitamin than food, and in these countries there is plenty of sunlight, but the children are often kept wrapped up (e.g. Lawson *et al.*, 1987).

Rickets is not a typical feature of PEM, because the classical changes in the long bones do not occur in the absence of growth. Bhattacharyya and Dutta (1976) in Calcutta described 'atrophic' rickets in children with PEM, with gross decalcification and thinning of the bone cortex, but without the classical cupping and spreading of the metaphyses. These changes became evident in the process of healing. In a survey of 200 cases of children with rickets in Tehran (Salimpour, 1975), malnutrition tended to disguise the characteristic biochemical changes of rickets (Table 4.2). Reddy and Srikantia (1967) also described normal alkaline phosphatase levels in malnourished children with rickets.

Table 4.2   Biochemical findings in children with rickets in Tehran

Age of children	0–12 months			13–36 months		
Grade of malnutrition[a]	I	II	III	I	II	III
No. of children	7	11	8	6	7	13
% with convulsions	43	17	0	33	0	8
Mean serum Ca, mg/dl	6.87	8.16	8.26	9.78	9.19	8.67
Mean serum P, mg/dl	3.81	2.52	2.57	3.54	3.46	2.56
Alkaline phosphatase, BLB units/ml[b]	12.4	7.3	8.0	10.2	5.7	12.1

From Salimpour (1975)
[a] Gomez classification
[b] Bessey *et al.* (1946)

It seems reasonable to conclude that Ca deficiency may well be common in PEM. It does not immediately follow that this is a cause of stunting in linear growth, because the process of stunting may begin within three months of birth, whereas the supply of Ca should be adequate as long as the child is fully breast-fed.

Magnesium

It was clearly established in the 1960s, as a result of the work of Montgomery (1960, 1961) in Jamaica, Linder *et al.* (1963) in South Africa and Caddell (1965) in Nigeria that magnesium deficiency is common in PEM. The basic clinical effect of the deficiency is an increase in neuromuscular excitability (Halpern, 1985), characterized by muscular twitching, squirming athetoid movements, rigidity, sometimes a positive Chvostek sign, sometimes convulsions. Caddell (1969) described ECG changes (premature ventricular beats and low-voltage T waves) and suggested that inadequate treatment of severe PEM with Mg could lead to fatal arrhythmias. Tetany is sometimes seen, but this may reflect the hypocalcaemia that results from Mg depletion (Shils, 1988).

In Jamaica we were first alerted to the possibility of Mg deficiency because the clinical signs became more common after we had begun to give supplementary potassium as a routine. The reason is that K^+ and Mg^{++} have antagonistic effects on excitability. In symptomatic cases the diagnosis is not difficult if one is aware of the problem. If the child has convulsions, the differential diagnosis is from hypoglycaemia, meningitis and cerebral malaria. Treatment of the acute deficiency is by intramuscular injection of a magnesium salt (Chapter 12).

When, as in the majority of cases, there are no symptoms diagnosis of Mg deficiency rests on biochemical measurements. There are differences of opinion about the value of measurements on serum. In experimentally induced Mg deficiency in adult volunteers, the serum concentration fell to very low levels after six or more weeks (Shils, 1969a). Montgomery (1960), on the other hand, found it of little value in PEM and concluded that the best diagnostic test was a low urinary Mg output. Caddell and Olson (1973) agree; they found plasma Mg normal or low-normal on admission, but hypomagnesaemia developed on treatment unless Mg was given. Like Montgomery they regarded a low Mg content of urine as a useful guide to Mg status. In Shils' experiment urinary Mg fell to almost undetectable levels after only a few days on the deficient diet, long before there was any change in serum Mg concentration. Balance studies in children with PEM showed a low urinary Mg output and substantial retention when supplements were given (Montgomery, 1961). Harris and Wilkinson (1971) used a loading test, in which $MgCl_2$ was given by slow intravenous injection and urine collected for 24 hours. A child was regarded as depleted if the output was less than 40 per cent of the dose. This method of diagnosis is clearly too invasive for general use.

Measurements on tissues, taken by biopsy or post-mortem, showed a decreased concentration of Mg in muscle, whether related to weight or to nitrogen, but not in liver, brain, heart or kidney (Alleyne *et al.*, 1970). It is presumably this reduction in muscle that causes many of the clinical signs.

There are important relationships between the two intracellular cations, K^+ and Mg^{++}, apart from their effects on excitability. It has been shown in experimental animals that Mg deficiency led to loss of K from muscle (Whang and Welt, 1963). In the study of Shils (1969a) the Mg deficient diet produced a reduction of about 25 per cent in total exchangeable K, a degree of deficit comparable to that found in PEM. At the same time there was evidence of retention of Na and a striking fall in urinary Ca (Shils, 1969*b*; 1988). These findings are clearly very relevant to the electrolyte changes in PEM. We believe that in PEM Mg deficiency and depletion are so important and so common that treatment should be given as a routine, without any attempt to make a specific diagnosis (Chapter 12).

The causes of Mg deficiency in PEM are similar to those of K deficiency: an inadequate intake and increased losses in the stools if there is diarrhoea. There is the further problem, which does not apply to K, that the absorption of Mg as well as of Ca may be impaired by factors in the food which make it insoluble, such as phytic acid. The requirement for Mg in the first year of life has been estimated at about 15 mg/day, assuming 20 per cent absorption (Fomon, 1974). Since the Mg content of human milk is of the order of 40 mg/l (Fomon, 1974) the requirement should be amply met as long as breast feeding is adequate. After weaning, green vegetables are an important source, since Mg plays the same role for chlorophyll in plants as Fe does for haemoglobin in animals.

When children are recovering from PEM and growing rapidly, ample amounts of Mg are necessary for restoring tissue depletion (Caddell, 1969). Nichols *et al.* (1978) carried out an extensive series of balance studies in recovering children. On the assumption that 50 per cent of dietary Mg was absorbed, and that two-thirds of this was retained, they estimated that satisfactory catch-up growth required an intake of 2.7 mmol (66 mg) Mg/kg/day. That is far more than would be supplied by a recovery diet based on skimmed milk powder (Chapter 12), and therefore supplementary Mg is essential. As mentioned above, the same problem arises with food used for relief operations. As for K, inadequacy of Mg may limit the rate of restoration of lean tissue and even contribute to death.

Phosphorus

Surprisingly little attention has been paid to the metabolism of phosphorus (P) in PEM, in spite of the fact that P deficiency is well-known in farm animals. Metcoff's studies of PEM in Mexico in the 1960s showed no decrease of intracellular phosphate concentration (Metcoff, 1975). Low concentrations of serum and urinary P have been found in children with PEM in Jamaica (Golden, 1988). The literature is otherwise silent on this subject.

In north-east Thailand there is, or used to be, a remarkably high prevalence of bladder-stones in infants and young children, associated particularly with the consumption of 'sticky' rice. This condition has been attributed to P deficiency, since urinary P concentrations were low and supplements of orthophosphate decreased the output of oxalic and uric acids (Valyasevi *et al.*, 1967*a*, *b*). However, there is no evidence of any particular association of bladder-stones with PEM. A possible role of P deficiency in stunting has been discussed by Fraser (1988).

The requirement for phosphorus is closely related to the rate of growth. Between six and 36 months the child accumulates 60–70 mg P/day (Fomon, 1974), of which about 40 per cent is used for tissue growth and 60 per cent for bone growth. In studies in Jamaica on children aged three to 17 months recovering from malnutrition, 70 per cent of dietary P was absorbed both from breast milk and from a cow's milk mixture. At the very least, therefore, the daily requirement would be 100 mg P, if all absorbed P was retained and utilized. In fact, some of our children fed on human milk retained 100 per cent of absorbed P (Waterlow and Wills, 1960). Fomon suggests that the 'advisable' intake should be about 130 mg/day, which would require almost a litre/day of mature human milk, with a P content of 120–150 mg/l. These calculations suggest that in the exclusively breast-fed infant the P intake may easily become limiting. However, nearly all plant and animal foods contain on a weight basis much more P than human milk. According to the values given by Sherman (1947), a daily supplement of 5 g cereal and 10 g green vegetables per kg body weight would contribute an extra amount of P of the order of 25 mg/kg.

There seems a clear case for studies of the possibility of P deficiency in PEM, particularly as a factor that might be limiting growth.

References

Alleyne, G. A. O. (1968). Studies on total body potassium in infantile malnutrition: the relation to body fluid spaces and urinary creatinine. *Clinical Science* **34**: 199–209.

Alleyne, G. A. O. (1970). Studies on total body potassium in malnourished infants: factors affecting potassium repletion. *British Journal of Nutrition* **24**: 205–212.

Alleyne, G. A. O., Halliday, D., Waterlow, J. C. (1969). Chemical composition of organs of children who died from malnutrition. *British Journal of Nutrition* **23**: 783–790.

Alleyne, G. A. O., Millward, D. J., Scullard, G. H. (1970). Total body potassium, muscle electrolytes and glycogen in malnourished children. *Journal of Pediatrics* **76**: 75–81.

Alleyne, G. A. O., Hay, R. W. *et al.* (1977). *Protein-energy malnutrition*. Edward Arnold, London,

Aykroyd, W. R., Krishnan, B. G. (1937). The effect of skimmed milk, soya bean and other foods in supplementing typical Indian diets. *Indian Journal of Medical Research* **24**: 1093–1115.

Aykroyd, W. R., Krishnan, B. G. (1939). A further experiment on the value of calcium lactate for Indian children. *Indian Journal of Medical Research* **27**: 409–412.

Bessey, A. O., Lowry, O. H., Brock, M. J. (1946). A method for the rapid determination of alkaline phosphatase in 5 cubic millimetres of serum. *Journal of Biological Chemistry* **164**: 321–329.

Bhattacharyya, A. K., Dutta, K. N. (1976). Atrophic rickets. *Indian Journal of Radiology* **30**: 267–270.

Black, D. A. K., Milne, M. D. (1952). Experimental potassium depletion in man. *Clinical Science* **11**: 397–415.

Caddell, J. L. (1965). Magnesium in the therapy of protein-calorie malnutrition of childhood. *Journal of Pediatrics* **66**: 392–413.

Caddell, J. L. (1969). Magnesium deficiency in protein-calorie malnutrition: a follow-up study. *Annals of New York Academy of Sciences* **162**: 874–890.

Caddell, J. L., Olson, R. E. (1973). An evaluation of the electrolyte status of malnourished Thai children. *Journal of Pediatrics* **83**: 124–135.

Campbell, A. K. (1990). Calcium as an intracellular regulator. *Proceedings of the Nutrition Society* **49**: 51–56.

Clausen, T. (1986). Regulation of active Na$^+$-K$^+$ transport in skeletal muscle. *Physiological Reviews* **66**: 542–580.

Clausen, T., Kjeldsen, K. (1987). Effects of potassium deficiency on Na, K homoeostasis and Na,K-ATPase in muscle. In Klausner, R. (ed) *Current topics in membranes and transport*. Academic Press, London, **28**: 403–419.

Clausen, T., van Hardefeld, C., Everts, M. E. (1991). The significance of cation transport in the control of energy metabolism and thermogenesis. *Physiological Reviews* **71**: 733–774.

Clements, M. R., Johnson, L., Fraser, D. R. (1987). A new mechanism for induced vitamin D deficiency in calcium deprivation. *Nature* **325**: 62–65.

Darrow, D. C. (1946). Retention of electrolyte during recovery from severe dehydration due to diarrhoea. *Journal of Pediatrics* **28**: 515–540.

Dørup, I., Clausen, T. (1989). Effects of potassium deficiency on growth and protein synthesis in skeletal muscle and the heart of rats. *British Journal of Nutrition* **62**: 269–284.

Dubois, J., Cremer, M., Vis, A. L. (1968). Etude des troubles electrolytiques accompagnant le kwashiorkor marastique. III. Perturbation de la composition corporelle. *Revues Françaises Etudes Cliniques Biologiques* **13**: 976–983.

Flear, C. T. G., Singh, C. M. (1973). Hyponatraemia and sick cells. *British Journal of Anaesthesia* **45**: 976–994.

Fomon, S. J. (1974). *Infant nutrition* 2nd edn. W. B. Saunders, Philadelphia.

Forbes, G. B. (1987). *Human body composition*. Springer-Verlag, New York.

Fraser, D. R. (1981). Biochemical and clinical aspects of vitamin D function. *British Medical Bulletin* **37**: 37–42.

Fraser, D. R. (1988). Nutritional growth retardation: experimental studies with special reference to calcium. In Waterlow, J. C. (ed) *Linear growth retardation in less developed countries*. Nestlé Nutrition/Raven Press, New York, pp. 127–134.

Garrow, J. S. (1962). The treatment and prognosis of infantile malnutrition in Jamaican children. *West Indian Medical Journal* **11**: 217–227.

Garrow, J. S. (1965). Total body potassium in kwashiorkor and marasmus. *Lancet* **2**: 455–458.

Garrow, J. S. (1967). Loss of brain potassium in kwashiorkor. *Lancet* **2**: 643–645.

Garrow, J. S., Smith, R., Ward, E. E. (1968). *Electrolyte metabolism in severe infantile malnutrition*. Pergamon Press, Oxford.

Golden, M. H. N. (1988). In discussion of paper by Fraser (1988). p. 138.

Gross, P. A., Ketteler, M. *et al.* (1987). The charted and uncharted waters of hyponatremia. *Kidney International* **32**: Suppl. 21, 567–575.

Halliday, D. (1967). Chemical composition of the whole body and individual tissues of two Jamaican children whose death resulted primarily from malnutrition. *Clinical Science* **33**: 365–370.

Halpern, M. J. (1985). Magnesium physiopathology: II. Magnesium deficiency and depletion. In Halpern, M. J., Durlach, J. (eds) *Magnesium deficiency: physiopathology and treatment*. Karger, Basel, pp. 9–23.

Hansen, J. D. L. (1956). Electrolyte and nitrogen metabolism in kwashiorkor. *South African Journal of Laboratory Clinical Medicine* **2**: 206–231.

Harris, I., Wilkinson, A. W. (1971). Magnesium depletion in children. *Lancet* **2**: 735–736.

Jackson, M. J. (1990). Intracellular calcium, cell injury and relationships to free radicals and fatty acid metabolism. *Proceedings of the Nutrition Society* **49**: 77–81.

Kingston, M. (1973). Electrolyte disturbances in Liberian children with kwashiorkor. *Journal of Pediatrics* **83**: 859–866.

Kjeldsen, K., Nørgaard, A., Clausen, T. (1984). Effect of K depletion on ^{3}H-ouabain binding and Na-K-contents in mammalian skeletal muscle. *Acta Physiologica Scandinavica* **122**: 103–117.

Krishna, G. G., Chusid, P., Hoeldtke, R. D. (1987). Mild potassium depletion promotes renal sodium retention. *Journal of Laboratory and Clinical Medicine* **109**: 724–730.

Laskey, M. A., Prentice, A. M. *et al.* (1990). Breast-milk calcium concentrations during prolonged lactation in British and rural Gambian mothers. *Acta Paediatrica Scandinavica* **79**: 507–512.

Lawson, D. E. M., Cole, T. J. *et al.* (1987). Aetiology of rickets in Egyptian children. *Human Nutrition:Clinical Nutrition* **41C**: 199–208.

Linder, G. C., Hansen, J. D. L., Karabus, C. D. (1963). The metabolism of magnesium and other inorganic cations and of nitrogen in acute kwashiorkor. *Pediatrics* **31**: 552–568.

MacIntyre, I. (1986). Hormonal regulation of extracellular calcium. *British Medical Bulletin* **42**: 343–352.

Mann, M. D., Hansen, J. D. L. (1972). The interpretation of total body potassium results in young children. *South African Medical Journal* **46**: 37–39.

Mann, M. D., Bowie, M. D., Hansen, J. D. L. (1975*a*). Total body potassium, potassium retention and potassium intake in protein energy malnutrition. *South African Medical Journal* **49**: 613–615.

Mann, M. D., Bowie, M. D., Hansen, J. D. L. (1975*b*). Potassium retention in acute diarrhoeal disease. *South African Medical Journal* **49**: 1835–1838.

Marie, P. J., Pettifor, J. M. *et al.* (1982). Histological osteomalacia due to dietary calcium deficiency in children. *New England Journal of Medicine* **307**: 584–588.

Matthews, E. K. (1986). Calcium and membrane permeability. *British Medical Bulletin* **42**: 391–397.

Mellander, O., Vahlquist, B., Mellbin, T. (1959). Breastfeeding and artificial feeding. *Acta Paediatrica Scandinavica* **48**: Suppl. 116.

Metcoff, J. (1975). Cellular energy metabolism in protein-calorie malnutrition. In Olson, R. E. (ed) *Protein-calorie malnutrition*. Academic Press, New York, pp. 65–85.

Michaelson, K. M., Clausen, T. (1987). Inadequate supplies of potassium and magnesium in relief food—implications and countermeasures. *Lancet* **1**: 1421–1423.

Montgomery, R. D. (1960). Magnesium metabolism in infantile protein malnutrition. *Lancet* **2**: 74–76.

Montgomery, R. D. (1961). Magnesium balance studies in marasmic kwashiorkor. *Journal of Pediatrics* **59**: 119–123.

Morgan, D. B., Thomas, T. H. (1979). Water balance and hyponatraemia. *Clinical Science* **56**: 517–522..

Nanda, S., Nanda, S. *et al.* (1984). Calcium metabolism in marasmus. *Indian Pediatrics* **21**: 891–895.

Nichols, B. L., Alleyne, G. A. O. *et al.* (1969). Relationship between muscle potassium and total body potassium in infants with malnutrition. *Journal of Pediatrics* **74**: 49–57.

Nichols, B. L., Alvarado, J. *et al.* (1978). Magnesium supplementation in protein-calorie malnutrition. *American Journal of Clinical Nutrition* **31**: 176–188.

Olson, R. E. (ed) (1975). *Protein-calorie malnutrition*. Academic Press, New York.

Patrick, J. (1978). Interrelations between the physiology of sodium, potassium and water and human nutrition. *Journal of Human Nutrition* **32**: 405–418.

Patrick, J., Golden, M. H. N. (1977). Leucocyte electrolytes and sodium transport in protein energy malnutrition. *American Journal of Clinical Nutrition* **30**: 1478–1481.

Pettifor, J. M., Ross, P. *et al.* (1979). Calcium deficiency in rural black children in South Africa—a comparison between rural and urban communities. *American Journal of Clinical Nutrition* **32**: 2477–2483.

Prentice, A., Laskey, M. A. *et al.* (1990). Bone mineral content of Gambian and British children aged 0–36 months. *Bone and Mineral* **10**: 211–224.

Reddy, V., Srikantia, S. G. (1967). Serum alkaline phosphatase in malnourished children with rickets. *Journal of Pediatrics* **71**: 595–597.

Salimpour, R. (1975). Rickets in Tehran: a study of 200 cases. *Archives of Disease in Childhood* **50:** 63–66.

Sherman, H. C. (1947). *Calcium and phosphorus in foods and nutrition.* Columbia University Press, New York.

Shils, M. E. (1969a). Experimental human magnesium depletion. *Medicine* **48:** 61–85.

Shils, M. E. (1969b). Experimental production of magnesium deficiency in man. *Annals of the New York Academy of Sciences* **162:** 847–855.

Shils, M. E. (1988). Magnesium in health and disease. *Annual Reviews of Nutrition* **8:** 429–460.

Tindall, S. F., Clark, R. G. (1976). Hyponatraemia in surgical practice. *British Journal of Surgery* **63:** 150 (abstract).

Valyasevi, A., Halstead, S. B., Dhanamitta, S. (1967a). Studies of bladder-stone disease in Thailand. VI. Urinary studies in children 2–10 years old, resident in a hypo- and hyperendemic area. *American Journal of Clinical Nutrition* **20:** 1362–1368.

Valyasevi, A., Dhanamitta, S. (1967b). Studies of bladder-stone disease in Thailand. VII. Urinary studies in newborn and infants of hypo- and hyperendemic areas. *American Journal of Clinical Nutrition* **20:** 1369–1377.

Vis, H., Dubois, R. et al. (1965). Etude des troubles electrolytiques accompagnant le kwashiorkor marastique. *Revues Françaises Etudes Cliniques Biologiques* **10:** 729–741.

Walker, A. R. P. (1972). The human requirement of calcium: should low intakes be supplemented? *American Journal of Clinical Nutrition* **25:** 518–530.

Waterlow, J. C., Wills, V. G. (1960). Balance studies in malnourished Jamaican infants. 2. Comparison of absorption and retention of nitrogen and phosphorus from human milk and a cow's milk mixture. *British Journal of Nutrition* **14:** 199–205.

Waterlow, J. C., Bunje, H. J., (1966). Observations on mountain sickness in the Colombian Andes. *Lancet* **2:** 655–661.

Whang, R., Welt, L. B. (1963). Observations in experimental magnesium depletion. *Journal of Clinical Investigation* **42:** 305–313.

Widdowson, E. M., Spray, C. M. (1951). Chemical development in utero. *Archives of Disease of Childhood* **25:** 205–214.

5
Effects of PEM on structure and functions of organs

Cardiac function

Alleyne (1966) began his classical paper on cardiac function in severely malnourished children with the words '. . . the heart does not escape the wasting that affects other organs'. This has been shown at autopsy, by chest X-ray and by echo-cardiography (Bergman *et al.*, 1988). Histological studies, summarized by Alleyne *et al.* (1977), have shown only non-specific changes.

Alleyne's work was followed by that of Tanman (1971) in Turkey and later by the very extensive studies of Viart (1977*a*, 1978) in Zaïre. The three sets of results are summarized and compared in Table 5.1. Considering the differences in age, weight and clinical picture, the extent of agreement is remarkable.

From the point of view of the body as a whole, the most important variable is the cardiac output. The values are expressed here as litres/min/m^2, because that ratio is given or can be derived in all three papers. Alleyne's values are higher than those of Tanman or Viart, perhaps for technical reasons, but all three studies show a decrease in cardiac output of 30 per cent in the malnourished compared with the recovered state. The increase on recovery is achieved partly through a rise in pulse rate but mainly through a larger stroke volume. Viart (1978) also measured systemic and pulmonary artery pressures by cardiac catheterization and found them to be significantly reduced, while peripheral resistance was increased.

Alleyne drew attention to the low rates of basal metabolism in these children (Chapter 6) and to the fact that in hypothyroidism a linear relationship had been demonstrated between cardiac output and oxygen consumption. The implication was that cardiac output was appropriate to the metabolic load. Viart (1978), following the same line of thought, considered that in most of his patients the circulation was adjusted to the demand, and that the functional reserve of the heart was sufficient to meet the very low circulatory load. There was a positive correlation (r = 0.68) between cardiac output and red cell volume, which supports this contention. However, a few children

Table 5.1 Cardiac function in children with PEM before and after treatment as reported by different authors

	Jamaica*	Turkey†	Zaïre§
Mean age, months	12.4	9.6	54
Initial weight, % for height	71	67	80
Heart rate, beats/min			
initial (I)	110	105	107
recovered (R)	131	112	115
I/R, %	84	94	93
Stroke volume, ml/beat/m²			
initial	28[a]	20	18
recovered	33.4[a]	26.5	28
I/R, %	84	75.5	64
Cardiac output, l/min/m²			
initial	3.0[a]	2.2	2.1
recovered	4.35[a]	3.15	3.1
I/R, %	69	69	68
Cardiac output, ml/min/kg			
initial	–	129	98
recovered	–	170	137
I/R, %	–	76	71

[a] Original data were related to metre³; corrected to metre² by multiplying by mean height (0.63 m).
Data from *Alleyne (1966); †Tanman (1971); §Viart (1977a).

who subsequently died showed on admission clinical and haemodynamic features of severe peripheral circulatory failure: low cardiac output, high systemic resistance and reduced filling pressure, as seen in endotoxic or hypovolaemic shock. These children had low plasma albumin concentrations; there seemed to be a threshold at 1.5 g/dl, which represented a transition from an adapted state to one of frank circulatory failure.

I think the idea that the children who did not die were adapted to a reduced metabolic load is questionable. As in the case of BMR (Chapter 2), in these malnourished children it is probably inappropriate to express cardiac output as the classical cardiac index, l/min/m², because what matters is the mass of tissue that has to be perfused. Table 5.1 shows that on a weight basis there is still a reduction of some 25 per cent in cardiac output in the malnourished state. Because of the distortion of body composition (Chapter 3), with a relative increase in actively metabolizing tissues (brain and viscera) in the malnourished child, for normal function to be preserved the cardiac output per kg should be greater than in the healthy child, rather than less. If it is assumed that 'active' tissue forms 40 per cent of body weight in the child with PEM, compared with 30 per cent in the normal (Chapter 3), then the perfusion of 'active' tissue would be reduced by about 50 per cent. Therefore, it might well be argued that, far from the cardiac output being adjusted to the metabolic demand, the metabolic rate is low because the heart cannot supply enough blood to the tissues. In support of this argument is Viart's finding (1978) that the oxygen extraction from the blood—the arteriovenous difference in O_2 content—was 20 per cent greater before treatment than after recovery (5.1 *versus* 4.1 vol %), and in five patients who died it was even higher (6.3 vol %).

Viart (1977a) concluded that the heart itself played no direct role in the circulatory disturbances observed before treatment, but from his findings he could not prove that the contractility of the malnourished myocardium was normal. It seems very likely that myocardial function is impaired in severe PEM, since the stress of an increase in circulatory volume as a result of intravenous infusions is much more likely to cause heart failure in a malnourished than in a normal child. The huge increase in venous pressure after an infusion, demonstrated by Kerpel-Fronius (1960) and illustrated in Fig. 5.1, is evidence of a heart that cannot cope with an increased load. In Uganda deaths from cardiac failure occurred when the diet contained excessive amounts of sodium (Wharton *et al.*, 1967).

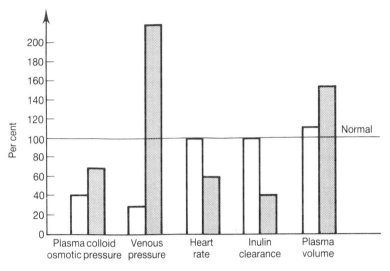

Fig. 5.1   Effects of a saline infusion on cardiac function in children with PEM. ▭ , before infusion; ▬ , after infusion. The horizontal line represents normal values and the columns show percentages of normal. Reproduced by permission from Kerpel-Fronius (1960).

Plasma and red cell volumes

Previous books and reviews of PEM have given little attention to plasma and red cell volumes; however, the subject is important, because if there is hypovolaemia it will tend to stimulate retention of water and salt and promote the formation of oedema; if the intravascular volumes are too large there will be danger of overloading the heart. The usual problem arises about the basis of reference. In this context Fondu (1977) expressed the opinion that 'reference to body weight is a major source of misunderstanding in childhood malnutrition'. Nevertheless, for the reasons already given, for most purposes it seems most meaningful to relate plasma and red cell volumes to body weight, preferably after loss of oedema, because what matters is the amount of blood available for perfusing the tissues. Therefore the results set out in Tables 5.2 and 5.3 are in terms of ml/kg actual weight, or oedema-free weight where stated by the authors. The primary measurements are the haematocrit and either the plasma volume by dye dilution or ^{131}I or the red cell volume, by cells labelled with ^{51}Cr.

Table 5.2 Plasma volume (ml/kg) in children with PEM before and after treatment

Author	Country		Plasma volume, ml/kg			
			Before	After	Healthy controls	Method
Gollan (1944)	Europe (wartime)		79	–	38	dye
Gomez *et al.* (1950)	Mexico		83	–	62	dye
Kerpel-Fronius and Varga (1949)	Hungary		42	–		dye
Cohen and Hansen (1962)	S. Africa		63	47		[131]I
Srikantia and Reddy (1963)	India		49	50.5		dye
Alleyne (1966)	Jamaica		63	49		dye
Viteri *et al.* (1968)	Guatemala		46	45		[51]Cr
Viart (1976)	Zaïre		42	–	46.5	[51]Cr
Viart (1977*b*)	Zaïre		41	49	47.4	[51]Cr
Fondu (1977)	Zaïre		45	54		[51]Cr
Olson (1979)	Thailand		46	50		–
		Mean	48.5	49.2		
		SD	8.1	2.6		
Without Cohen and Hansen and Alleyne:		Mean	44.3			
		SD	2.6			

Plasma volume in healthy children is 47–50 ml/kg (e.g. Russell, 1949).

Table 5.3 Red cell volume (ml/kg) in children with PEM before and after treatment

Author		Red cell volume, ml/kg		
		Before	After	Healthy controls
Srikantia and Reddy (1963)		17.5	20	
Alleyne (1966)		17	23.5	
Viteri *et al.* (1968)		16	19.5	
Viart (1976)		15.7	–	23.3
Viart (1977*b*)		15.4	18.0	23.3
Fondu (1977)		20	19	–
	Mean	16.9	20.0	
	SD	1.6	1.9	

Red cell volume in healthy children is about 30 ml/kg (Russell, 1949)

In the analysis that follows two early studies, those of Gomez *et al.* (1950) and of Gollan (1948), have been excluded, because for reasons that are not clear their results are completely out of line with those of all the others. Several points emerge from the tables.

Plasma volume   Comparison of the plasma volume (PV) after recovery with standard values gives an indication of the reliability of the methods. The recovery values are remarkably consistent and on average a little higher than those of healthy controls. If this difference is real, it is probably because, as several of the studies showed, when growth begins the PV increases more rapidly than the body weight, and by the time that the recovery measurements were made, weight gain was still incomplete.

With the exception of two studies, those of Alleyne (1966) and Cohen and Hansen (1962), the initial values are also remarkably consistent, and on average about 10 per cent lower than those after recovery. It is difficult to explain the high initial PVs found in Jamaica and South Africa. Alleyne observed an inverse relation between PV per kg body weight and weight for height, and it is possible that the children in these two series were initially more undernourished. Another possibility is that the early treatment was more vigorous, with a more rapid regeneration of plasma albumin and expansion of the intravascular volume.

Red cell volumes   Initially these were consistently low and during treatment the increase in red cell mass only slightly surpassed that in body weight. In contrast to plasma volume, after two months or so of treatment the normal RCV per kg had not yet been achieved.

It is remarkable how consistent the results are considering the differences between the groups of children. As far as the clinical descriptions go, it is probable that oedema was most severe in the Zaïre children. Their average age was four years, with a range from one and a half to eight years, whereas the children in the other studies were almost all less than two years old. The Zaïre series (Viart, 1976) is far larger than any of the others. Of 42 children, 11 died. Mean blood and plasma volumes were no different in those who died compared with the survivors, nor were they different in children less than three years old compared with the group as a whole. (In passing, it may be remarked how valuable it is when results are published in full, so that an interested reader can make this kind of analysis.)

Finally, it is worth considering whether the slightly low initial plasma volumes do represent a significant degree of hypovolaemia. It may be argued that the malnourished child wastes around its skeletal structures, of which the vascular tree, composed largely of collagen and elastin, could be regarded as a part. On this basis, height would be an appropriate indicator of the capacity of the vascular bed. In the 13 cases which Viart (1977*b*) followed for 60 days there was virtually no increase in height over that period, but on average the absolute plasma volume increased by a factor of 1.57 and the blood volume by a factor of 1.5. If, in parallel with the height, the capacity of the vascular bed remained unchanged, either it must have been overfilled after treatment or underfilled initially. The former seems unlikely, since the values are similar to those in healthy children. It is therefore possible that the vascular bed was underfilled initially, and it is noteworthy that all these children were oedematous, some severely so. Although none of the children in this particular sub-group died, the concept of hypovolaemia is consistent with the clinical evidence of peripheral circulatory failure mentioned in the previous section.

Anaemia

The typical child with PEM has a moderate anaemia, with a haemoglobin concentration of perhaps 8–10 g/dl; the red cells are normal in size, with a normal or somewhat low haemoglobin content; the bone marrow may show normal erythropoiesis or it may be fatty and hypoplastic. Vilter (1975) called it a 'lazy marrow'.

According to WHO, some 50 per cent of children between six months and five years old in less developed countries are anaemic (Hb < 11 g/dl) (De

Maeyer and Adiels-Tegman, 1985), and it is generally considered that the principal cause is iron deficiency, compounded by blood loss from malaria and intestinal parasites. It would be logical to suppose that the same factors are responsible for anaemia in PEM. The difficulty in accepting this explanation is that there is no consistent evidence of Fe deficiency. Serum Fe concentrations are normal and transferrin saturation increased, partly because of the reduction in transferrin concentration that is characteristic of PEM (Ramdath and Golden, 1989). Serum ferritin levels, which, in the absence of infection, are considered to be a good measure of Fe stores, are not reduced and are often raised. The bone marrow contains normal or increased amounts of stainable Fe and measurements on the liver by biopsy or post-mortem have shown abnormally high concentrations of Fe, particularly in marasmus (Waterlow, 1948; McLaren *et al.*, 1968). Therefore it is necessary to look for other causal factors.

The most extensive studies of anaemia in PEM are those of Fondu and his colleagues in Zaïre, summarized by Fondu *et al.* (1978*a*), with a wide-ranging review of the literature. Several possible causal factors emerge from the findings of this group: dietary factors other than Fe that may limit haemopoiesis; adaptation to reduced oxygen demand; increased red cell destruction and chronic infection.

Factors limiting haemopoiesis

Protein   Waterlow (1948) made the obvious suggestion that in severe PEM deficiency of protein might limit haemoglobin production, so that Fe, although available, could not be utilized. However, Finch (1975) drew attention to the experimental evidence that in depleted animals haemoglobin formation has a high priority and that the necessary amino acids can be raided from other tissues. The argument is similar to the proposition that in marasmus muscle wasting helps to maintain the capacity of the liver for albumin synthesis (Chapter 6). It may be premature to rule out the possibility of deficiency of specific amino acids such as histidine (Laidlaw and Kopple, 1987) and glycine (Jackson, 1989), in which haemoglobin is particularly rich.

Vitamins   Deficiencies of ascorbic acid and riboflavin have been considered as candidates for the role of limiting factors, but there is very little support for them. Folic acid deficiency is in a different category, being sometimes superimposed on the typical anaemia of PEM. The marrow is megaloblastic, or it may be initially hypoplastic, with megaloblastic changes occurring when the child starts to grow. Folic acid deficiency as a complication of PEM has been described in a number of countries, e.g. Jamaica (McIver and Back, 1960), Guatemala (Viteri *et al.*, 1968), India (Swarup-Mitra *et al.*, 1976) and the Sudan (Omer *et al.*, 1973), but it is by no means constant and no evidence of it was found in the studies in Zaïre. When anaemia is very severe, with haemoglobin concentration as low as 5 g/dl, the possibility of folic acid deficiency should always be considered. Vitamin B_{12}, on the other hand, has never been found to be limiting.

Copper   Cases of PEM have been described in Peru in which anaemia failed to respond to iron supplements, but did respond to copper (Cordano *et al.*, 1964; Graham and Cordano, 1976). McLaren *et al.* (1968) suggested that copper deficiency might be limiting the utilization of iron, since they found reduced concentrations of copper in the liver.

Adaptation

It has been suggested that because the metabolic rate in PEM is depressed, adequate oxygenation of the tissues can be maintained with a reduced haemoglobin concentration. A decrease in oxygen extraction by the tissues should in theory lead to a fall in the level of 2-3 diphosphoglycerate (2-3 DPG) in the red cells. This in turn should result in oxygen being more tightly bound to haemoglobin, with an increase in the oxygen pressure needed for half-saturation (P_{50}) (Finch, 1975). In fact Fondu and Mandelbaum (1975) found no change in 2-3 DPG content of the red cells and normal values of P_{50}. Moreover, according to the adaptation hypothesis, an excess of oxygen supply over demand should lead to a reduced output of erythropoietin by the kidney. The immediate cause of the anaemia would therefore be a lack of stimulus for red cell production. In fact, however, the evidence suggests that erythropoietin production is increased rather than decreased (Fondu *et al.*, 1978*b*; Suttajit, 1975).

Destruction of red cells

Several authors have observed a decreased life-span of red cells in PEM. Fondu *et al.* (1978*a*) found a mean life-span of 18 days on admission, rising to 30 days after two months. The latter figure is probably an underestimate, because it does not allow for dilution by newly formed red cells during recovery. It was suggested that in the initial stages erythrocyte fragility might be increased as a result of deficiencies of selenium and vitamin E (see Chapter 9).

A further cause of anaemia might be suppression of erythropoiesis by chronic infection, but this is not a factor in most cases of PEM, and the rapid response to nutritional treatment seems to rule out this possibility.

It is therefore difficult to reach a definite conclusion about the cause of anaemia in PEM. Fondu *et al.* (1978*a*) believed that the initial event was a decrease in red cell life-span, followed by a reduction in erythropoietic activity as a result of a fall in tissue metabolism. Finch (1975), on the other hand, concluded that the primary cause was Fe deficiency. There is in any case general agreement that during the recovery phase, when the red cell mass should be rapidly increasing, Fe stores become exhausted and the supply of Fe may become limiting. At this stage Fe supplements are necessary, but they are not needed in the early stages and may even be dangerous (Chapter 10).

Iron deficiency is important in the wider context of mild or moderate PEM. The Fe content of breast milk is low and the young infant has to rely to a large extent on Fe stores laid down *in utero*. When the time comes for weaning, the Fe in the usual cereal foods is poorly absorbed. The subject of Fe absorption has been extensively studied (e.g. Layrisse *et al.*, 1969; Narasinga Rao, 1981), but mainly in adults rather than young children. The haem Fe in animal products is much better absorbed than the inorganic Fe in plant foods, in which interfering factors such as phytic acid may further reduce the availability of Fe. Ashworth *et al.* (1973) found that infants recovering from malnutrition absorbed only about 5 per cent of the Fe in maize meal, and even a slight infection such as a cold reduced the absorption practically to zero (Beresford *et al.*, 1971).

The final question is whether moderate degrees of anaemia in the young have any functional importance. In adults a close relationship has been found between haemoglobin level and physical work capacity (Viteri and Torun, 1974), but it seems doubtful whether a moderate degree of anaemia would be enough to limit the physical activity of young children. A study in Bangladesh suggested that Fe deficiency might limit growth in height, since those drinking well-water containing more than 1 mg/l Fe were significantly taller than children whose water contained less Fe (Briend *et al.*, 1990).

Of greater importance is the possibility that Fe deficiency and anaemia may impair mental development, a subject on which at present there is much concern. The evidence is not entirely consistent, probably because of differences in study design, ages of children and duration of follow-up, but it cannot be ignored. For example, Lozoff *et al*. (1987) in a study on children aged one to two years in Costa Rica, found that children with Fe deficiency anaemia showed significantly lower mental and motor test scores than controls, even after eliminating interfering factors such as family background, parental IQ and home environment. After three months of treatment the scores were still low in infants who had more severe or chronic Fe deficiency. Palti *et al*. (1983) recorded defects in intellectual performance in moderately anaemic children (Hb < 10 g/dl), which persisted at least up to the age of five years. From the practical standpoint this effect on mental development, if confirmed, is clearly a most serious problem, more important than the exact mechanism of anaemia in severe PEM.

Liver

Fatty liver has been accepted as an important feature of kwashiorkor ever since the early description by Williams (1935). The huge and immensely fatty livers seen in the West Indies in the early days made such an impression that, ignorant of the work on kwashiorkor in Africa, I proposed the name 'fatty liver disease' for the syndrome (Waterlow, 1948). In Jamaica there was a significant association between fatty liver and oedema (Waterlow *et al.*, 1957), though it was not invariable; fatty liver was more often found without oedema than the opposite. Workers in three very different environments—in Budapest during the siege of the last war (Veghelyi, 1950), in Uganda (Davies, 1954) and in Jamaica (Waterlow *et al.*, 1957)—have reported that the development of fatty liver preceded the appearance of oedema. However, over a longer time-scale they both represent relatively recent events: in children with fatty liver growth in length was less retarded than in those diagnosed as marasmus (Chapter 1). In Jamaica there was also a positive correlation between liver fat and weight for age, indicating that fatty liver was less common and less severe in infants who showed the most severe growth failure.

Table 5.4 shows some of the characteristics of the livers in Jamaican children who died. In those days hepatomegaly was assessed clinically by the distance of the liver edge below the costal margin; sometimes it may even extend beyond the umbilicus. Nowadays the size of the liver can be estimated *in vivo* by ultrasound (J. Doherty, personal communication). The total protein content of the liver was reduced in the children diagnosed as kwashiorkor, but to a lesser extent than in those with marasmus. The water content was increased but we do not know the location of the excess water. Certainly the

Table 5.4 Some characteristics of the liver in children who died of PEM or infection

	Kwashiorkor	Marasmus	Malnutrition with infection	Infection[a] without malnutrition
No. of cases	16	9	6	20
No. with:				
oedema	14	0	4	3
hepatomegaly[b]	11	3	2	7
fatty liver[c]	15	3	3	9
Mean liver weight:				
% expected[d]	153	69	99	113
total excess fat, g	145	38	57	53
total liver protein,				
% expected	67	51	64	80
liver water/protein	7.1	5.4	5.7	5.5

[a] Children dying of acute infections (13), tuberculosis (4), miscellaneous (3)
[b] Liver edge 1½ fingers' breadth or more below costal margin
[c] Fat more than 15% of net weight
[d] Expected liver weight for age, from tables of Coppoletta and Wolbach (1933)
Summarized from Waterlow *et al.* (1957)

histological appearance does not suggest any expansion of the extracellular space, particularly when the hepatocytes are distended with fat.

The distribution and amount of fat in the liver are important for under-standing the cause of this remarkable change. Information on the histology is available from several series of biopsies (Davies, 1948; Waterlow, 1948; McLaren *et al.*, 1968; Datta Chaudhuri *et al.*, 1972) as well as from autopsies (Waterlow, 1948; Veghelyi, 1950; Gillman and Gillman, 1951; Davies, 1954). All the reports agree that when the fatty infiltration is not universal through-out the liver lobule it is predominantly periportal and in large droplets. This picture differentiates the fatty liver of kwashiorkor from the fatty change produced by infections, which is initially centrolobular, although in severe and chronic infections such as tuberculosis it may spread throughout the lobule. Davies (1954) recorded that 'observation of centrolobular or of irregu-lar fat deposition in a biopsy specimen has on several occasions directed the attention of clinicians to a hitherto unsuspected infective element'. In the fatty degeneration produced by exposure to hepatotoxins such as carbon tetrachloride (a powerful producer of free radicals—see Chapter 10), the fat is in small droplets and again mainly centrolobular. These differences are important for diagnosis. For example, a parallel has been drawn between the fatty liver of kwashiorkor and that of Reye's syndrome, but this is misleading. Reye described the changes as those of fatty degeneration, affecting both liver and kidneys (Reye *et al.*, 1963). In the liver 'every cell in every lobule is packed with fatty droplets; large globules displacing the nucleus are not characteristic' (Reye and Morgan, 1963).

Histological grading of the amount of fat is not very accurate; Bras *et al.* (1957) found it impossible to distinguish histologically between concentrations of 25 per cent and 50 per cent. Quantitative measurements on biopsies have been made in only two studies, by Chatterjee and Mukherjee (1968) in India and by Waterlow (1975) in Jamaica, with generally similar results. The find-ings in Jamaica are shown in Fig. 5.2. In extreme cases fat may account for

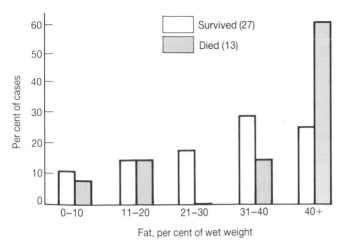

Fig. 5.2 Relation between the fat content of liver and mortality in children with PEM in Jamaica. J. C. Waterlow, unpublished data.

more then 50 per cent of the wet weight, compared with which the increases produced by noxious agents are trivial. The figure shows that very severe fatty infiltration is not necessarily fatal; nevertheless, the more the fat the greater the mortality. Eventually, as the fat accumulates the secretion of bile appears to be blocked and a raised serum bilirubin indicates a bad prognosis. An increase in serum aminotransferases suggests some degree of cell damage; McLean (1966) showed a correlation between the level of glutamate-pyruvate aminotransferase and mortality rate (Table 5.5).

Electron microscopy has revealed mitochondrial abnormalities in the livers of children with PEM who died (S. E. H. Brookes, personal communication), and measurements made on biopsies showed a defect in oxidative phosphoryl-ation (Waterlow, 1961), but the possibility could not be ruled out that this was an artefact caused by the fat.

The excess fat in the liver consists of triglycerides. The reason why it accumulates has not been definitely established, partly because it has not been easy to reproduce the lesion experimentally. In the rat low protein diets result in only small increases in liver fat, and amounts comparable to those

Table 5.5 Relation of mortality to activity of serum glutamate-pyruvate aminotransferase (GPT) on admission

GPT activity units	No. of patients	No. of deaths	Mortality (%)
0– 50	16	0	0
51–100	47	0	0
101–150	27	1	4
151–200	17	2	12
201–250	8	2	25
251–500	18	5	28
> 500	4	4	100

GPT activity in healthy Jamaican children = 45 ± 24 (SD)
From McLean (1966).

found in kwashiorkor have been achieved in this animal only with diets low in choline or methionine. It is perhaps worth reconsidering whether these deficiencies, particularly of methionine, could have any relevance in man. Veghelyi (1950) observed that B vitamins, especially nicotinic acid, increased the deposition of fat in the liver and on the basis of Handler's work suggested that this might be because nicotinic acid 'annihilates the lipotropic effect of methionine by using up the methyl groups of the latter substance'. Both Davies (1948, 1954) and Veghelyi (1950) inclined to the view that the fatty liver might be secondary to atrophy of the exocrine pancreas (see pp. 65, 66). However, the idea, derived from experiments on dogs, that the pancreas produces a lipotropic substance ('lipocaic') seems never to have been substantiated.

Ramalingaswami and co-workers in India found a better model in the rhesus monkey. In this animal a low protein diet produced a 25-fold increase in liver triglycerides (Kumar *et al.*, 1972). Heard *et al.* (1958) reported that in pigs on a low protein diet increasing the energy intake promoted the deposition of fat in the liver. Veghelyi (1950) had observed that liver disease never appeared in subjects whose calorie intake was inadequate. These various observations parallel the dietary conditions that produce hypoalbuminaemia and oedema (Chapter 11).

The origin of the excess liver fat has been reviewed by Truswell (1990). One explanation is that it is derived from the fat depots (Lewis *et al.*, 1964). Datta Chaudhuri *et al.* (1972) observed that the degree of fatty change in the liver was inversely proportional to the degree of wasting of subcutaneous tissues. On this hypothesis, marasmic children do not have fatty livers because their fat stores are empty. If fat was being transported from the periphery to the liver, one would expect an increase in serum free fatty acid (FFA) concentrations in kwashiorkor but not in marasmus. Such an increase has been reported by some authors but not by others. In the series of Flores *et al.* (1970) FFA levels were normal in kwashiorkor and low in marasmus. The hypothesis is difficult to substantiate because FFA concentrations are very sensitive to the recent food intake.

A second and more likely explanation, first proposed by Truswell *et al.* (1969) in South Africa and almost simultaneously by Flores *et al.* (1970) in Chile, is a failure of fat transport out of the liver because of impaired synthesis of the apolipoprotein B which is essential for the secretion of triglycerides from the liver into the plasma. Most authors have found that fasting serum triglyceride levels are low in kwashiorkor and peak after a few days of treatment, as if the accumulation of fat in the liver was being unblocked, although there are exceptions to this pattern (Flores *et al.*, 1974). Truswell and Hansen (1969) reported an inverse relationship between serum triglyceride and the histologically graded amount of liver fat. The key point in this hypothesis is the consistent finding of low serum concentrations of β-lipoproteins, which increase on recovery. In experiments on rats on a low protein diet the synthesis rate of apolipoproteins was reduced (Seakins and Waterlow, 1972). Preliminary measurements on malnourished children (unpublished) showed that lipoprotein synthesis was depressed even more than that of albumin. The evidence, therefore, seems to be strong that the fatty liver results from a block in the transport of fat out of the liver. A selective deficiency of hepatic triglyceride lipase, as described by Agbedana *et al.* (1979) would enhance the block, by preventing the formation of free fatty acids which could then be oxidized.

The lipoproteins contain cholesterol as well as triglyceride. Truswell *et al.* (1969) showed that the concentrations of total cholesterol and β-lipoprotein cholesterol were initially low in children with fatty livers; on treatment, like the triglycerides, they rose to a peak well above normal levels. Truswell (1990) has therefore proposed that measurement of total serum cholesterol, which can be done as a routine in most laboratories, would be useful for the diagnosis of fatty liver and for following its response to treatment.

There is at present no specific treatment for the fatty liver, which may take several weeks to resolve, but if the child does not die at an early stage the persistence of some degree of liver enlargement need not be cause for concern. Experimental evidence summarized by Truswell (1990) suggests that a generous protein intake may speed up clearance of the excess fat. This would fit in with the hypothesis of protein deficiency as a causal factor. On the recovery diet that was used in the 1960s in Jamaica, providing 3 g protein/kg/ day, the fat content decreased from the average initial value of 30 per cent to 10 per cent after a month (Waterlow, 1975).

It was thought at one time that fatty liver in infancy might lead on to cirrhosis and even carcinoma in later life (Waterlow, 1948; Walters and Waterlow, 1954), but long-term follow-ups by Srikantia *et al.* (1958) and by Cook and Hutt (1967) showed that at least in cases of kwashiorkor who had been treated, the liver recovered completely or presented only negligible abnormalities. Cook and Hutt caution that the sequel may be different if kwashiorkor remains untreated for a long time, or if an extra stress is imposed, such as that of malaria. Alleyne *et al.* (1977) concluded that 'all the evidence points to the complete resolution of the acute effects of PEM on the liver'. However, Veghelyi (1950) recorded fine fibrosis of the liver in a few children who died some years after complete recovery; in two others there was evidence of sub-acute necrosis with scarring. I believe, nevertheless, that cirrhosis of the liver in children or young adults, as observed in India (Ramalingaswami and Nayak, 1970) and the West Indies (Bras and Hill, 1956; Rhodes, 1957) has a different pathogenesis, although malnutrition may make the organ more vulnerable to the effects of toxins and infections. In Calcutta follow-up studies showed no evidence of cirrhosis (Chaudhuri and Bhattacharyya, 1962).

Pancreas

As long ago as 1957 Bras *et al.* listed no less than 12 papers from different parts of the world describing pancreatic lesions in malnourished subjects. In children the most important change is atrophy of the acinar cells with loss of zymogen granules. This atrophy could be so severe that Davies (1954) described children with kwashiorkor as 'having virtually undergone a pancreatectomy as regards the acinar tissue'. Similar atrophic changes were found in the salivary glands. Bras *et al.* (1957) observed a close association between the pancreatic changes and fatty liver and, as noted in the previous section, Davies suggested that there might be a causal relationship.

Changes in the islets have not been observed in PEM, but the atrophy of the exocrine pancreas may lead on to a fine fibrosis of the organ (Davies, 1948; Veghelyi, 1950; Bras *et al.*, 1957). It is not known whether this predisposes to the more extensive fibrosis and calcification of the pancreas that are sometimes found in older children and adults and that may give rise to what has been called malnutrition-related insulin-dependent diabetes (WHO, 1980). This question is clearly of importance, in view of the high prevalence of diabetes in some tropical countries.

Functionally, as might be expected, the production of pancreatic enzymes is impaired. In Veghelyi's marasmic infants, studied during the siege of Budapest, a reduction in enzyme activity in the duodenal juice preceded the development of fatty liver and oedema, lipase being most affected, then trypsin and then amylase. The activities were rapidly restored when the children were treated with milk. Similar results were reported by Thompson and Trowell (1952).

The production rate of pancreatic enzymes has been measured in adults with infusions of ^{14}C-labelled amino acids (O'Keefe *et al.*, 1989). This method cannot be applied in children unless stable isotopes are used, which has not yet been done. Therefore we do not know the actual production rate of pancreatic enzymes in PEM, but judging by the low activities in the duodenal fluid, it must be greatly reduced. It is therefore remarkable that there appears to be so little effect on the digestion and absorption of foodstuffs. Since the turnover of the proteins secreted by the pancreas is very fast (O'Keefe *et al.*, 1989), it is logical to suppose that the rate of production of the enzymes increases rapidly, once amino acids become available for their synthesis.

Gastrointestinal tract

The changes in the gut in PEM are well described by James (1971), Alleyne *et al.* (1977), and by Viteri and Schneider (1974, 1980). The gut mucosa responds rather sensitively to changes in food intake; it atrophies when food is in short supply and hypertrophies when it is overloaded, as after resection of part of the bowel. In fact, mild degrees of atrophy are often seen in clinically normal children and adults in tropical countries. Brasseur (1986) observed moderate atrophy in about 40 per cent of apparently healthy children between five and 20 months old in Kivu, Zaïre. In PEM the villi tend to be flattened and broadened, but the crypts are well preserved. Brunser *et al.* (1968), in a pioneer paper on this subject, reported that in kwashiorkor the mucosa was completely flat, as in coeliac disease, while the crypts were elongated. In marasmus, by contrast, the architecture of the mucosa was normal, but it was thinner than in kwashiorkor and the mitotic index was much lower. Loeb *et al.* (1976) listed 11 studies of the gut mucosa in PEM from different parts of the world and reported great variability in the degree of atrophy found. In Equatorial Africa Gendrel *et al.* (1986) found a negative correlation between villus height and severity of PEM, whereas in Venezuela the morphological changes showed no relationship to the degree of PEM (Römer *et al.*, 1983). These differences may be accounted for by differences in the impact of infection, or in the time at which the biopsies were done, since with treatment the normal villus structure is restored very quickly.

The villi are normally covered with columnar epithelial cells which have high levels of absorptive capacity. Cuboidal secretory cells are normally only found in the crypts, rapidly maturing to columnar cells as they rise up the villus. In malnutrition, however, there is delay in replacement of the cells exfoliated from the villus tips, with the result that the villi are coated with cuboidal cells. Electron microscopy shows accumulation of lipid in the villus cells, similar to that seen in congenital β-lipoprotein deficiency (Martins Campos *et al.*, 1979). Perhaps the mechanism is the same as that which causes fatty liver.

The atrophy of the villus cells affects particularly the brush borders in which are located a variety of enzymes—disaccharidases, amino-peptidases, alkaline phosphatase and Na^+-K^+-ATPase. Many authors have measured activities of the disaccharidases, lactase, sucrase and maltase in biopsy samples of the jejunal mucosa and found them all to be decreased, lactase most and maltase least. In the series described by James (1970) in Jamaica the decreases were greater in kwashiorkor than in marasmus. The other brush-border enzymes appear to have been little studied, although Sökücü (1987) reported that enterokinase activity was decreased.

The practical question is how far these structural and functional changes, together with the decreased production of pancreatic enzymes mentioned earlier, actually affect the absorption of food. In this connection the perfusion studies of James (1971) are very interesting. Table 5.6 shows that the amount of sugar absorbed by only 40 cm of jejunum was about half that likely to be provided in the early stages of treatment, if given in frequent small feeds. This does not indicate a severe degree of malabsorption.

Another approach is by oral tolerance tests. These have shown that after test doses of glucose, galactose or lactose the peak of blood sugar was less and it was achieved more slowly in malnourished children than in controls (Gabr *et al.*, 1968*a*; Brasseur *et al.*, 1985). This suggests that there was some degree of malabsorption of sugars, but lactase deficiency was not incriminated because the results were the same with glucose and lactose. Alleyne *et al.*, (1977) discussed the possible contribution of congenital lactase deficiency to lactose malabsorption in PEM, and concluded that it is not very important. Gabr *et al.* (1968*b*) measured the time-course of radioactivity in the blood after a test dose of ^{131}I-labelled triolein and found no difference between children with kwashiorkor and normal children.

The acid test of the efficiency of absorption is by measurements of balance. Early balance studies, summarized by Waterlow *et al.* (1960), were mostly

Table 5.6 Rate of absorption of monosaccharide in a 40 cm length of jejunum by malnourished children before and after treatment

Sugar infused:	glucose	glucose	glucose	lactose	sucrose
Rate of infusion, mmol/hour	12.5	25	50	25	26.3
Rate of absorption, mmol/hour					
malnourished	7.4	11.0	16.0	7.3	11.6
treated	9.6	19.4	33.7	15.4	18.2

An early recovery diet might provide 100 kcal/kg, of which 60 per cent was from carbohydrate. If a child weighing 6 kg was given this food at very frequent intervals, the rate of intake of carbohydrate would be 21 mmol monosaccharide/hour.
Data of James (1971).

done while the children were recovering. Few have been conducted in severe PEM at an early stage after admission to hospital, before the mucosa has had time to regenerate. The results obtained by Torun *et al.* (1984), shown in Table 5.7, are therefore particularly important. These children are described as having severe PEM, and many had diarrhoea, which seems, however, to have been mild. This did not prevent very satisfactory absorption of nitrogen, fat and total energy. Even the damaged gut mucosa evidently has an adequate functional reserve. The picture, however, changes when diarrhoea is more severe. Children in Bangladesh with rotavirus infection absorbed only 45 per cent of their intake of nitrogen, 42 per cent of fat and 55 per cent of total energy (Molla *et al.*, 1982).

Bacterial colonization of the upper intestine is common in PEM, though it varies in degree. As Gracey (1981) has pointed out, inter-country comparisons are difficult because of differences in methodology; certainly the bacterial counts in jejunal fluid recorded by James in Jamaica were much lower than those found in Guatemala, Indonesia or the Gambia (James, 1977).

Several factors promote bacterial overgrowth: decreased gastric acidity, reduced motility of the gut, increased transit time, and impaired absorption of sugars, providing a good culture medium. The bacteria in turn enhance malabsorption, possibly through an effect of microbial toxins on the Na^+-K^+-ATPase pump responsible for the sodium-linked absorption of water and glucose. The absorption of fat is also affected; the bacteria deconjugate bile salts to bile acids, impairing the formation of the micelles of bile salts, phospholipids and triglycerides that are essential for normal fat absorption (Viteri and Schneider, 1974). As a result of diarrhoea bile salts are poorly absorbed and are lost in the faeces. Jackson (1986) has suggested that this may result in a drain on the supply of the amino acids glycine and taurine, which are conjugated with bile acids to form bile salts. Excretion of hydrogen in the breath is increased in PEM (Caballero *et al.*, 1983). This results from fermentation of unabsorbed carbohydrate in the ileum and colon.

The classical test of absorptive capacity, the measurement of D-xylose excretion in the urine after an oral test dose, is not considered very useful in PEM because the result may be affected by uncontrolled factors such as renal function, intestinal motility or incomplete urine collection. Moreover, in asymptomatic children in Bangladesh there was no relation between the absorption of xylose and that of macronutrients (Brown *et al.*, 1981). A modification of the xylose test uses two sugars given simultaneously: lactulose, a disaccharide that is normally neither absorbed nor metabolized, and a

Table 5.7   Absorption of energy, nitrogen and calcium during early recovery from PEM

	Percent of intake absorbed	
	Days 2–5	After day 8
Energy	90	94
Nitrogen	88	91
Calcium	44	39

Diet initially provided 100 kcal/kg/day; later 150 kcal/kg/day. Majority of children had some diarrhoea, with increased number and weight of stools.
From Torun *et al.* (1984).

monosaccharide that is absorbed but not metabolized, such as rhamnose or mannitol. The ratio of the two sugars, L/R or L/M, is then measured in the urine. In patients with villus atrophy this ratio was greatly increased as a result of changes in both components (Menzies *et al.*, 1979; Ford *et al.*, 1985). The monosaccharide is normally absorbed by the transcellular pathway, and its absorption was decreased as a consequence of the reduced area of the mucosa. Lactulose cannot enter healthy enterocytes, but it crosses the atrophic mucosa through leaks between the epithelial cells. The result therefore depends both on the functional capacity of the gut and on its structural integrity. Table 5.8 shows results obtained in children in the Gambia (Behrens *et al.*, 1987). The L/M ratio was increased seven-fold in children with chronic diarrhoea. This reflected mainly an increase in the entry of lactulose rather than a decrease in that of mannitol. The L/M ratio fell as diarrhoea resolved.

Leakiness of the intestinal epithelium may allow abnormal penetration of intact proteins. The subject has been reviewed by Gardner (1984), who suggested that 'passage of small amounts of large protein molecules across the intestinal epithelium is an essential component of the normal immune reaction'. However, increased permeability with entry of larger amounts of foreign protein may be expected to give rise to local immune reactions, as in cow's milk protein intolerance. It is a matter of debate whether this could be the underlying mechanism in some cases of protracted diarrhoea (Chapter 17). Such a process would tend to be self-perpetuating, with damage to the epithelium leading to abnormal entry of macromolecules and further epithelial damage.

Table 5.8 Intestinal permeability in Gambian children, measured by the urinary excretion of the non-metabolizable sugars lactulose (L) and mannitol (M)

Condition of children	L/M ratio
Normal children	0.42
Underweight (60–80% weight for age)	0.52
Marasmus	1.3
Acute diarrhoea	1.4
Chronic diarrhoea	2.85
Measles	1.4

Data of Behrens *et al.* (1987).

Kidney

In contrast to the liver, changes in histopathology of the kidney in PEM are not very prominent and seem to be non-specific. Hyalinization of the glomeruli and cloudy swelling and necrosis of tubular cells have been recorded in severe cases (Davies, 1948; Bhattacharyya, 1975). In a later paper Davies (1956) said that the characteristic lesion was fatty change in the cells of the convoluted tubules.

Examination by electron microscopy of glomerular ultra-structure in Jamaican children with oedematous malnutrition has shown what has been described as effacement of the foot processes (Golden *et al.*, 1990). This is the morphological expression of absence or reduction of the normal anionic charge of the basement membrane, on which the integrity of the filtration system depends. The anionic charge arises from the sulphate groups of the basement membrane proteoglycans. It is an interesting possibility that this lesion might reflect a defect in the process of sulphation—a possibility that comes up in other contexts, e.g. in relation to cartilage growth (Chapter 13).

Golden *et al.* point out that this lesion is similar to that seen in minimal-change nephrotic syndrome, but in their patients there was no albuminuria. Davies (1956) mentions that albuminuria is slight and inconstant, with different findings in different countries. Said *et al.* (1973) examined the urine of children with PEM by immunoelectrophoresis and reported increasing proteinuria as the disease progressed, but never reaching the level found in the nephrotic syndrome. In severe kwashiorkor a variety of proteins were found in the urine and in some cases the pattern matched closely that of the proteins in serum.

Changes in renal function in PEM were investigated in detail by Alleyne (1967). His findings, as well as those of earlier authors, have been discussed in several reviews (Klahr and Alleyne, 1973; Alleyne *et al.*, 1977) and are summarized in Table 5.9. No more work on this subject seems to have been done since then. The inability to excrete a sodium load, which has also been recorded by Gordillo *et al.* (1957), Kerpel-Fronius (1960) and Mönckeberg (1988), is striking and important in relation to the pathogenesis of oedema (Chapter 11). Alleyne measured sodium excretion before and after expansion of the extracellular fluid volume with hypotonic saline. This was done in three malnourished children before and after recovery. Initially the sodium load produced a less than two-fold increase in sodium excretion; after recovery the same load was followed by a ten-fold increase in excretion. Unfortunately this study did not include a comparison between children with and without oedema.

The most likely cause of this defect is potassium deficiency, although in measurements on kidneys post-mortem Alleyne found only a small reduction in potassium content, 2 mmol K/g N compared with 2.5 mmol K/g N in normal children. In an earlier study by Smith (1959) on the ability of children with PEM to excrete acid a significant negative correlation was found between minimum urine pH and the potassium content of muscle (μmol K/mg DNAP). The possible role of potassium deficiency in the production of oedema is considered in Chapter 11.

Table 5.9 Changes in renal function in PEM

Reductions in:
  kidney weight, parallel to reduction of body weight
  [a] glomerular filtration rate
  [a] renal plasma flow
  ability to excrete acid
  ability to excrete sodium
  ability to produce a concentrated urine
Some evidence of impaired tubular function:
  aminoaciduria
  occasional phosphaturia

[a] In these studies a specific comparison was made between children with and without oedema. No differences were found.
Data of Alleyne (1967) and Klahr and Alleyne (1973)

Skin and hair

Changes in the skin were prominent in the early description of kwashiorkor. The classical picture called 'crazy pavement' or 'flaky paint' dermatosis resembles in some ways that of pellagra, with hyperpigmentation distributed mainly but not exclusively on exposed parts. Gillman and Gillman (1951) gave a detailed description of the development of the lesions in their extreme form. They begin with reddish spots which become black, hard, scaly and raised. Fusion of these spots is followed by desquamation, exfoliation and cracking of the skin surface. Often there is ulceration in the genital and peri-anal regions, in the body creases and on exposed surfaces.

This severe form of dermatosis is quite variable and is absent in many children who show the other cardinal characteristics of kwashiorkor. Bhattacharyya (1972), working in Calcutta, said that the classical dermatosis was never seen in the absence of oedema, although oedema often occurred without dermatosis. The skin changes were also related to the presence of fatty liver. In their cases 'the presence of a considerable amount of subcutaneous fat seemed to be essential for the development of kwashiorkor dermatosis'. In the Calcutta series the mortality in cases of kwashiorkor with skin lesions was twice as high as in those without (21 per cent *versus* 9 per cent) (Bhattacharyya, 1986). In Mexico, by contrast, the presence of skin lesions did not imply a bad prognosis (Gomez *et al.*, 1956).

The variability of the severe dermatosis suggests that it might be caused by an associated specific deficiency. Long ago it was proposed that kwashiorkor was really infantile pellagra, but no evidence has ever been produced, either biochemical or by therapeutic tests, of a deficiency of nicotinic acid. Another possible factor might be vitamin A deficiency, but in the Calcutta series of 700 cases of PEM, in which 10 per cent overall had eye signs of vitamin A deficiency, there was no relationship with skin lesions (Bhattacharyya, 1983). A possible role for tryptophan deficiency has not been investigated. Golden and Golden (1985) pointed out the clinical similarity to acrodermatitis enteropathica, a condition in which there is congenital impairment of zinc absorption. They showed that children with skin ulceration had significantly lower plasma zinc levels and when the lesions were symmetrical, treatment of one side with topical zinc produced more rapid healing than on the untreated side (Golden *et al.*, 1980). A comparative study of the incidence of the dermatosis in children with PEM in different parts of the world might throw more light on the aetiology, but systematic information of this kind is not available.

Very often in PEM there are less marked changes, variously described as 'xerosis' or 'mosaic skin', in which the skin is dry, thin, shiny or wrinkled. In such cases the basic histological feature is atrophy of the basal layers of the epidermis with hyperkeratosis. These changes, which are perhaps analogous to those in the gut epithelium, appeared histologically to be much the same, whatever the clinical picture (J. C. Waterlow, unpublished observations).

From the metabolic point of view the skin is an important but neglected organ. Writing of marasmic children, the French paediatrician Nobécourt (1912) said 'the envelope is too big for the body that it encloses'—a picture only too familiar in famines today. This appearance presumably results from loss of subcutaneous fat, because the evidence summarized below suggests that the skin itself loses protein just as other tissues do. Quantitative data, however, are scarce. According to Kerpel-Fronius and Frank (1949), in normal children the skin weight is about 15 per cent of body weight. In two malnourished children analysed by Halliday (1967) the skin (including fat) accounted for 16 per cent of body weight, 22 per cent of total body collagen and 15 per cent of total non-collagen protein. Thus the loss of skin tissue was parallel to the overall loss of body weight. In experiments on rats on a low protein diet, the skin lost more protein than any other tissue, even muscle (Waterlow and Stephen, 1966). One might expect a relatively greater loss in the rat than in the child, because of its higher surface to volume ratio.

The complex structure of the skin makes analysis of it difficult. It can either be divided anatomically into dermis and epidermis, or chemically into collagen and non-collagen protein. Biopsies of the skin in children with kwashiorkor showed a large reduction in the total collagen content with an increase in the proportion of labile collagen (Vasantha, 1969), which suggests a block in the formation of collagen cross-links (Table 5.10). Therefore in absolute terms there must have been a substantial loss of skin collagen. We have argued (Chapter 3) that in PEM the collagen scaffolding of the body remains more or less intact while other tissues waste around it, but the skin may be to some extent a special case. Collagen is not, as used to be thought, completely inert (Waterlow *et al.*, 1978; Laurent, 1988), and the collagens in different tissues have different characteristics. It may be reasonable, therefore, to regard the skin, like muscle, as a store of protein which can be drawn upon for the maintenance of other tissues.

Table 5.10 Collagen content of the skin in kwashiorkor

	Total collagen (µg hydroxyproline per 100 mg wet tissue)	Labile collagen (% of total collagen)
Normal	2418	4.8
Kwashiorkor:		
without skin lesions	1360	12.3
with skin lesions	767	21.4
after treatment	1898	6.9

After Vasantha (1969)

Vasantha (1969; Vasantha *et al.*, 1970) made two other important observations, although their significance is not entirely clear. In kwashiorkor, particularly in those with dermatosis, there was a relative increase in the amount of labile collagen, suggesting an inhibition in collagen maturation. Secondly, the proportions, as a percentage of total dermal N, of proline, hydroxyproline, glycine and tyrosine were significantly decreased. Proline, hydroxyproline which is formed from proline, and glycine are the most abundant amino acids in collagen. They have been classified by Jackson (1989) as conditionally essential (Chapter 6), and it may be that in PEM an inadequate supply of these amino acids is limiting collagen synthesis.

The epidermis contains only a small proportion of the total protein of the skin, but it is probable that it is responsible for the greater part of its metabolic activity, at least in relation to protein turnover (Waterlow and Stephen, 1966). In rats two weeks after a dose of labelled amino acid (Neale and Waterlow,

1974) the whole skin had taken up as much of the label as the liver. The skin was found to have a fractional rate of protein synthesis of 60 per cent/day (Preedy and Waterlow, 1981), from which it can be calculated that in the rat the skin accounted for as large a fraction of whole-body protein turnover as the liver. Protein synthesis in the skin was also relatively resistant to starvation, compared with muscle. No comparable data are available for man.

The cells of the basal layer of the epidermis, like those of the gut epithelium, are continually being renewed, although not so rapidly. It has been estimated that in normal adult man it takes 10–14 days for a basal cell to reach the cornified layer, by which time it is effectively dead (Wright, 1980). It is not known whether this process is slowed down in PEM, although changes in the hair provide some suggestive evidence.

One of the classical signs in PEM is that the hair becomes thin, sparse and easily pulled out, although these changes, like those in the skin, are quite variable. The hair follicles are morphologically part of the epidermis and presumably share in its high rate of protein and cell turnover. Bradfield and co-workers took advantage of this fact to use the morphology and composition of the hair bulb as indicators of early PEM. In PEM a higher proportion of bulbs were in the resting than in the growing phase (Bradfield *et al.*, 1968), and the diameter of the hair root was closely correlated with weight for age (Bradfield and Jelliffe, 1970). The protein and DNA content per hair were also correlated with the size of the hair bulb, and were reduced in malnourished children. It was suggested that measurement of hair bulb diameter could be used as a sensitive field test of 'protein deficiency', at least for groups, if not for individuals (Bradfield, 1972). However, more profound changes in the bulb were found in marasmus than in kwashiorkor; differences were attributed to chronicity rather than to 'specific differences in relative protein-calorie density' (Bradfield *et al.*, 1969).

Hypopigmentation of the skin and hair is often seen in PEM, and Brock and Autret (1951) considered that discolouration of the normally black hair was essential for the diagnosis of kwashiorkor. In fact, this change, like all the others discussed in this section, is by no means always present. In some children with severe PEM the hair remains black; in others who seem quite well-nourished all the hair may be reddish-brown. Sometimes a light-coloured band is seen, which is thought to represent an earlier episode of malnutrition. Excellent illustrations of the hair changes are given by Jelliffe (1966) and Pereira (1990).

It was suggested many years ago that the cause of dyspigmentation of the hair might be a deficiency of cystine, which is a principal component of keratin, but analysis of hair showed no evidence of a decrease in sulphur-amino acid content. Another possibility would be a deficiency of tyrosine, which is a precursor of the pigment melanin, but this appears not to have been investigated.

In conclusion, the skin is a large organ which can perhaps provide a reserve of protein; the epidermis, at least, is metabolically active and therefore vulnerable to malnutrition. However, the skin is a neglected tissue, and few detailed studies have been made of the changes that are seen in PEM. We remain ignorant both of the epidemiology and of the pathophysiology of these lesions which, though very variable, are sometimes quite dramatic.

The nervous system

Although, as we have seen (Chapter 3), the brain is relatively protected in PEM, the protection is not absolute. The head circumference is less than in normal children of the same age, but apparently this does not fully reflect the reduction in brain tissue. Studies in Ethiopia by transillumination and echo-ventriculography showed that the size of the ventricles was increased in kwashiorkor but not in marasmus (Engsner *et al.*, 1974). This finding has been confirmed in India by CAT scan (Udani and Dastur, 1989) and appears to be reversible on treatment.

Brown (1966) in Uganda found the brain weight reduced in severely malnourished children who died. In a large series in Bombay the average deficit in brain weight in under-nourished compared with normally-nourished children was 19 per cent; it was considerably greater in children who died below the age of three months (Udani and Dastur, 1989). From animal experiments it seems unlikely that the brain actually loses weight in malnutrition: it is much more likely that it has simply failed to grow. In that case one might expect to find a correlation between deficits in the weight of the brain and the length of the body. Such a correlation is suggested by the measurements of Garrow *et al.* (1965) on children who died. If the 'brain-age' is calculated as the age of a normal child with the same brain weight as the malnourished child, the mean ratio of brain age: actual age in the five least stunted children of Garrow's series was 0.82 and in the five most stunted 0.66. If this approach is valid, stunting in linear growth is evidently accompanied by significant retardation in brain growth. Since marasmic children tend to be more stunted than those with kwashiorkor, one would expect their brain growth to be more retarded, but the data are too scanty to test the point.

The deficit in weight of the brain is accompanied by a deficit in total DNA, that is, in the number of brain cells (Fig. 5.3). Our ideas about the functional

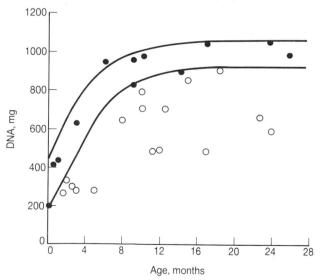

Fig. 5.3 DNA content of cerebrum in normal and marasmic children. ●, normal; ○, marasmic (Jamaica). Reproduced by permission from Winick *et al.* (1970).

significance of this finding are dominated by Dobbing's pioneer concept of vulnerable periods (Dobbing and Sands, 1973; Dobbing and Smart, 1974). According to this concept, malnutrition will only have an effect if it coincides with a time of rapid growth and differentiation. Dobbing pointed out that in relation to birth this time varies in different animal species; it varies in different regions of the brain and for different cell types. In man brain cell growth occurs in two distinct phases: a phase of very rapid growth between ten and 20 weeks of pregnancy, representing multiplication of neuronal cells, followed by a phase of slower growth resulting from multiplication of glial cells, which extends through the third trimester of pregnancy up to about six months of post-natal life (Dobbing and Sands, 1970). On the vulnerable period hypothesis PEM developing post-natally should have its greatest effect during the second phase of growth. Since glial cells are responsible for the production of myelin, it is not surprising that there is evidence of delayed myelin formation in PEM (Rosso *et al.*, 1970). There is also a reduction in polyamine content, though the significance of this is not clear (McAnulty *et al.*, 1977).

A number of workers have observed a decrease in conduction velocity in peripheral nerves, both sensory and motor, in severe PEM (Engsner *et al.*, 1974; Ghosh *et al.*, 1979; Chopra *et al.*, 1986) with a predominance of fibres of small diameter (Udani and Dastur, 1989). Finally, and perhaps most important from a functional point of view, there is evidence of a decrease in the density of neuronal synapses. Bedi (1987), using the laborious method of quantitative histology, documented a lower synapse : neurone ratio in some regions of the brain as a result of early post-natal malnutrition. Mönckeberg (1985) has reproduced a remarkable illustration of disappearance of dendrites in a neurone of a child who died from severe marasmus. However, recovery may be possible from the deficit in synapses.

Dobbing (1990) has discussed the functional implications of these reductions or retardations in the structural and chemical development of the brain. He concludes that nerve cell number, which in any case may not be significant for mental function, is 'out of the reach of malnutrition' in man, since almost all the adult nerve cell number is produced before mid-pregnancy. As for the other changes, he considers that 'not all are irreversible. Some appear to be so, but others recover slowly and some even seem to recover completely. If we knew which of them were significant for higher mental function, we would be in a better position to interpret these findings in behavioural terms' but 'effects on achievement can only be investigated directly'. Such direct investigations of the effects of malnutrition on the mental development of children are reviewed in Chapter 19. Handicaps in development certainly occur, but Dobbing regards it as naïve to suppose that these result from irreversible structural brain damage. On the other hand, slowing down of the brain's development during a child's formative years could well have a lasting effect on achievement in later life. Dobbing (1987) has marshalled the evidence that has been brought together from different disciplines.

References

Agbedana, E. O., Johnson, A. O. *et al.* (1979). Selective deficiency of hepatic trigly-ceride lipase and hypertriglyceridaemia in kwashiorkor. *British Journal of Nutrition* **43**: 351–356.

Alleyne, G. A. O. (1966). Cardiac function in severely malnourished children. *Clinical Science* **30**: 553–562.

Alleyne, G. A. O. (1967). The effect of severe protein calorie malnutrition on the renal function of Jamaican children. *Pediatrics* **39**: 400–411.

Alleyne, G. A. O., Hay, R. W. *et al.* (1977). *Protein-energy malnutrition.* Edward Arnold, London, p. 34.

Ashworth, A., Milner, P. F. *et al.* (1973). Absorption of iron from maize (*Zea mays, L.*) and soya beans (*Glycine hispida Max.*) in Jamaican infants. *British Journal of Nutrition* **29**: 269–278.

Bedi, K. S. (1987). Lasting neuroanatomical changes following undernutrition during early life. In Dobbing, J. (ed) *Early nutrition and later development.* Academic Press, London, pp. 1–36.

Behrens, R. H., Lunn, P. G. *et al.* (1987). Factors affecting the integrity of the intestinal mucosa of Gambian children. *American Journal of Clinical Nutrition* **45**: 1433–1441.

Beresford, C. H., Neale, R. J., Brooke, O. G. (1971). Iron absorption and pyrexia. *Lancet* **1**: 568–572.

Bergman, J. W., Human, D. G. *et al.* (1988). Effect of kwashiorkor on the cardio-vascular systems. *Archives of Disease in Childhood* **63**: 1359–1362.

Bhattacharyya, A. K. (1972). Concomitants of kwashiorkor dermatosis. *Bulletin of the Calcutta School of Tropical Medicine* **20**: 46–48.

Bhattacharyya, A. K. (1975). Studies on kwashiorkor and marasmus in Calcutta, 1957–74. II. Pathological, biochemical and metabolic studies. *Indian Pediatrics* **12**: 1115–1123.

Bhattacharyya, A. K. (1983). Xerophthalmia in kwashiorkor-marasmus syndrome (KMS). *Bulletin of the Calcutta School of Tropical Medicine* **31**: 41–44.

Bhattacharyya, A. K. (1986). Protein-energy malnutrition (kwashiorkor-marasmus syndrome): terminology, classification and evolution. *World Reviews of Nutrition and Dietetics* **47**: 80–133.

Bradfield, R. B. (1972). A rapid tissue technique for the field assessment of protein-calorie malnutrition. *American Journal of Clinical Nutrition* **25**: 720–729.

Bradfield, R. B., Jelliffe, E. F. P. (1970). Early assessment of malnutrition. *Nature* **225**: 283–284.

Bradfield, R. B., Bailey, M. A., Cordano, A. (1968). Hair-root changes in Andean Indian children during marasmic kwashiorkor. *Lancet* **2**: 1169–1170.

Bradfield, R. B., Cordano, A., Graham, G. G. (1969). Hair root adaptation to marasmus in Andean Indian children. *Lancet* **2**: 1395–1397.

Bras, G., Hill, K. R. (1956). Veno-occlusive disease of the liver: essential pathology. *Lancet* **2**: 161–163.

Bras, G., Waterlow, J. C., DePass, E. (1957). Further observations on the liver, pancreas and kidney in malnourished infants and children. The relation of certain histopathological changes in the pancreas and those in liver and kidney. *West Indian Medical Journal* **6**: 33–42.

Brasseur, D. (1986). *Influence de la malnutrition protéo-énergétique sur l'expression genetique de la lactase.* PhD Thesis, Université Libre, Brussels.

Brasseur, D., Hennart, P. H., Vis, H. L. (1985). "Malabsorption" of intact lactose. *Lancet* **1**: 100–101.

Briend, A., Hoque, B. A., Aziz, K. M. A. (1990). Iron in tubewell water and linear growth in rural Bangladesh. *Archives of Disease in Childhood* **65**: 224–227.

Brock, J. F., Autret, M. (1951). *Kwashiorkor in Africa.* World Health Organization Monograph Series No. 8. WHO, Geneva.

Brown, K. H., Khatun, M., Ahmed, M. G. (1981). Relationship of the xylose absorption status of children in Bangladesh to their absorption of macronutrients from the local diets. *American Journal of Clinical Nutrition* **34**: 1540–1547.

Brown, R. E. (1966). Organ weight in malnutrition with special reference to brain weight. *Developmental Medicine and Child Neurology* **8**: 512–522.

Brunser, O., Reid, A. *et al.* (1968). Jejunal mucosa in infantile malnutrition. *American Journal of Clinical Nutrition* **21**: 976–983.

Caballero, B., Solomons, N. W., Torun, B. (1983). Fecal reducing substances and breath hydrogen excretion as indicators of carbohydrate malabsorption. *Journal of Pediatric Gastroenterology and Nutrition* **2**: 487–490.

Chatterjee, K. K., Mukherjee, K. L. (1968). Phospholipids of the liver in children suffering from protein-calorie malnutrition. *British Journal of Nutrition* **22**: 145–151.

Chaudhuri, R. N., Bhattacharyya, A. K. (1962). Marasmus: treatment with whole milk as compared to skimmed milk. *Bulletin of the Calcutta School of Tropical Medicine* **10**: 56.

Chopra, J. S., Upinder, K. *et al.* (1986). Effect of protein-energy malnutrition on peripheral nerves: a clinical, electrophysiological and histopathological study. *Brain* **109**: 307–324.

Cohen, S., Hansen, J. D. L. (1962). Metabolism of albumin and γ-globulin in kwashiorkor. *Clinical Science* **23**: 351–359.

Cook, G. C., Hutt, M. S. R. (1967). The liver after kwashiorkor. *British Medical Journal* **3**: 454–457.

Coppoletta, J. M., Wolbach, S. B. (1933). Body length and organ weights of infants and children. *American Journal of Pathology* **9**: 55–70.

Cordano, A., Baertl, J. M., Graham, G. G. (1964). Copper deficiency in infancy. *Pediatrics* **34**: 324–336.

Datta Chaudhuri, A., Bhattacharyya, A. K., Mukherjee, A. M. (1972). The liver in pre-kwashiorkor and kwashiorkor-marasmus syndromes. *Transactions of the Royal Society of Tropical Medicine and Hygiene* **66**: 258–262.

Davies, J. N. P. (1948). The essential pathology of kwashiorkor. *Lancet* **1**: 317–320.

Davies, J. N. P. (1954). The exocrine enzyme secreting glands. In Trowell, H. C., Davies, J. N. P., Dean, R. F. A. *Kwashiorkor*. Academic Press, London, pp. 144–150. Reprinted 1982.

Davies, J. N. P. (1956). Renal lesions in kwashiorkor. *American Journal of Clinical Nutrition* **4**: 539–542.

DeMaeyer, E., Adiels-Tegman, O. (1985). The prevalence of anaemia in the world. *World Health Organization Statistical Quarterly* **38**: 302–316.

Dobbing, J. (1990). Early nutrition and later achievement. *Proceedings of the Nutrition Society* **49**: 103–118.

Dobbing, J., Sands, J. (1970). Timing of neuroblast multiplication in the developing brain. *Nature (London)* **226**: 639–640.

Dobbing, J., Sands, J. (1973). Quantitative growth and development of human brain. *Archives of Disease in Childhood* **48**: 757–767.

Dobbing, J., Smart, J. L. (1974). Vulnerability of developing brain and behaviour. *British Medical Bulletin* **30**: 164–168.

Engsner, G., Woldemariam, T. (1974). Motor nerve conduction velocity in marasmus and in kwashiorkor. *Neuropädiatrie* **1**: 34–48.

Engsner, G., Habte, D. *et al.* (1974). Brain growth in children with kwashiorkor. *Acta Paediatrica Scandinavica* **63**: 1–8.

Finch, C. A. (1975). Erythropoiesis in protein-calorie malnutrition. In Olson, R. E. (ed) *Protein-calorie malnutrition*. Academic Press, New York, pp. 247–256.

Flores, H., Pak, N. *et al.* (1970). Lipid transport in kwashiorkor. *British Journal of Nutrition* **24**: 1005–1011.

Flores, H., Seakins, A. *et al.* (1974). Serum and liver triglycerides in malnourished

Jamaican children with fatty liver. *American Journal of Clinical Nutrition* **27**: 610–614.

Fondu, P. (1977). A reassessment of intravascular volume measurements in protein-calorie malnutrition. *European Journal of Clinical Investigation* **7**: 161–165.

Fondu, P., Mandelbaum, I. N. (1975). Marasmic kwashiorkor anemia. III. Hemoglobin oxygen affinity. *Biomedicine* **22**: 291–297.

Fondu, P., Hariga-Muller, C. *et al.* (1978a). Protein-energy malnutrition and anaemia in Kivu. *American Journal of Clinical Nutrition* **31**: 46–56.

Fondu, P., Hâgâ P., Halvorsen, S. (1978b). The regulation of erythropoiesis in protein-energy-malnutrition. *British Journal of Haemotology* **38**: 29–36.

Ford, R. P. K., Menzies, I. S. *et al.* (1985). Intestinal sugar permeability: relationship to diarrhoeal disease and small bowel morphology. *Journal of Pediatric Gastroenterology and Nutrition* **4**: 568–574.

Gabr, M., Salam, E. A., Malek, A. (1968a). Lactose tolerance in marasmic infants. *Medical Journal of Cairo University* **36**: 23–36.

Gabr, M., Shukry, A. S. *et al.* (1968b). Studies on fat digestion and absorption in kwashiorkor. *Journal of Tropical Medicine and Hygiene* **71**: 187–192.

Gardner, M. L. (1984). Intestinal assimilation of intact peptides and proteins from the diet—a neglected field? *Biological Reviews* **59**: 289–331.

Garrow, J. S., Fletcher, K., Halliday, D. (1965). Body composition in severe infantile malnutrition. *Journal of Clinical Investigation* **44**: 417–425.

Gendrel, D., Gahouma, D. *et al.* (1986). Anomalies de la muqueuse jéjunale et malnutrition protéino-calorique chez le nourrisson en Afrique Équatoriale. *Annales Pédiatrie* **31**: 871–876.

Ghosh, S., Vaid, K. *et al.* (1979). Effect of degree and duration of PEM on peripheral nerves in children. *Journal of Neurology, Neurosurgery and Psychiatry* **42**: 760–763.

Gillman, J., Gillman, T. (1951). *Perspectives in human malnutrition.* Grune and Stratton, New York.

Golden, M. H. N., Golden, B. E. (1985). Problems with the recognition of human zinc responsive conditions. In Mills, C. F., Bremner, I., Chesters, J. K. (eds) *Trace element metabolism in man and animals, 5.* Commonwealth Agricultural Bureau, Aberdeen, pp. 933–938.

Golden, M. H. N., Golden, B. E., Jackson, A. A. (1980). Skin breakdown in kwashiorkor responds to zinc. *Lancet* **1**: 1256.

Golden, M. H. N., Brooks, S. E. H. *et al.* (1990). Effacement of glomerular foot processes in kwashiorkor. *Lancet* **336**: 1472–1474.

Gollan, F. (1948). Blood and extracellular fluid studies in chronic malnutrition in infancy. *Journal of Clinical Investigation* **27**: 352–363.

Gomez, F., Ramos Galván, R. *et al.* (1950). Estudios sobre el niño desnutrido. VII. El volumen sanguineo y del plasma en el prescolar desnutrido. *Boletin Medical Hospital Infantil (Mexico)* **7**: 514–520.

Gomez, F., Ramos-Galván, R. *et al.* (1956). Mortality in second and third degree malnutrition. *Journal of Tropical Pediatrics* **2**: 77–83.

Gordillo, G., Soto, S., Metcoff, J. (1957). Renal adjustments in malnutrition. *Pediatrics* **20**: 303–316.

Gracey, M. (1981). Nutrition, bacteria and the gut. *British Medical Bulletin* **37**: 71–75.

Graham, G. G., Cordano, A. (1976). Copper deficiency in human subjects. In Prasad, A. S. (ed) *Trace elements in human health and disease, 1.* Academic Press, New York, pp. 363–372.

Halliday, D. (1967). Chemical composition of the whole body and individual tissues of two Jamaican children whose death resulted primarily from malnutrition. *Clinical Science* **33**: 365–370.

Heard, C. R. C., Platt, B. S., Stewart, R. J. C. (1958). The effect on pigs of a low protein diet with and without additional carbohydrate. *Proceedings of the Nutrition Society* **17:** xli.

Jackson, A. A. (1986). Severe undernutrition in Jamaica. *Acta Paediatrica Scandinavica* Suppl. **323:** 43–51.

Jackson, A. A. (1989). Optimizing amino acid and protein supply and utilization in the newborn. *Proceedings of the Nutrition Society* **48:** 293–301.

James, W. P. T. (1970). Sugar absorption and intestinal motility in children when malnourished and after treatment. *Clinical Science* **39:** 305–318.

James, W. P. T. (1971). Effects of protein-calorie malnutrition on intestinal absorption. *Annals of the New York Academy of Sciences* **176:** 244–261.

James, W. P. T. (1977). Kwashiorkor and marasmus: old concepts and new developments. *Proceedings of the Royal Society of Medicine* **70:** 611–615.

Jelliffe, D. B. (1966). *Assessment of the nutritional status of the community.* World Health Organization Monograph Series No. 53. WHO, Geneva.

Kerpel-Fronius, E. (1960). Volume and composition of the body fluid compartments in severe infantile malnutrition. *Journal of Pediatrics* **56:** 826–833.

Kerpel-Fronius, E., Frank, K. (1949). Einige Besonderheiten der Korperzusammensetzung und Wasserverteilung bei der Sauglingsatrophie. *Annales Paediatrica* **173:** 321–330.

Kerpel-Fronius, E., Varga, F. (1949). Dynamics of circulation in infantile malnutrition. *Pediatrics* **4:** 301–308.

Klahr, S., Alleyne, G. A. O. (1973). Effects of chronic protein-calorie malnutrition on the kidney. *Kidney International* **3:** 129–141.

Kumar, V., Deo, M. G., Ramalingaswami, V. (1972). Mechanism of fatty liver in protein deficiency. *Gastroenterology* **62:** 445–451.

Laidlaw, S. J., Kopple, J. D. (1987). Newer concepts of the indispensable amino acids. *American Journal of Clinical Nutrition* **46:** 593–605.

Laurent, G. J. (1988). Dynamic state of collagen: pathways of collagen degradation in vivo and their possible role in regulation of collagen mass. *American Journal of Physiology* **251:** (Cell Physiol. 20), C1–C9.

Layrisse, M., Cook, J. D. *et al.* (1969). Food iron absorption: a comparison of vegetable and animal foods. *Blood* **33:** 430–443.

Lewis, B., Hansen, J. D. L. *et al.* (1964). Plasma free fatty acids in kwashiorkor and the pathogenesis of fatty liver. *American Journal of Clinical Nutrition* **15:** 161–168.

Loeb, H., Van Steierteghem, A. *et al.* (1976). Jejunal mucosa in infantile protein-calorie deficiency. *Acta Paediatrica Belgique* **29:** 19–23.

Lozoff, B., Brittenham, G. M. *et al.* (1987). Iron deficiency anemia and iron therapy effects on infant developmental test performance. *Pediatrics* **79:** 981–995.

McAnulty, P. A., Yusuf, H. K. M. *et al.* (1977). Polyamines of the human brain during normal fetal and postnatal growth and during postnatal malnutrition. *Journal of Neurochemistry* **28:** 1305–1310.

McIver, J. E., Back, E. H. (1960). Megaloblastic anaemia of infancy in Jamaica. *Archives of Disease in Childhood* **35:** 134–145.

McLaren, D. S., Fariz, R., Zekian, B. (1968). The liver during recovery from protein-calorie malnutrition. *Journal of Tropical Medicine and Hygiene* **71:** 271–281.

McLean, A. E. M. (1966). Enzyme activity in the liver and serum of malnourished children in Jamaica. *Clinical Science* **30:** 129–137.

Martins Campos, J. V., Neto, V. F. *et al.* (1979). Jejunal mucosa in marasmic children. Clinical, pathological and fine structure evaluation of the effect of protein-energy malnutrition and environmental contamination. *American Journal of Clinical Nutrition* **32:** 1575–1591.

Menzies, I. S., Laker, M. F. *et al.* (1979). Abnormal intestinal permeability to sugars in villous atrophy. *Lancet* **2:** 1107–1109.

Molla, A. Rahim, A. *et al.* (1982). Intake and absorption of nutrients in children with cholera and rotavirus infection during acute diarrhoea and after recovery. *Nutrition Research* **2**: 233–242.

Mönckeberg, F. (1985). Protein-energy malnutrition: marasmus. In Brunser, O., Carrazza, F. R. *et al.* (eds) *Clinical nutrition of the young child*. Raven Press, New York, pp. 121–132.

Mönckeberg, F. (ed) (1988). *Desnutricion infantil*. Instituto de Nutricion y Technologia de los Alimentos, Santiago, Chile.

Narasinga Rao, B. S. (1981). Physiology of iron absorption and supplementation. *British Medical Bulletin* **37**: 25–30.

Neale, R. J., Waterlow, J. C. (1974). Critical evaluation of a method for estimating amino acid requirements for maintenance in the rat by measurement of the rate of ^{14}C-labelled amino acid oxidation in vivo. *British Journal of Nutrition* **32**: 257–272.

Nobécourt, P. (1916). Des hypotrophies et des cachesies des nourrissons. *Archives de Médecine des Enfants* **19**: 113–136.

O'Keefe, S. J. D., Ogden, J. M. *et al.* (1989). Measurement of pancreatic enzyme synthesis in humans. *International Journal of Pancreatology* **4**: 13–27.

Olson, R. E. (1979). Reply to letter by Fondu *et al*. *American Journal of Clinical Nutrition* **31**: 720.

Omer, A., El Shazali, H. *et al.* (1973). Studies on the anaemia of kwashiorkor and marasmus in the Sudan. *Journal of Tropical Pediatrics and Environmental Child Health* **19**: 91–97.

Palti, H., Pevsner, B., Adler, B. (1983). Does anaemia in infancy affect achievement on developmental and intelligence tests? *Human Biology* **55**: 183–194.

Pereira, S. M. (1990). Clinical aspects and treatment. In Ballabriga, A., Brunser, O. *et al.* (eds) *Clinical nutrition of the young child*. Raven Press, New York, pp. 143–148.

Preedy, V. R., Waterlow, J. C. (1981). Protein synthesis in the young rat—the contribution of skin and bones. *Journal of Physiology* **317**: 45P.

Ramalingaswami, V., Nayak, M. C. (1970). Liver disease in India. *Progress in Liver Disease* **III**: 222–235.

Ramdath, D. D., Golden, M. H. N. (1989). Non-haematological aspects of iron nutrition. *Nutrition Research Reviews* **2**: 29–50.

Reye, R. D. K., Morgan, G. (1963). Encephalopathy and fatty degeneration of the viscera. *Lancet* **2**: 1061.

Reye, R. D. K., Morgan, G., Baral, J. (1963). Encephalopathy and fatty degeneration of the viscera—a disease entity in childhood. *Lancet* **2**: 749–752.

Rhodes, K. (1957). Two types of liver disease in Jamaican children: Part I. *West Indian Medical Journal* **6**: 1–29.

Römer, H., Urbach, R. *et al.* (1983). Moderate and severe protein-energy malnutrition in childhood: effects on jejunal mucosal morphology and disaccharidase activities. *Journal of Pediatric Gastroenterology and Nutrition* **2**: 459–464.

Russell, S. J. M. (1949). Blood volume studies in healthy children. *Archives of Disease in Childhood* **24**: 88–98.

Said, A., El-Hawary, M. F. S. *et al.* (1973). Protein-calorie malnutrition in Egypt. 1. Immuno-electrophoretic studies on urinary proteins. *American Journal of Clinical Nutrition* **26**: 1355–1359.

Seakins, A., Waterlow, J. C. (1972). Effect of a low-protein diet on the incorporation of aminoacids into rat serum lipoproteins. *Biochemical Journal* **129**: 793–795.

Smith, R. (1959). Urinary acidification defect in chronic infantile malnutrition. *Lancet* **1**: 764.

Sökücü, S. (1987). Enterokinase and disaccharidase activity of the small intestinal mucosa in infants with protein-energy malnutrition and in normal infants. *Turkish Journal of Pediatrics* **29**: 15–24.

Srikantia, S. G., Reddy, V. (1963). Plasma volume and total circulating albumin in kwashiorkor. *Journal of Pediatrics* **63**: 133–137.

Srikantia, S. G., Sriramachari, S., Gopalan, C. (1958). A follow-up study of fifteen cases of kwashiorkor. *Indian Journal of Medical Research* **46:** 121–128.

Suttajit, M. (1975). Discussion in Olson, R. E. (ed) *Protein-calorie malnutrition.* Academic Press, New York, pp. 269–271.

Swarup-Mitra, S., Sinha, A. K., Bhattacharyya, A. K. (1976). Anaemia in kwashiorkor and pre-kwashiorkor—haematological indices before treatment. *Archives of Child Health* **18:** 91–98.

Tanman, B. F. (1971). Changes of cardiac output and total body oxygen consumption in protein-calorie malnourished infants. *Proceedings of the 13th International Congress of Pediatrics.* Wiener Medical Akademie, Vienna, pp. 407–412.

Thompson, M. D., Trowell, H. C. (1952). Pancreatic enzyme activity in the duodenal contents of children with a type of kwashiorkor. *Lancet* **1:** 1031–1035.

Torun, B., Solomons, N. W. *et al.* (1984). The effect of dietary lactose on the early recovery from protein-energy malnutrition. *American Journal of Clinical Nutrition* **40:** 601–610.

Truswell, A. S. (1990). Malnutrition and carbohydrate and lipid metabolism. In Suskind, R. M., Suskind, L. L. (eds) *The malnourished child.* Nestlé, Vevey/Raven Press, New York, pp. 95–115.

Truswell, A. S., Hansen, J. D. L. (1969a). Fatty liver in protein-calorie malnutrition. *South African Medical Journal* **43:** 280–283.

Truswell, A. S., Hansen, J. D. L. *et al.* (1969b). Relation of serum lipids and lipoproteins to fatty liver in kwashiorkor. *American Journal of Clinical Nutrition* **22:** 568–576.

Udani, P. M., Dastur, D. K. (1989). Pediatric malnutrition—a global neurological problem. In Dastur, D. K., Shahani, M., Bharucha, E. P. (eds) *Neurological sciences: an overview on current problems.* Interprint, New Delhi, pp. 251–275.

Vasantha, L. (1969). Labile collagen content of the skin in kwashiorkor. *Clinica Chimica Acta* **26:** 277–280.

Vasantha, L., Srikantia, S. G., Gopalan, C. (1970). Biochemical changes in the skin in kwashiorkor. *American Journal of Clinical Nutrition* **23:** 78–82.

Veghelyi, P. V. (1950). Nutritional oedema. *Annales Paediatrica* **175:** 349–377.

Viart, P. (1976). Blood volume (^{51}Cr) in severe protein-calorie malnutrition. *American Journal of Clinical Nutrition* **29:** 25-37.

Viart, P. (1977a). Hemodynamic findings is severe protein-calorie malnutrition. *American Journal of Clinical Nutrition* **30:** 334–348.

Viart, P. (1977b). Blood volume changes during treatment of protein-calorie malnutrition. *American Journal of Clinical Nutrition* **30:** 349–354.

Viart, P. (1978). Hemodynamic findings during treatment of protein-calorie malnutrition. *American Journal of Clinical Nutrition* **31:** 911–926.

Vilter, R. W. (1975). The anaemia of protein-calorie malnutrition. In Olson, R. E. (ed) *Protein-calorie malnutrition.* Academic Press, New York, pp. 257–261.

Viteri, F. E., Schneider, R. E. (1974). Gastrointestinal alterations in protein-calorie malnutrition. *Medical Clinics of North America* **58:** 1487–1505.

Viteri, F. E., Schneider, R. (1980). Gastrointestinal functions in children with mild to severe protein-energy malnutrition and during recovery. In Wharton, B. (ed) *Topics in paediatrics 2: nutrition in childhood.* Pitman Medical, London, pp. 63-71.

Viteri, F. E., Torun, B. (1974). Anaemia and physical work capacity. *Clinical Haematology* **3:** 609–626.

Viteri, F. E., Alvarado, J. *et al.* (1968). Haematological changes in protein-calorie malnutrition. *Vitamins and Hormones* **26:** 573–615.

Walters, J. H., Waterlow, J. C. (1954). *Fibrosis of the liver in West African Children.* Medical Research Council Special Report Series No. 285. HM Stationery Office, London.

Waterlow, J. C. (1948). *Fatty liver disease in the British West Indies.* Medical Research Council Special Report Series No. 263. HM Stationery Office, London.

82   *Protein-energy malnutrition*

Waterlow, J. C. (1961). Oxidative phosphorylation in the livers of normal and malnourished human infants. *Proceedings of the Royal Society B* **155:** 96–114.

Waterlow, J. C. (1975). Amount and rate of disappearance of liver fat in malnourished infants in Jamaica. *American Journal of Clinical Nutrition* **28:** 1330–1336.

Waterlow, J. C., Stephen, J. M. L. (1966). Adaptation of the rat to a low-protein diet: the effect of a reduced protein intake on the pattern of incorporation of L-[^{14}C] lysine. *British Journal of Nutrition* **20:** 461–484.

Waterlow, J. C., Bras, G., DePass, E. (1957). Further observations in the liver, pancreas and kidney in malnourished infants and children. II. The gross composition of the liver. *Journal of Tropical Pediatrics* **2:** 189–198.

Waterlow, J. C., Cravioto, J., Stephen, J. M. L. (1960). Protein malnutrition in man. *Advances in Protein Chemistry* **15:** 131–238.

Waterlow, J. C., Garlick, P. J., Millward, D. J. (1978). *Protein turnover in mammalian tissues and in the whole body*. North Holland, Amsterdam, pp. 510–523.

Wharton, B. A., Howells, G. R., McCance, R. A. (1967). Cardiac failure in kwashiorkor. *Lancet* **2:** 384–387.

Williams, C. D. (1935). Kwashiorkor: a nutritional disease of children associated with a maize diet. *Lancet* **2:** 1151–1152.

Winick, M., Rosso, P., Waterlow, J. C. (1970). Cellular growth of cerebrum, cerebellum and brain stem in normal and marasmic children. *Experimental Neurology* **26:** 393–400.

World Health Organization (1980). *Expert Committee on diabetes mellitus, 2nd report*. Technical Report Series No. 646. WHO, Geneva.

Wright, N. A. (1980). The kinetics of human epidermal cell populations in health and disease. In Rook, A. J., Savin, J. A. (eds) *Recent advances in dermatology* Vol. 5. Churchill-Livingstone, Edinburgh and London, pp. 317–343.

6
Metabolic changes

Energy metabolism

In the words of Kerr *et al.* (1978*a*), even severely wasted infants have a remarkable flexibility of energy homoeostasis. These authors studied the pattern of substrate utilization in malnourished and recovered children in the fasted state. When glycogen stores were exhausted, which occurred much more rapidly than in adults, fat became the predominant source of energy even in marasmic children. Oxidation of fat was more efficient, since urinary excretion of ketone bodies was much less in the malnourished than in the recovered state. Only a very small proportion of energy was derived from the oxidation of protein: 4 per cent in the malnourished and 7 per cent after recovery. The rate of glucose production was the same in malnourished and recovered children (Kerr *et al.*, 1978*b*) and there was no evidence of any defect in gluconeogenesis. It was suggested that children who develop hypoglycaemia (Chapter 8) may represent a specially sensitive sub-group.

It seems, therefore, that the most important adjustment made by the child with PEM is quantitative rather than qualitative; a reduction in total energy expenditure, the greater part of which is accounted for by the basal metabolism.

Metabolic rate (MR) in PEM

The 'basal' metabolic rate in young children is usually measured while they are asleep, three to five hours after the last meal. Since these conditions are not strictly basal, it is better to use the term MR. The MR is about 10 per cent higher during the transition from non-rapid to rapid eye movement sleep (Butte, 1990), but it is hardly possible to control for this in practice.

Different methods of expressing the metabolic rate in malnourished children were discussed in Chapter 2. Here body weight will generally be used as the basis.

It is an interesting and unresolved question whether the MR measured in infants several hours after the last meal includes the energy cost of growth. Butte (1990) suggests that it does, because growth hormone is released during sleep. However, as was shown in Fig. 2.1, there is no evident relationship between MR and growth rate. Brooke and Ashworth (1972) showed a positive correlation between the rate of growth and the increase in oxygen consumption after a meal (Fig. 6.1), and suggested that growth occurs in bursts, stimulated by food. This fits in with the demonstration in adults of a diurnal rhythm of protein metabolism related to meals (Clugston and Garlick, 1982). Similarly, in low birth-weight infants there was a correlation between resting energy expenditure and the rate of protein gain (Cazeflis *et al.*, 1985). In this study metabolic rate was apparently measured immediately after completion of a meal and therefore would include the thermic effect of food.

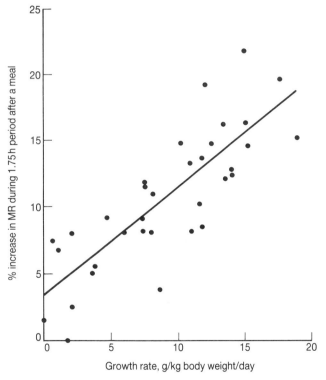

Fig. 6.1 Relation of postprandial increase in metabolic rate over 1.75 hours after a meal to rate of weight gain in children recovering from malnutrition. Reproduced by permission from Brooke and Ashworth (1972).

Seventy years ago Talbot (1921) in a classic paper showed that in marasmic children the MR, whether related to weight or surface area, was higher than in normal children. The explanation that he proposed was that because of loss of subcutaneous fat and increase in surface/volume ratio, malnourished babies had to produce more heat to maintain body temperature. When measurements of MR began to be made in children with severe PEM the results confirmed Talbot's findings in some but not all cases. Montgomery (1962) in Jamaica reported that the greater the weight deficit, the higher the MR/kg. In marasmics who were only 40 per cent of expected weight, the MR/

kg was twice that of controls. Mönckeberg *et al.* (1964) in Chile found that the MR/kg was slightly higher in marasmic than in normal infants, whereas Ablett and McCance (1971) in Uganda showed that in kwashiorkor the MR/kg was 25 per cent lower than in controls.

When metabolic rates in malnourished children are related not to weight but to height or to the 3/4 power of weight, the picture changes and the deficits are magnified (Table 6.1). However, it was argued in Chapter 2 that there is no sound physiological basis for these methods of expression.

Table 6.1 Metabolic rate (MR) in malnutrition expressed in various ways in relation to metabolic rate in normal or recovered children

Reference	MR, malnourished/recovered × 100		
	MR/kg	MR/100 cm	MR/kg$^{0.75}$
Brooke and Cocks (1974)	84	60	68
Ablett and McCance (1971)	75	64	71
Mönckeberg *et al.* (1964)	103	56	–

Montgomery (1962) was apparently the first to suggest that Talbot's and his own seemingly paradoxical findings resulted from the distorted pattern of organs and tissues described in Chapter 3. He made some tentative calculations to show that if a marasmic and a normal child have the same MR/kg, because of his larger brain the marasmic must have a 30 per cent lower MR of tissues other than brain. A similar computation was made by Brooke and Cocks (1974), who calculated that in a malnourished child weighing about 60 per cent of normal, the oxygen uptake of non-muscle tissues per kg non-muscle weight was decreased by 22 per cent. Holliday (1978) made a calculation based on organ weights and their specific rates of oxygen uptake to explain the higher MR/kg in children than in adults. This promising approach could be applied in principle, using the organ weights recorded by Garrow *et al.* (1965) in malnourished children, but it is limited by our lack of knowledge about the size and metabolic activity of important tissues such as the gastrointestinal tract and the lymphatic system.

Another approach to the problem is based not on differences in organ patterns but on differences in body composition. Many studies have been made in adults in which MR is related to lean body mass (LBM) rather than total body weight, in order to avoid the diluting effect of fat. This should also make the results more uniform. Surprisingly, when Butte (1990) measured LBM in four-month old infants, the relationship of MR to LBM was no closer than that to body weight.

Since the LBM contains a considerable proportion of inert structural tissue, the ideal way of expressing the MR should be to relate it to active cell mass. As discussed in Chapter 3, in the absence of specific K deficiency, active cell mass can be estimated from total body, K. Table 6.2 shows results expressed in this way. The reduction in MR was less in the oedematous children; they had a lower TBK/kg, and if this was the result of loss of K from cells rather than dilution by oedema fluid, it would lead to an underestimate of the active cell mass.

On treatment the MR rises rapidly and often overshoots the control level,

Table 6.2 Metabolic rate (MR) in relation to total body potassium (TBK) in malnourished and recovered children

	Weight for height (%)	TBK (mmol/kg)	MR (kcal/mmol K/day)	
Controls	98	46.6	1.21	
Marasmic, initial	71	48.2	1.05	} $P < 0.001$
recovered	98	45.0	1.39	
Oedematous, initial	77	41.4	1.14	} $P < 0.05$
recovered	98	46.8	1.33	

Calculated from Brooke and Cocks (1974)

long before there could have been much deposition of lean tissue (Varga, 1959; Montgomery, 1962) (Fig. 6.2). This suggests that the first stage in recovery is restoration of the normal rate of cellular respiration, preceding the deposition of new tissue (Waterlow, 1990).

There is some evidence from studies *in vitro* that respiration at the level of the cell is indeed depressed in malnutrition. Nichols *et al.* (1968) showed a correlation between the overall MR *in vivo* and the respiratory rate *in vitro* of muscle homogenates from biopsy samples. Both rates were lower in children with moderate K deficits, which might reflect the reduction in sodium pump (Na^+-K^+-ATPase) activity that occurs in K deficiency, at least in muscle (Chapter 4). However, a recent review by Clausen *et al.* (1991) indicates that the activity of the ion pumps accounts for a much smaller part of the whole-body metabolic rate than used to be thought. In biopsies from fatty livers of

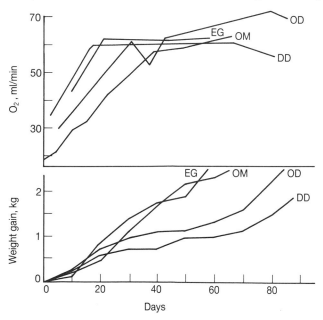

Fig. 6.2 Changes in metabolic rate and weight gain in four marasmic children during recovery from malnutrition. Reproduced by permission of the American Society for Clinical Investigation from Montgomery (1962).

children with PEM the rate of oxidative phosphorylation was reduced, although this could have been an artefact caused by the presence of fat in the homogenates. The pioneer studies of Metcoff and his colleagues in Mexico revealed that children with PEM had reduced concentrations of oxidative enzymes in muscle and of intermediary metabolites in leucocytes (Metcoff *et al.*, 1966; Yoshida *et al.*, 1967). Continuing this line of work Parra *et al.* (1973) found significant reductions of ATP, creatine phosphate and glycogen in muscle biopsies, compared with the levels after three weeks of recovery. All this evidence taken together suggests a reduced state of cellular oxidation in severe PEM. One might suppose that a cell in this condition is on the way to death.

Another possible reason for diminished oxygen uptake could be an inadequate oxygen supply to the tissues as a result of impaired cardiac function (Chapter 5), perhaps combined with anaemia. Figure 6.3 shows that a given increase in whole-body oxygen consumption was associated with a much greater increase in pulse rate in the malnourished state than after recovery (Spady *et al.*, 1976). This suggests that the heart may have difficulty in coping with any extra demand. A practical consequence is that if MR is being estimated from the heart rate, the child has to be frequently recalibrated during recovery.

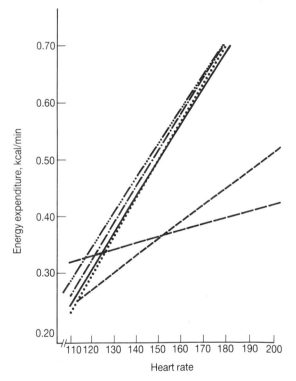

Fig. 6.3 Relation between energy expenditure and heart rate in a child recovering from malnutrition. ——————, day 0; ————, day 3; ••••• , day 43; ——···—, day 65; —·—·, day 73; ——————, day 82. As the child recovered the slope becomes steeper, implying more efficient utilization of energy per heart beat. Reproduced by permission of the American Society for Clinical Nutrition from Spady *et al.* (1976).

Impaired heat production and hypothermia

A consequence of the reduction in MR (i.e. in heat production) is that the child with PEM has difficulty in maintaining a normal body temperature. In a series described by Brooke (1972) in Jamaica nearly half the children had rectal temperatures below 35.5°C in their first week in hospital. In Uganda 25 per cent of children with rectal temperatures below 36.5°C died (Brenton *et al.*, 1967). Figure 6.4 shows that the child with severe PEM has difficulty in regulating its body temperature, which follows the ambient temperature more closely than in a normal child. As mentioned earlier, the thermic response to a meal is also reduced until the child begins to gain weight (Brooke and Ashworth, 1972).

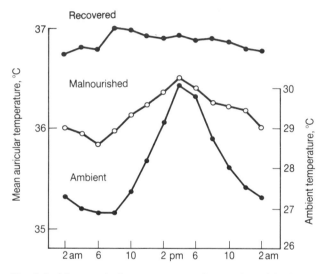

Fig. 6.4 Mean auricular temperature of ten malnourished children before and after recovery, and the mean ambient temperature. Reproduced by permission from Brooke (1972).

If the MR is not only low, but is unable to react to stimuli in a normal way, one would expect a reduced ability to produce a fever in response to infection. This is indeed the case; as a result, not only is it more difficult to diagnose the presence of an infection, but if fever has any protective value the child who cannot produce it is handicapped. Duggan *et al.* (1986) showed that in children with measles the MR/kg was some 25 per cent lower than after recovery. During the period of infection the food intake was also lower, as a result of anorexia, but since the measurements were post-prandial, that should not have affected the MR.

In The Gambia mildly undernourished infants (about 80 per cent weight for age at one year) had no increase in MR when they were ill, compared with when they were well (Eccles *et al.*, 1989).

In simplistic terms, therefore, in severe PEM not only is the machine run down, but its responses are sluggish and inadequate. These facts have very important implications for treatment (Chapter 12).

Nitrogen metabolism

In severe PEM, as we have seen (Chapter 5), the gut mucosa and exocrine pancreas show a considerable degree of atrophy and the production of digestive enzymes is decreased; nevertheless, there seems to be enough reserve capacity for the hydrolysis of such proteins as are provided by the food. In the absence of diarrhoea the capacity for absorbing the resulting amino acids and small peptides is retained, even though for the most part this is achieved by active transport, requiring energy. This section is therefore concerned with the metabolism of nitrogen after it has entered the body and reached the tissues.

Protein turnover

'Turnover' of protein is a general term which covers the two opposing processes, synthesis and breakdown of protein (Waterlow *et al.*, 1978). In the steady state, in an organism that is not growing, the rate of protein synthesis is equal to that of breakdown, just as the rate of nitrogen intake is equal to the rate of output. The growing state, when N is being retained, is described by the simple relationship:

synthesis − breakdown = net retention = input − output. It follows that the same rate of N retention can occur at different rates of synthesis/breakdown, just as it can occur at different rates of input/output. Thus the conventional measurement of N balance tells us nothing about the dynamics of protein turnover (Fig. 6.5). Under normal conditions the rate of protein synthesis is four or five times the rate of dietary protein intake. These concepts are quite important for understanding what happens in PEM.

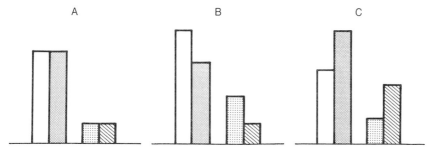

Fig. 6.5 Schematic relationships of protein synthesis, protein breakdown and nitrogen balance in the steady state (A), during rapid growth (B) and in response to infection (C). The rates of protein synthesis (S) and breakdown (B) bear no necessary relation to rates of nitrogen intake (I) or excretion (E) but S − B is always equal to I − E (N balance). ☐, synthesis; ▨, breakdown; ▦, intake; ▧, excretion.

Protein or nitrogen turnover appears to be as essential for life as oxygen uptake, which can be regarded as a form of turnover, though why this dynamic state of protein should be necessary is still not at all clear. There is in fact a numerical relationship between the two turnovers, both within a species, as when infants are compared with adults, and between species (Waterlow, 1984).

In the 1960s we already knew that oxygen consumption was depressed in severe PEM. When there continued to be a high mortality, in spite of strenuous efforts to treat dehydration, electrolyte imbalance and infection, we wondered whether the cause of death might be a parallel depression of protein synthesis. Such a state could be irreversible, because the machinery for synthesizing proteins involves enzymes that are themselves proteins. To test this hypothesis it was necessary to devise a method of measuring whole-body protein synthesis with the stable nitrogen isotope ^{15}N (Picou and Taylor-Roberts, 1969; Waterlow *et al.*, 1978). Figure 6.6 illustrates some results obtained by this method. Initially the synthesis rate, at about 4 g/kg/day, was some two-thirds of that found in normal children of the same age. Because of the differences in body composition already discussed in relation to the BMR, this result almost certainly underestimates the true depression of the rate of protein synthesis in the essential visceral organs. Perhaps one could say that the original hypothesis was partially but by no means completely supported.

An important question is the relation of protein turnover to protein intake. The turnover rates shown in Fig. 6.6 were all measured at the same level of intake, so the depression of turnover in acute PEM reflects the nutritional state rather than the immediate diet. The effect of the level of intake was further investigated by Jackson *et al.* (1983), whose results are summarized in Table 6.3. The rate of protein synthesis was reduced by about 25 per cent on the low protein diet, and there was an indication of a preferential reduction of protein synthesis in muscle. That could be regarded as an adaptive response.

No measurements have been made of rates of protein synthesis in individual tissues in children with PEM, but animal experiments have shown that on low protein diets or during fasting there is a large reduction in the rate of protein synthesis in muscle (Millward *et al.*, 1976). This could be regarded as an adaptation which protects the amino acid supply to other more essential

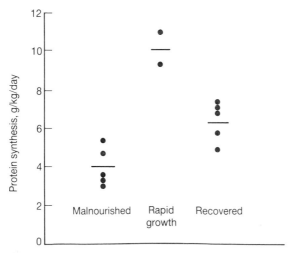

Fig. 6.6 Rates of whole-body protein synthesis in children in the acute phase of PEM, during the rapid growth phase and after recovery. From data of Golden *et al.* (1977*a*).

Table 6.3 Rates of whole-body protein synthesis in young children at different levels of protein and energy intake

Protein intake (g/kg/day)	Energy intake (kcal/kg/day)	Protein synthesis (g/kg/day)	Number of subjects
1.7	100	5.5	5
	90	5.5	5
	80	6.0	5
0.7	100	4.1	2
	90	4.25	2
	80	3.6	2

Data from Jackson *et al.* (1983)

tissues. In rats after several days fasting there is an increase in muscle protein breakdown, so that muscle is in negative N balance.

A method for estimating the rate of muscle protein breakdown *in vivo* was introduced by Young *et al.* (1973), based on the fact that myofibrillar proteins contain a methylated amino acid, 3-methylhistidine (3MH). The methylation occurs after the incorporation of histidine into protein. The modified amino acid cannot be utilized for protein synthesis, so when liberated in the free form by protein breakdown it is excreted quantitatively in the urine. Since there are also small amounts of 3MH in the proteins of gut and skin, as well as in those of muscle, the urinary excretion may not give a true picture of muscle protein breakdown (Rennie and Millward, 1983), but it is probably a reasonable indicator. In children with PEM the daily excretion of 3MH per kg body weight was only one-third of normal (Nagabhushan and Narasinga Rao, 1978). These findings fit in with the experimental results and support the idea that when dietary protein is low muscle responds in a way that protects the amino acid supply to the essential organs.

During recovery from PEM the rate of whole-body protein synthesis increases dramatically to levels well above normal, in just the same way as the rate of O_2 consumption increases (Fig. 6.2). A linear relationship has been found between rates of protein synthesis and of weight gain. In children during the rapid growth phase of recovery, both rates are similar to those in premature infants (Pencharz *et al.*, 1981). From the relationship shown in Fig. 6.5, if protein synthesis and nitrogen balance are both measured, the rate of protein breakdown can be determined by difference. In this way it has been shown that during rapid growth there is an increase in protein breakdown, though not of the same extent as the increase in synthesis (Fig. 6.7). Thus to retain 1 g protein about 1.5 g have to be synthesized. An increase in protein breakdown appears to be a general phenomenon of rapid growth (Millward, 1978). It is energetically wasteful, because protein synthesis requires energy (Waterlow and Millward, 1989), but presumably the advantage of it is to allow remodelling of tissues during growth.

It is probable that during recovery some tissues have priority over others; albumin, for example, clearly has a high priority. Skeletal growth seems only to take off after normal weight for height has been restored (Walker and Golden, 1988). This might be because the soft tissues have the first call on the sulphur amino acids that are necessary for the formation of cartilage, or of the glycine and proline that are needed for collagen formation (Chapter 13).

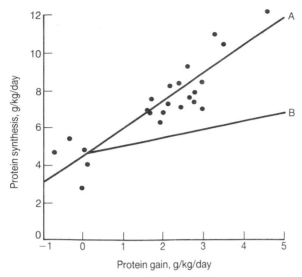

Fig. 6.7   Relation between rates of protein synthesis and breakdown and rates of net protein gain in children recovering from malnutrition. A, measured rate of protein synthesis; B, calculated rate of protein breakdown. For each g protein gained, about 1.5 g protein has to be synthesized, over and above the basal level of synthesis, and of this 0.5 g is broken down. Drawn from data of Golden *et al.* (1977*b*).

Effects of infection

Infection and trauma are other situations in which protein breakdown is increased, but here there is a negative N balance. As has long been known, the loss of nitrogen is part of the usual metabolic response to injury and infection; however, as Table 6.4 shows, if the child is malnourished the response appears to be blunted, as if conservation of N takes priority over any benefits that the normal response may confer. It is generally supposed that the extra N lost in infection is derived from muscle. In the relatively well-nourished children with measles in Table 6.4 (group I), there was a

Table 6.4   Effects of infection and malnutrition on nitrogen metabolism in Nigerian children

Group[a]	I	II	III	IV
No. of children	5	6	6	5
Weight for height, %	87	75	65	63
Temperature, °C	39.3	37.4	37.6	36.3
Plasma albumin, g/dl	3.76	3.77	1.87	1.66
N balance, mg/kg/9 hours[b]	−208	−59	+12	+23
Protein breakdown, g/kg/9 hours	5.2	4.5	2.3	1.2
3MH excretion, mmol/kg/9 hours	5.90	1.96	1.58	0.96

[a] Group   I: mildly malnourished, acute measles
           II: moderately malnourished, acute systemic infections other than measles
          III: severely malnourished with persistent subacute infection; five out of six had oedema
           IV: severely malnourished without clinical infection; four out of five had oedema
[b] Balances and turnover rates measured over 9 hours
Data of Tomkins *et al.* (1983)

massive excretion of both 3MH and creatinine, suggesting an actual destruction of muscle tissue, but this was not found in the other groups. In the malnourished children, muscle protein breakdown accounted for only a small proportion (25 per cent or less) of the protein breakdown in the whole body.

Another element in the response of protein metabolism to infection is production by the liver of a group of proteins called 'acute phase (AP) proteins', stimulated by polypeptide hormones (cytokines) that are released by macrophages (for reviews see Grimble, 1989, 1990). Table 6.5 lists some of the more important AP proteins. They have been divided by Kushner (1988) into three groups: those normally present in minute amounts, whose concentration may increase 1000 times; those whose concentration increases two to four times; and those which show only a small increase, if any. Some of the AP proteins have clear-cut functions, e.g. fibrinogen in blood-clotting, haptoglobin in binding free haemoglobin, caeruloplasmin (a copper-containing protein) and metallothionein (a zinc-containing protein) in the scavenging of free radicals (Chapter 10). Others may have a role in immunoregulation (Dinarello, 1984). Malnutrition or deficiency of specific nutrients may affect the acute phase response in two ways: by reducing the production of cytokines or by modulating the response of target tissues (Grimble, 1989). Bhaskaram and Sivakumar (1986) showed that in kwashiorkor production of one of the cytokines, interleukin 1, was reduced. Jackson (1991) has suggested that specific deficiencies of amino acids such as cysteine, glycine or serine may limit the production of some AP proteins which are proportionately very rich in these amino acids.

The increased synthesis of the AP proteins in the liver is accompanied by a decrease in the plasma concentrations of the classical nutritionally important proteins such as albumin and transferrin, so that these are sometimes called 'negative AP' proteins. Whether this decrease results from reduced synthesis or increased breakdown is not known. The peak concentrations in the AP response are usually found at 48 hours or later (Colley *et al.*, 1983). If we ignore breakdown of the newly synthesized AP proteins, it is possible to calculate a minimum synthesis rate of the AP proteins in response to an acute injury (Table 6.5). An estimate for those proteins which are present in the largest amounts gives a rough figure of 1.2 g protein synthesized per kg per day, which is six times the normal rate of albumin synthesis in adult man.

Table 6.5 Calculated amounts of acute phase proteins synthesized in response to infection

Protein	Normal plasma concentration (g/l)	Maximum increase in 48 hours	New synthesis (g/kg/24 hours)[a]
C-reactive protein	0.01	× 1000	0.25
Serum amyloid A	0.01	× 1000	0.25
α_1-acid glycoprotein	1	× 4	0.1
α_1-antitrypsin	2	× 4	0.2
Fibrinogen	2	× 4	0.2
Haptoglobin	2	× 4	0.2
			Total 1.2

[a] Plasma volume taken as 50 ml/kg
From data of Fleck (1989) and Colley *et al.* (1983)

This may well constitute a serious drain on the capacity of the liver to synthesize the negative AP proteins, through competition for available amino acids.

Loss of nitrogen from the gut

Faecal nitrogen as measured by balances includes the endogenous loss of N from the gut as well as unabsorbed N from food. Except when the food contains a large amount of fibre, there is little evidence of malabsorption of amino acids (Chapter 5). The endogenous N loss can only be measured on a protein-free diet, and this has not been done in children with PEM. Torres-Pinedo (1976) perfused the jejunum in infants after an episode of acute diarrhoea and showed that the amounts of protein and DNA in the perfusion fluid increased on recovery, indicating a greater turnover rate of enterocytes. However, it is not possible to translate these results into amounts lost in the stools.

In chronic inflammatory disease of the gastrointestinal tract there is an exudation of protein from the plasma to the gut lumen (protein-losing enteropathy). in early studies of this source of loss various non-absorbable radioactively labelled plasma protein analogues or markers, e.g. ^{59}Fe-dextran or ^{131}I-PVP were injected intravenously and the radioactivity measured in the stools. In a preliminary study Cohen *et al.* (1962) found a seven-fold increase in the excretion of ^{131}I-PVP in kwashiorkor and considered that this might be significant in the pathogenesis of hypoalbuminaemia. Leakage of plasma protein into the gut appears to be particularly great during and after an attack of measles (Dossetor and Whittle, 1975).

The radioactive markers have been superseded by the non-invasive method of determining the faecal excretion of α_1-antitrypsin, because this protein is naturally present in plasma, and is not broken down in the gut. The results can therefore be expressed as plasma clearances (ml/day). Sarker *et al.* (1986), using this method, found that on the first day of post-measles diarrhoea the average clearance was 129 ml/day, falling to about 50 ml/day after three weeks, which is still high compared with the normal of about 20 ml/day. The initial loss would represent about 25 per cent of the intravascular albumin mass; this is a very large amount, and could explain the observation made by many workers of oedema appearing after an attack of measles (Chapter 11). However, there is some controversy about the extent to which faecal α_1-antitrypsin is an accurate marker of loss of plasma proteins (Quigley *et al.*, 1987). In PEM uncomplicated by infection faecal protein loss appears to be of little importance (Cohen *et al.*, 1962; Shukry *et al.*, 1965).

Mechanisms for economizing nitrogen

When dietary amino acids are in short supply a number of mechanisms for economy come into play (Waterlow, 1986). First, there is a decrease in activity of enzymes responsible for the irreversible oxidation of essential amino acids, such as the branched-chain amino acids, so that a larger proportion of those entering the free amino acid pool from protein breakdown can be reutilized for protein synthesis. Secondly, there is a co-ordinated decrease in activity of the four enzymes of the urea cycle, and at the same time an increase in activity of the amino-acyl-tRNA transferases, which catalyse the first step in protein synthesis. These enzyme changes have been found in malnourished children as well as in experimental animals (Stephen and Waterlow, 1968). The effect of them is that amino acids are diverted into the pathway of protein synthesis and away from oxidation to urea. This is a beautiful example of an adaptive change, but the mechanism regulating the shift in fluxes from one pathway to another is not understood. This mechanism would not be expected to function efficiently when energy is also limiting and protein has to be used as an energy source.

Another adaptive process that helps to conserve nitrogen is an increase in the recycling and reutilization of urea. In normal subjects on a usual protein intake about 30 per cent of the urea produced in the liver enters the colon, where it is split by bacteria to ammonia. The ammonia is either used by the bacteria for their own protein synthesis, or transported to the liver, where part of it is recycled to urea and part retained and probably incorporated into amino acids. Picou and Phillips (1972), using ^{15}N-labelled urea, were the first to make quantitative studies of urea recycling and utilization in children. They showed that children, whether malnourished or recovered, retained a larger proportion of urea production on a low than on a high protein intake. This work has been extended by Jackson *et al.* (1990); they compared children during the rapid growth phase of recovery on diets providing 10.6 and 8.8 per cent protein energy. The results in Fig. 6.8 show that on the lower protein intake significantly larger amounts of urea N were recycled and retained. It is important for our understanding of protein requirements (Chapter 15) that even this relatively small difference in protein intake should have such a clear effect when, as during rapid growth, demands for protein are high.

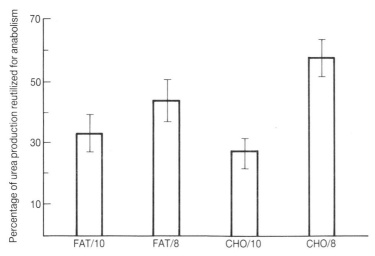

Fig. 6.8 Percentage of urea production that is retained and used for anabolism during the rapid growth phase of recovery from PEM. Isocaloric diets (170 kcal/kg/day) provided protein at either 10.6 or 8.8 per cent of total energy, and were high in either fat (arachis oil) or carbohydrate (maize starch). Reproduced by permission from Jackson (1989).

It might be supposed that conservation of ammonia N derived from urea would only be useful when the limiting factor in the diet is total N rather than essential amino acids. Current controversies about amino acid requirements

(Millward *et al.*, 1989) suggest that this situation may be more common than has been thought. Moreover, there is preliminary evidence in the literature that essential amino acids synthesized by bacteria in the colon could be absorbed and available for protein synthesis (Tanaka *et al.*, 1980), but this needs to be confirmed.

It is also possible that amino acids synthesized from urea N by bacteria are absorbed directly from the colon into the bloodstream. Heine *et al.* (1987) found that when ^{15}N-labelled yeast protein was instilled into the colon in children with a colostomy, 90 per cent of the ^{15}N was absorbed and retained. Earlier, Tanaka *et al.* (1980) produced preliminary evidence suggesting that essential amino acids synthesized by bacteria in the colon could be absorbed and available for protein synthesis. The extent to which such mechanisms come into play is probably quite variable, depending on the nature of the bacterial flora and the energy available to them (Jackson *et al.*, 1990). Factors of this kind might explain in part differences in the efficiency with which dietary protein is utilized.

Amino acid metabolism

It was proposed at one time that changes in the pattern of free amino acids in plasma might be useful in distinguishing between kwashiorkor and marasmus (see Chapter 7). However, such changes are difficult to interpret, because the concentration of a free amino acid at any moment depends on the resultant of four factors: on the one hand, input from food and, in the case of the non-essential amino acids, from *de novo* synthesis; on the other hand, removal by oxidation or uptake into protein.

Nevertheless, there are certain changes in PEM that are of interest. Of all the essential amino acids, the concentrations of the branched chain amino acids (BCA) are most severely reduced. This occurs in spite of evidence from animal experiments that on low protein diets there is an adaptive reduction in the rate of oxidation of these amino acids. Since the concentration of BCAs in protein is relatively high and their free pools are small, it could well be that these amino acids are the first to become limiting for protein synthesis. It has indeed been suggested from experiments *in vitro* that the BCA leucine has a specific role in the regulation of protein synthesis in muscle, although this was not confirmed by measurements *in vivo* (McNurlan *et al.*, 1982).

Dean and Whitehead (1963) demonstrated in the urine of children with kwashiorkor intermediary metabolites of histidine, phenylalanine and tyrosine. They suggested that there might be failures of enzyme activity similar to those found in some inborn errors of metabolism, with the difference that the abnormalities were reversed on treatment. These interesting findings appear never to have been followed up. It is tempting to suppose that they may be examples of a more widespread impairment of enzyme activity. If the machinery of intermediary metabolism is run down, then it is not surprising that too early overloading with a high protein-high energy diet may have disastrous effects, as discussed from a practical point of view in Chapter 12. The tissues need time to adjust from a situation in which the 'bottom line' is economy to one in which there is profuse expenditure on new growth.

Nitrogen metabolism in PEM is also an example of a practical problem stimulating a substantial amount of basic research.

Albumin metabolism

The metabolism of plasma albumin in PEM and the mechanism of hypo-albuminaemia are of special interest. There is a long history of experiments, listed by Golden (1985), in which animals of various kinds were maintained on low protein diets. Sometimes oedema appeared and sometimes it did not. The rat is not a very good animal for this kind of experiment, because it does not readily consume a low protein diet, but the pig eats it voraciously and becomes oedematous (Widdowson, 1968). However, the question of oedema comes later (Chapter 11). Here the focus is on the dietary production of hypoalbuminaemia. The early studies of Weech and his colleagues (1939) are very illuminating. They demonstrated a large reduction in plasma albumin concentration in dogs fed a diet of carrots, rice, lard, sugar and a salt mixture containing a substantial amount of potassium. It was noted that the decline in plasma albumin was not more rapid when the dogs were fasted than when they had an adequate energy intake. Weech considered that these experimental findings reproduced very closely their earlier observations on famine oedema in China (Weech and Ling, 1931).

The most direct demonstration of the effects of diet and nutritional state on plasma albumin metabolism comes from measurements of albumin synthesis. Cohen and Hansen (1962) reported that in children with kwashiorkor the synthesis rate of albumin was reduced, whereas there was no change in that of γ-globulin. They measured albumin breakdown from the decay curve of albumin labelled with radioactive iodine, and assumed a steady state in which synthesis and breakdown were equal. Plasma albumin concentration and the intravascular (IV) albumin mass were decreased in the malnourished state and restored on recovery. Normally about 40 per cent of total albumin is intravascular, about 60 per cent extravascular (EV). In the malnourished children the EV pool bore the larger share of the loss. These observations were confirmed and extended by James and Hay (1968), who showed that in both malnourished and recovered children a period of seven to ten days on a low protein diet produced an immediate fall in the rate of albumin synthesis, followed a little later by a fall in the rate of breakdown, which may be regarded as a compensatory response (Fig. 6.9). They also found, like Cohen and Hansen, that albumin was moving from the EV to the IV compartment. These mechanisms for maintaining albumin mass prevented a fall in albumin concentration during the short periods of low protein feeding. We do not know whether, if those periods had been longer, it would have been possible to maintain the compensation.

The effect of low protein feeding on albumin synthesis has been amply confirmed by animal experiments, both *in vivo* and *in vitro* (for references see Waterlow *et al.*, 1978). It has also been shown that the reduction is mediated by a fall in production of messenger RNA, implying an inhibition of gene expression (Pain *et al.*, 1978; Sakuma *et al.*, 1987).

Other factors affect plasma albumin levels. As mentioned in the previous section, injuries and infections are accompanied by a fall in plasma albumin and an increased production of the acute phase proteins, which may divert amino acids away from albumin synthesis.

Liao *et al.* (1986) measured the rate of albumin synthesis during acute inflammation produced experimentally, with very striking results. After 36

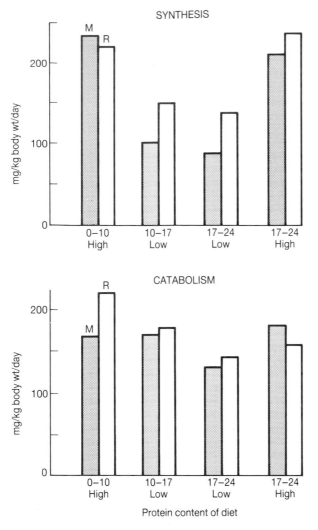

Fig. 6.9   Effect of protein content of the diet on albumin synthesis and breakdown in malnourished (▨) and recovered (☐) children. Drawn from data of James and Hay (1968).

hours the rate of synthesis of albumin was 38 per cent of the control and that of secreted proteins other than albumin (many of which will be acute phase proteins) 268 per cent of the control. Albumin messenger RNA was reduced to 25 per cent of the control level. Another possible mechanism of hypo-albuminaemia is an increased loss of albumin from the capillaries. Fleck *et al.* (1985) showed that in septic shock the transcapillary escape rate may be increased three- or four-fold, and they regard this as a major cause of hypoalbuminaemia. A further route of albumin loss is through the gut but, as discussed above, this is probably not very important in the absence of diarrhoea.

Protein intake and its effects on albumin metabolism cannot be considered in isolation from energy intake. There is quite impressive experimental support for the concept that a relatively high energy intake actually promotes the development of hypoalbuminaemia. Samonds and Hegsted (1978) fed a low protein diet to monkeys and found that an 'excessive' energy intake contributed to rather than protected against the development of hypoalbuminaemia, whereas restriction of energy intake prevented it. Graham *et al.* (1966) observed this process in reverse. In treating malnourished children they found that an energy intake that promoted rapid weight gain adversely affected serum albumin levels, whereas inadequate energy intakes favoured the synthesis of albumin. In rats albumin synthesis was less depressed by fasting than by low protein diets (Quartey-Papafio *et al.*, 1980).

The interrelationships of energy and protein intake were examined in more detail by Lunn and Austin (1983) in rats. They showed that on the same low protein intake the serum albumin concentration varied inversely with the energy intake, and that for hypoalbuminaemia to occur it was necessary for energy consumption to be greater than the rat's energy requirement.

The hypothesis developed in the 1970s, supported by animal experiments such as those of Coward and co-workers (1977), was that in the face of severe energy restriction insulin output decreases and that of corticosteroids increases (Chapter 9). These effects acting together lead to decreased synthesis and increased breakdown of muscle protein (Millward *et al.*, 1983), so that more amino acids become available for protein synthesis in the liver. In rats administration of cortisone increased the amount of liver protein and the albumin concentration, presumably at the expense of muscle (Lunn *et al.*, 1976).

On the other hand, according to the hypothesis, in the early stages of the development of hypoalbuminaemia, protein rather than energy is limiting; insulin levels are high and those of cortisol low—a pattern that promotes the uptake of amino acids into muscle at the expense of protein synthesis in the liver. We return to this subject in Chapter 11.

References

Ablett, J. G., McCance, R. A. (1971). Energy expenditure of children with kwashiorkor. *Lancet* **2:** 517–519.

Bhaskaram, P., Sivakumar, B. (1986). Interleukin-1 in malnutrition. *Archives of Disease in Childhood* **61:** 182–185.

Brenton, D. P., Brown, R. E., Wharton, B. A. (1967). Hypothermia in kwashiorkor. *Lancet* **1:** 410–413.

Brooke, O. G. (1972). Influence of malnutrition on the body temperature of children. *British Medical Journal* **1:** 331-333.

Brooke, O. G., Ashworth, A. (1972). The influence of malnutrition on the postprandial metabolic rate and respiratory quotient. *British Journal of Nutrition* **27:** 407–415.

Brooke, O. G., Cocks, T. (1974). Resting metabolism rate in malnourished babies in relation to total body potassium. *Acta Paediatrica Scandinavica* **63:** 817–825.

Butte, N. F. (1990). Basal metabolism of infants. In Schürch, B., Scrimshaw, N. S. (eds) *Activity, energy expenditure and energy requirements of young children.* Nestlé Foundation, Lausanne, pp. 117–138.

Cazeflis, C., Schütz, Y. *et al.* (1985). Whole body protein synthesis and energy expenditure in very low birth weight infants. *Pediatric Research* **19**: 679–687.

Clausen, T., van Hardefeld, C., Everts, M. E. (1991). The significance of cation transport in the control of energy metabolism and thermogenesis. *Physiological Reviews* **71**: 733–774.

Clugston, G. A., Garlick, P. J. (1982). The response of protein and energy metabolism to food intake in lean and obese man. *Human Nutrition: Clinical Nutrition* **36C**: 57–70.

Cohen, S., Hansen, J. D. L. (1962). Metabolism of albumin and γ-globulin in kwashiorkor. *Proceedings of the Nutrition Society of South Africa* **3**: 26–31.

Cohen, H., Metz, J., Hart, D. (1962). Protein-losing gastroenteropathy in kwashiorkor. *Lancet* **1**: 52 (letter).

Colley, C. M., Fleck, A. *et al.* (1983). Early time course of the acute-phase protein response in man. *Journal of Clinical Pathology* **36**: 203–207.

Coward, W. A., Whitehead, R. G., Lunn, P. G. (1977). Reasons why hypoalbuminaemia may or may not appear in protein-energy malnutrition. *British Journal of Nutrition* **38**: 115–126.

Dean, R. F. A., Whitehead, R. G. (1963). The metabolism of aromatic amino acids in kwashiorkor. *Lancet* **1**: 188–191.

Dinarello, C. A. (1984). Interleukin-1. *Review of Infectious Diseases* **6**: 51–95.

Dossetor, J. F. B., Whittle, H. C. (1975). Protein-losing enteropathy and malabsorption in acute measles enteritis. *British Medical Journal* **2**: 592–593.

Duggan, M. B., Alwar, J., Milner, R. D. G. (1986). The nutritional cost of measles in Africa. *Archives of Disease in Childhood* **61**: 61–66.

Eccles, M. P., Cole, T. J., Whitehead, R. G. (1989). Factors influencing sleeping metabolic rates in infants. *European Journal of Clinical Nutrition* **43**: 485–492.

Fleck, A. (1989). Clinical and nutritional aspects of changes in acute-phase proteins during inflammation. *Proceedings of the Nutrition Society* **48**: 347–354.

Fleck, A., Raines, G. *et al.* (1985). Increased vascular permeability: a major cause of hypoalbuminaemia in disease and injury. *Lancet* **1**: 781–783.

Garrow, J. S., Fletcher, K., Halliday, D. (1965). Body composition in severe infantile malnutrition. *Journal of Clinical Investigation* **44**: 417–425.

Golden, M. H. N. (1985). The consequences of protein deficiency in man and its relationship to the features of kwashiorkor. In Blaxter, K. L., Waterlow, J. C. (eds) *Nutritional adaptation in man*. John Libbey, London, pp. 169–188.

Golden, M. H. N., Waterlow, J. C., Picou, D. (1977*a*). Protein turnover, synthesis and breakdown before and after recovery from protein-energy malnutrition. *Clinical Science* **53**: 473–477.

Golden, M., Waterlow, J. C., Picou, D. (1977*b*). The relationship between dietary intake, weight change, nitrogen balance and protein turnover in man. *American Journal of Clinical Nutrition* **30**: 1345–1348.

Graham, G. G., Cordano, A., Baertl, J. M. (1966). Studies in infantile malnutrition. IV. The effect of protein and calorie intake on serum proteins. *American Journal of Clinical Nutrition* **18**: 11–15.

Grimble, R. F. (1989). Cytokines: their relevance to nutrition. *European Journal of Clinical Nutrition* **43**: 217–230.

Grimble, R. F. (1990). Nutrition and cytokine action. *Nutrition Research Reviews* **3**: 193–210.

Heine, W., Wutzke, K. D. *et al.* (1987). Evidence for colonic absorption of protein nitrogen in infants. *Acta Paediatrica Scandinavica* **76**: 741–744.

Holliday, M. A. (1978). Body composition and energy needs during growth. In Falkner, F., Tanner, J. M. (eds) *Human growth vol. 2: Postnatal growth*. Plenum Press, New York, pp. 117–139.

Jackson, A. A. (1989). Optimizing amino acid and protein supply in the newborn. *Proceedings of the Nutrition Society* **48**: 293–301.

Jackson, A. A. (1991). The glycine story. *European Journal of Clinical Nutrition* **45:** 59–66.
Jackson, A. A., Golden, M. H. N. *et al*. (1983). Whole body protein turnover and nitrogen balance in young children at intakes of protein and energy in the region of maintenance. *Human Nutrition: Clinical Nutrition* **37C:** 433–446.
Jackson, A. A., Doherty, J. *et al*. (1990). The effect of the level of dietary protein, carbohydrate and fat in urea kinetics in young children during rapid catch-up weight gain. *British Journal of Nutrition* **64:** 371–385.
James, W. P. T., Hay, A. M. (1968). Albumin metabolism: effect of the nutritional state and the dietary protein intake. *Journal of Clinical Investigation* **47:** 1958–1972.
Kerr, D. S., Stevens, M. C. G., Robinson, H. M. (1978*a*). Fasting metabolism in infants. I. Effect of severe undernutrition on energy and protein utilization. *Metabolism* **27:** 411–435.
Kerr, D. S., Stevens, M. C. G., Picou, D. I. (1978*b*). Fasting metabolism in infants. II. The effect of severe undernutrition and infusion of alanine on glucose production estimated with U-^{13}C-glucose. *Metabolism* **27:** 831–848.
Kushner, I. (1988). The acute phase response: an overview. *Methods in Enzymology* **163:** 373–383.
Liao, W. S., Jefferson, L. S., Taylor, J. M. (1986). Changes in plasma albumin concentration, synthesis rate and mRNA levels during acute inflammation. *American Journal of Physiology* **251:** C928–C934.
Lunn, P. G., Austin, S. (1983). Excess energy intake promotes the development of hypoalbuminaemia in rats fed on low protein diets. *British Journal of Nutrition* **49:** 9–16.
Lunn, P. G., Whitehead, R. G. *et al*. (1976). The effect of cortisone acetate on the course of development of experimental protein-energy malnutrition in rats. *British Journal of Nutrition* **36:** 537–550.
McNurlan, M. A., Fern, E. B., Garlick, P. J. (1982). Failure of leucine to stimulate protein synthesis *in vivo*. *Biochemical Journal* **204:** 831–838.
Metcoff, J., Frenk, S. *et al*. (1966). Cell composition and metabolism in kwashiorkor (severe protein-calorie malnutrition in children). *Medicine (Baltimore)* **45:** 365–390.
Millward, D. J. (1978). The regulation of muscle protein turnover in growth and development. *Biochemical Society Transactions* **6:** 494–499.
Millward, D. J., Odedra, B., Bates, P. C. (1983). The role of insulin, corticosterone and other factors in the acute recovery of muscle protein synthesis on refeeding food-deprived rats. *Biochemical Journal* **216:** 583–587.
Millward, D. J., Garlick, P. J. *et al*. (1976). The relative importance of muscle protein synthesis and breakdown in the regulation of muscle mass. *Biochemical Journal* **156:** 185–188.
Millward, D. J., Jackson, A. A. *et al*. (1989). Human amino acid and protein requirements: current dilemmas and uncertainties. *Nutrition Research Reviews* **2:** 109–132.
Mönckeberg, F., Beas, F. *et al*. (1964). Oxygen consumption in infant malnutrition. *Pediatrics* **33:** 554–561.
Montgomery, R. D. (1962). Changes in the basal metabolic rate of the malnourished infant and their relation to body composition. *Journal of Clinical Investigation* **41:** 1653-1663.
Nagabhushan, V. S., Narasinga Rao, B. S. (1978). Studies on 3-methylhistidine metabolism in children with protein-energy malnutrition. *American Journal of Clinical Nutrition* **31:** 1322–1327.
Nichols, B. L., Barnes, D. J. *et al*. (1968). Relation between total body and muscle respiratory rates in malnutrition. *Nature (London)* **217:** 475–476.
Pain, V. M., Clemens, M. J., Garlick, P. J. (1978). The effect of dietary protein deficiency on albumin synthesis and the concentration of active albumin messenger RNA in rat liver. *Biochemical Journal* **172:** 129–135.
Parra, A., Garza, C. *et al*. (1973). Changes in growth hormone, insulin and thyroxin

values and in energy metabolism of marasmic infants. *Journal of Pediatrics* **82:** 133–142.

Pencharz, P. B., Masson, M. *et al.* (1981). Total-body protein turnover in human premature neonates: effect of birth weight, intra-uterine nutritional status and diet. *Clinical Science* **61:** 207–215.

Picou, D., Phillips, M. (1972). Urea metabolism in malnourished and recovered children receiving a high or low protein diet. *American Journal of Clinical Nutrition* **25:** 1261–1266.

Picou, D., Taylor-Roberts, T. (1969). The measurement of total protein synthesis and catabolism and nitrogen turnover in infants in different nutritional states and receiving different amounts of dietary protein. *Clinical Science* **36:** 283–296.

Quartey-Papafio, P., Garlick, P. J., Pain, V. M. (1980). Effect of dietary protein on liver protein synthesis. *Biochemical Society Transactions* **8:** 357.

Quigley, E. M. M., Ross, I. N. *et al.* (1987). Reassessment of faecal α-1-antitrypsin excretion as screening test for protein loss. *Journal of Clinical Pathology* **40:** 61-66.

Rennie, M. J., Millward, D. J. (1983). Controversies in medicine: 3-methylhistidine excretion and the urinary 3-methylhistidine/creatinine ratio are poor indicators of skeletal muscle protein breakdown. *Clinical Science* **65:** 217–225.

Sakuma, K., Ohyama, T. *et al.* (1987). Low protein-high energy diet induces repressed transcription of albumin mRNA in rat liver. *Journal of Nutrition* **117:** 1141–1148.

Samonds, K. W., Hegsted, D. M. (1978). Protein deficiency and energy restriction in young cebus monkeys. *Proceedings of the National Academy of Sciences* **75:** 1600–1604.

Sarker, S. A., Wahed, M. A. *et al.* (1986). Persistent protein-losing enteropathy in post-measles diarrhoea. *Archives of Disease in Childhood* **61:** 731–743.

Shukry, A. S., Gabr, M. *et al.* (1965). Protein-losing gastroenteropathy in kwashiorkor. *Journal of Tropical Medicine and Hygiene* **68:** 269–271.

Spady, D. W., Payne, P. R. *et al.* (1976). Energy balance during recovery from malnutrition. *American Journal of Clinical Nutrition* **29:** 1073–1078.

Stephen, J. M. L., Waterlow, J. C. (1968). Effect of malnutrition on activity of two enzymes concerned with amino acid metabolism in human liver. *Lancet* **1:** 118–119.

Talbot, F. B. (1921). Severe infantile malnutrition: the energy metabolism with the report of a new series of cases. *American Journal of Diseases in Children* **22:** 358–370.

Tanaka, N., Kubo, K. *et al.* (1980). A pilot study on protein metabolism in the Papua New Guinea highlanders. *Journal of Nutrition Science and Vitaminology* **26:** 247–259.

Tomkins, A. M., Garlick, P. J. *et al.* (1983). The combined effects of infection and malnutrition on protein metabolism in children. *Clinical Science* **65:** 313–324.

Torres-Pinedo, R. (1976). Intestinal exfoliated cells in infant diarrhoea: changes in cell renewal and disaccharidase activities. In Elliott, K., Knight, J. (eds) *Acute diarrhoea in childhood.* CIBA Foundation Symposium No. 42. Elsevier, Amsterdam, pp. 193–204.

Varga, F. (1959). The respective effects of starvation and changed body composition on energy metabolism in malnourished infants. *Pediatrics* **23:** 1085–1090.

Walker, S. P., Golden, M. H. N. (1988). Growth in length of children recovering from severe malnutrition. *European Journal of Clinical Nutrition* **42:** 395–404.

Waterlow, J. C. (1984). Protein turnover with special reference to man. *Quarterly Journal of Experimental Physiology* **69:** 409–438.

Waterlow, J. C. (1986). Metabolic adaptation to low intakes of energy and protein. *Annual Reviews of Nutrition* **6:** 495–526.

Waterlow, J. C. (1990). Energy-sparing mechanisms: reductions in body mass, BMR and activity: their relative importance and priority in undernourished infants and children. In Schürch, B., Scrimshaw, N. S. (eds) *Activity, energy expenditure and energy requirements of infants and children*. Nestlé Foundation, Lausanne, pp. 239–252.

Waterlow, J. C., Millward, D. J. (1989). Energy cost of turnover of protein and other cellular constituents. In Wieser, W., Gnaiger, E. (eds) *Energy transformations in cells and organisms*. Thieme Verlag, Stuttgart, pp. 277–282.

Waterlow, J. C., Garlick, P. J., Millward, D. J. (1978). *Protein turnover in mammalian tissues and in the whole body*. North Holland Publishing Co., Amsterdam.

Weech, A. A. (1939). The significance of the albumin fraction of the serum. *Bulletin of the New York Academy of Medicine* 15: 63–91.

Weech, A. A., Ling, S. M. (1931). Nutritional edema. Observations on the relation of the serum proteins to the occurrence of edema and to the effect of certain inorganic salts. *Journal of Clinical Investigation* 10: 869–887.

Widdowson, E. M. (1968). The place of experimental animals in the study of human nutrition. In McCance, R. A., Widdowson, E. W. (eds) *Calorie deficiencies and protein deficiencies*. Churchill, London, pp. 225–236.

Yoshida, T., Metcoff, J. *et al.* (1967). Intermediary metabolites and adenine nucleotides in leukocytes of children with protein-calorie malnutrition. *Nature* 214: 525–526.

Young, V. R., Haverberg, L. N. *et al.* (1973). Potential use of 3-methylhistidine excretion as an index of progressive reduction in muscle catabolism during starvation. *Metabolism* 22: 1429–1441.

7

Biochemical measurements for the assessment of PEM

Introduction

This subject which nowadays attracts little interest was discussed in some detail by Waterlow and Alleyne (1971). Biochemical 'tests' or measurements on blood and urine which have been popular at various times have had several objectives:

i.   as early and sensitive indicators of the development of PEM;
ii. as indicators of severity and prognosis;
iii. as aids to distinguishing between kwashiorkor and marasmus;
iv. to provide information about underlying processes;
v.   for indirect assessment of food intake.

Often the purposes of a measurement fall into more than one category. Those of the first three, concerned with diagnosis and prognosis, are comparable to the measurements made in routine clinical biochemistry and it seems legitimate to apply the word 'tests' to them. Measurements of the fourth kind will be considered in relation to the metabolic disturbances discussed in other chapters. Under the fifth heading, urinary nitrogen excretion has been used to provide a measure of protein intake.

   In the days when it was generally supposed that kwashiorkor could be equated with protein deficiency and marasmus with energy deficiency, as typified by the book *Calorie deficiencies and protein deficiencies* (McCance and Widdowson, 1968), the third and fourth purposes that I have tried to distinguish are merged.

Early detection of PEM and the search for 'sensitive' tests

The underlying idea is that growth failure, the principal indicator of malnutrition in community surveys, is non-specific and perhaps insensitive. Repeated infections cause growth failure, but it is by no means certain that they do this simply by producing secondary malnutrition, through anorexia, malabsorption, etc. Therefore we need an independent test for 'subclinical' PEM, analogous to the measurements of vitamin concentrations in blood that have been used to detect subclinical vitamin deficiencies. Ideally, as Whitehead (1969) said about biochemical tests of subclinical protein deficiency—a very popular subject at that time: 'any abnormality must first be shown to have significance or potential significance in terms of essential bodily function'. Moreover, such tests, to be of any use, must be applied in the field; once clinical PEM becomes obvious, they are unnecessary for diagnosis.

Whitehead in Uganda and McLaren in Lebanon were the pioneers of this approach, which may be called biochemical epidemiology. The test that has been most widely used since the early days is plasma albumin concentration.

Plasma albumin

One would expect the measurement of plasma albumin to be useful in view of the sensitivity of albumin synthesis to amino acid supply (Chapter 6). Whitehead and co-workers in Uganda (1971) measured plasma albumin in children attending an outpatient clinic. Their results are shown in Table 7.1. They concluded that a value less than 3.0 g/dl should certainly be regarded as abnormal. In a later study they showed that periods of hypoalbuminaemia were closely associated with episodes of infection and emphasized the multifactorial causation of kwashiorkor (Frood *et al.*, 1971).

Table 7.1 Appearance of symptoms or signs of oedema[a] in children attending an outpatient clinic

Serum albumin (g/dl)	No. of cases	No. (%) with symptoms or signs
> 3.5	18	1 (6)
3.1–3.5	33	2 (6)
2.6–3.0	27	14 (52)
2.0–2.5	16	11 (60)
< 2.0	4	4 (100)

[a] Symptoms or signs: pitting oedema; moonface; history of 'swelling'
From Whitehead *et al.* (1971)

Other studies have not been so encouraging. In Central America albumin level showed no relation at all to nutritional status, but here the predominant form of malnutrition was deficit in linear growth rather than in weight for height (Viteri *et al.*, 1973).

In a large survey of one- to three-year old children in the Ivory Coast, albumin and a number of other potential indicators were measured (Pique *et al.*, 1982). The authors concluded that it was possible 'to identify a significant number of children who are apparently healthy but in fact are in a borderline state which exposes them to increased risk'. However, the sample had to be very large to achieve this result.

Other plasma proteins

The most sensitive test would be the one which, for any degree of malnutrition, as assessed clinically or by anthropometry, showed the greatest deviation from normal and the greatest increase on recovery. Having established this by studies on patients it would then in theory be possible to apply the results in the field.

McFarlane and co-workers in Nigeria were the first to suggest that transferrin provided 'the most accurate assessment of the true nutritional state and showed the largest changes in response to treatment' (Antia *et al.*, 1968; McFarlane *et al.*, 1969). Reeds and Laditan (1976) confirmed this conclusion. In their series there was quite a good correlation between transferrin level and weight for height which extended even to moderate degrees of weight deficit. An interesting example of the extension of a 'test' from the clinic to the field is the finding in Tanzania that serum transferrin levels in mothers at delivery were significantly related to the birth weight of the baby, whereas the albumin level showed no such relation (Malentlema and Eddy, 1972).

Other candidates as a more sensitive test than albumin were prealbumin (Ingenbleek *et al.*, 1972) and retinol-binding protein (transthyretin), which is linked to prealbumin as a carrier of vitamin A (Rees Smith *et al.*, 1973). Table 7.2 shows the levels of these proteins in the malnourished state as a percentage of those on recovery. There is little difference between the various proteins other than albumin. Ingenbleek *et al.* (1975) cautioned that the sensitivity of transferrin concentration to iron deficiency may limit its value as a measure of protein deficiency. All these proteins are synthesized in the liver, and the reason suggested for their being more sensitive than albumin is that they have shorter half-lives (Shetty *et al.*, 1979). Fibronectin, like transferrin, is a glycoprotein, but its shorter half-life does not apparently make its response more sensitive (Yoder *et al.*, 1987).

Table 7.2   Comparison of changes in different serum proteins in severe PEM

Protein	Initial concentration as % of concentration after recovery (3 weeks)
Albumin	54
Transferrin	29
Thyroxin-binding prealbumin	28
Retinol-binding protein	30

The reductions were reported to be greater in kwashiorkor than in marasmus.
From Ingenbleek *et al.* (1975)

Measures of severity and prognosis

If a test is used for clinical assessment the extent of deviation from normal should be related to severity, as judged independently by weight deficit, degree of oedema, etc., and finally by outcome—death or survival. McLaren *et al.* (1967) proposed a system of scoring, calculated according to weight for age, the degree of oedema and the plasma albumin concentration, but they did not report any relationship to outcome. Significant correlations were found by Reeds and Laditan (1976) between transferrin level and deficits in both weight for length and length for age.

Since muscle mass could be regarded as a more sensitive indicator than body weight of the overall extent of tissue depletion (Chapter 3), Viteri and Alvarado (1970) suggested that the creatinine height index would be a useful measure of the severity of PEM. This index is the 24-hour creatinine excretion of the subject compared with the 24-hour creatinine excretion of a normal child of the same height. The method is discussed in some detail in Alleyne *et al.* (1977). The idea is logical, but the disadvantage is that it needs a 24-hour urine collection.

In several studies the albumin level provided a good indication of prognosis. Montgomery (1963) in Jamaica reported a gradation of mortality rate with decreasing serum albumin. Mortality was 6 per cent at concentrations above 3 g/dl and 29 per cent when the serum albumin was 1.5 g/dl or less. For Viart (1977) in Zaïre a level of 1.5 g/dl represented a threshold, below which the mortality rate rose sharply. Hay *et al.* (1975) reported that in a series of some 400 children in Uganda there was a linear correlation between mortality and the logarithm of serum albumin concentration. By contrast, in a smaller series in Nigeria no difference in albumin level was found between children who died and those who survived, but there was a difference in serum transferrin (Reeds and Laditan, 1976). These authors concluded that 'it would seem appropriate to measure routinely the serum concentration of transferrin in all hospital cases of severe PEM'.

Other indicators of prognosis, which relate to particular causes of death, are hyponatraemia (Chapter 4) and raised serum concentrations of bilirubin and aminotransferases (Chapter 12).

Biochemical distinction between kwashiorkor and marasmus

Originally the underlying idea was that if kwashiorkor represents protein deficiency and marasmus energy deficiency, it might be possible by biochemical tests to distinguish which process was operating most strongly at an early stage, before the clinical characteristics became apparent. The levels of the plasma proteins discussed above were generally lower in kwashiorkor than marasmus, which seemed to confirm the basic hypothesis. In the early days a number of us attempted to extend this approach and to identify functional impairment of particular organs. It was suggested that organs with a high rate of protein turnover, such as liver and pancreas, would be most severely affected by protein deficiency. One might then expect to find decreases in the concentration in the blood of proteins produced in these organs, such as albumin and pseudocholinesterase in the liver and amylase in the pancreas. It might even be possible by this means to assess the degree of protein deficiency. Such was the hope; the results of these studies have been reported in previous reviews (Waterlow *et al.*, 1960; Waterlow and Alleyne, 1971). In fact, it was naïve to suppose that these changes in circulating proteins could provide a quantitative measure of protein deficiency, because there is no independent standard of protein depletion against which to assess them (Chapter 2).

Another difficulty with these measurements is that they are sensitive to interfering factors. Thus reductions in plasma albumin and β-lipoprotein were found to be closely associated with periods of infection (Truswell *et al.*, 1963; Frood *et al.*, 1971).

A complementary approach developed when amino acid analyses became available. Holt and co-workers (1963) arranged for blood samples from children with PEM to be collected in a number of countries and sent to New York for measurement of their amino acid profiles. The idea was that different clinical features, more prominent in some places than in others, might be associated with different specific amino acid deficiencies, which would be identified by the aminogram. In fact the picture was very uniform: reduced concentrations of the essential amino acids (E) and relatively high levels of the non-essentials (N). Whitehead and Dean (1964) devised a simple measurement on serum by paper chromatography that could be used in the field to give an estimate of the N/E ratio, based on representative amino acids of each group. Full details are given in Alleyne *et al.* (1977). The ratio was typically low in marasmus and high in kwashiorkor. However, a serious difficulty in applying this test was that, because of the high turnover rate of free amino acids in the plasma, the results are affected by recent food intake, which cannot easily be standardized in the field.

For these practical reasons, added to what seemed to be the demise of the protein deficiency theory of kwashiorkor (Chapter 11), there has been little interest in these biochemical tests in recent years. One exception, however, is the work of Schelp and co-workers, which is founded on a different idea.

Serum contains a number of proteins that are inhibitors of proteinases, such as α_1-anti-trypsin, α_1-anti-chymotrypsin and α_2-macroglobulin. The hypothesis was that muscle proteins are continuously being broken down to provide amino acids for essential organs. This is one of the body's homoeostatic mechanisms. The proteinase inhibitors tend to damp down this process, and an increase in their concentration would imply a breakdown of homoeostasis. In their first study Schelp *et al.* (1977) found increases in anti-chymotrypsin in children with oedema and hepatomegaly, but in a second paper (Schelp *et al.*, 1978) they reported much less clear-cut results. As with the acute phase proteins (Chapter 6), the synthesis of the proteinases is increased in response to infection.

Further development along the lines described in this chapter has also been limited by severely practical considerations. A basic objective was to find tests that could be applied in the field for the early diagnosis of PEM. Further experience, e.g. that of Pique *et al.* (1982) in the Ivory Coast, has shown that a large number of subjects is needed to establish any definite differences between 'normal' and 'malnourished' children. For such a study, even with simplified methods biochemical measurements greatly increase the work load, and the likelihood of obtaining useful information about individuals is not strong enough to justify taking blood samples from children in the community. These objections apply with much less force to urine samples.

Estimates of protein intake from the partition of urinary nitrogen

In children on a low protein intake urinary nitrogen excretion is low (Waterlow, 1963). Collection of 24-hour urine specimens is not practicable except in a metabolic ward, but much information can be gained from the proportions of different N compounds in a single specimen of urine. Reduction in total N is achieved almost entirely at the expense of urea, so that the ratio of urea N: total N may be as low as 50 per cent in children with PEM, compared with the normal of 80–90 per cent.

A more sensitive index is the ratio of urea N:creatinine. Table 7.3 shows results obtained by Simmons (1972) in Kenya in different tribal groups. This way of estimating protein intake is based on sound physiological principles and is being increasingly used in nutritional surveys (Bingham, 1987). Although there are diurnal fluctuations of urea production and plasma urea concentration in relation to intakes, they are damped by the large size of the urea pool, so that a rough and ready standardization of timing, by collecting urine in the morning before a meal, appears to be sufficient. The rate of creatinine excretion is very regular throughout the 24 hours, but it is important to achieve an adequate rate of urine flow. However, creatinine excretion will be reduced and the ratio of urea: creatinine increased if children are malnourished and have a low muscle mass (Chapter 3).

Table 7.3   Urea:creatinine ratio in urine from children in four rural areas of Kenya

Group	Protein intake (% of recommended intake)	Urea N/creatinine (mg/mg)
Controls	–	15.3
Masumbi	117	11.2
Nyasani	112	10.7
West Koguta	88	9.2
Uthiuni	77	6.6

Data of Simmons (1972).

Since measurements of both urea and creatinine are simple and can be done in any routine laboratory, this ratio seems to be an eminently practical way of assessing protein intake, at least for comparative purposes and particularly in communities with a fairly regular pattern of diet.

References

Alleyne, G. A. O., Hay, R. W. *et al.* (1977). *Protein-energy malnutrition.* Edward Arnold, London.
Antia, A. V., McFarlane, H., Soothill, J. F. (1968). Serum siderophilin in kwashiorkor. *Archives of Disease in Childhood* **43**: 459–462.
Bingham, S. (1987). The dietary assessment of individuals; methods, accuracy, new techniques and recommendations. *Nutrition Abstracts and Reviews* (Series A) **57**: 705–742.

Frood, J. D. L., Whitehead, R. G., Coward, W. A. (1971). Relationship between pattern of infection and development of hypoalbuminaemia and hypo-β-lipoproteinaemia in rural Ugandan children. *Lancet* **2**: 1047–1049.

Hay, R. W., Whitehead, R. G., Spicer, C. C. (1975). Serum albumin as a prognostic indicator in protein-calorie malnutrition. *Lancet* **2**: 427–429.

Holt, L. E., Snyderman, S. E. *et al.* (1963). The plasma aminogram in kwashiorkor. *Lancet* **2**: 1343–1348.

Ingenbleek, Y., De Visscher, M., De Nayer Ph. (1972). Measurement of prealbumin as index of protein-calorie malnutrition. *Lancet* **2**: 106–109.

Ingenbleek, Y., Van der Schrieke H-G. *et al.* (1975). Albumin, transferrin and the thyroxine-binding prealbumin/retinol-binding protein (TBPA-RBP) complex in assessment of malnutrition. *Clinica Chimica Acta* **63**: 61–67.

McCance, R. A., Widdowson, E. M. (eds) (1968). *Calorie deficiencies and protein deficiencies.* Churchill, London.

McFarlane, H., Ogbeide, M. I. *et al.* (1969). Biochemical assessment of protein-calorie malnutrition. *Lancet* **1**: 392–395.

McLaren, D. S., Pellett, P. L., Read, W. (1967). A simple scoring system for classifying the severe forms of protein-calorie malnutrition of early childhood. *Lancet* **1**: 533-535.

Malentlema, T. N., Eddy, T. P. (1972). Serum transferrin of pregnant mothers related to birth weight of their infants. *British Medical Journal* **3**: 386–387.

Montgomery, R. D. (1963). The relation of oedema to serum protein and pseudo-cholinesterase levels in the malnourished infant. *Archives of Disease in Childhood* **38**: 343–348.

Pique, G., Roy, C., Gateff, C. (1982). Étude de certains parametres biologiques dans les malnutritions protéino-caloriques subcliniques de l'enfant Ivorien. *Médicine Tropicale* **42**: 649–658.

Reeds, P. J., Laditan, A. O. (1976). Serum albumin and transferrin in protein-energy malnutrition. Their use in the assessment of marginal undernutrition and the prognosis of severe undernutrition. *British Journal of Nutrition* **36**: 255–263.

Rees Smith, F. B., Goodman, D. S. *et al.* (1973). Serum vitamin A, retinol-binding protein and prealbumin concentrations in protein-calorie malnutrition. I. A functional defect in hepatic retinol release. *American Journal of Clinical Nutrition* **26**: 973–981.

Schelp, F. P., Migasena, P. *et al.* (1977). Serum proteinase inhibitors and other serum proteins in protein-energy malnutrition. *British Journal of Nutrition* **38**: 31–38.

Schelp, F. P., Migasena, P. *et al.* (1978). Are proteinase inhibitors a factor for the derangement of homoeostasis in protein-energy malnutrition? *American Journal of Clinical Nutrition* **31**: 451–456.

Shetty, P. S., Watrasiewicz, K. E. *et al.* (1979). Rapid turnover transport proteins: an index of subclinical protein-energy malnutrition. *Lancet* **2**: 230–232.

Simmons, W. K. (1972). Urinary urea nitrogen/creatinine ratio as indicator of recent protein intake in field studies. *American Journal of Clinical Nutrition* **25**: 539–542.

Truswell, A. S., Hansen, J. D. L. *et al.* (1963). Serum proteins in infants with severe gastroenteritis. *South African Medical Journal* **37**: 527–534.

Viart, P. (1977). Haemodynamic findings in severe protein-calorie malnutrition. *American Journal of Clinical Nutrition* **30**: 334–348.

Viteri, F. E., Alvarado, J. (1970). The creatinine height index: its use in the estimation of the degree of protein depletion and repletion in protein-calorie malnourished children. *Pediatrics* **46**: 696–706.

Viteri, F. E., Mata, L. J., Béhar, M. (1973). Métodos de evaluacion del estado nutritionel proteino-calorico en pre-escolares de condiciones socio-economicas diferentes. *Archivos Latinoamericanos de Nutricion* **23**: 23–31.

Waterlow, J. C. (1963). The partition of nitrogen in the urine of malnourished infants. *American Journal of Clinical Nutrition* **12**: 235–240.

Waterlow, J. C., Alleyne, G. A. O. (1971). Protein malnutrition in children: advances in knowledge in the last ten years. *Advances in Protein Chemistry* **25**: 117–241.

Waterlow, J. C., Cravioto, J., Stephen, J. M. L. (1960). Protein malnutrition in man. *Advances in Protein Chemistry* **15**: 131–238.

Whitehead, R. G. (1969). The assessment of nutritional status in protein malnourished children. *Proceedings of the Nutrition Society* **28**: 1–16.

Whitehead, R. G., Dean, R. F. A. (1964). Serum amino acids in kwashiorkor: II. An abbreviated method of estimation and its application. *American Journal of Clinical Nutrition* **14**: 320–330.

Whitehead, R. G., Frood, J. D. L., Poskitt, E. M. E. (1971). Value of serum albumin measurements in nutritional surveys. *Lancet* **2**: 287–289.

Yoder, M. C., Anderson, D. C. *et al.* (1987). Comparison of serum fibronectin, prealbumin and albumin concentrations during nutritional repletion in protein-calorie malnourished infants. *Journal of Pediatrics, Gastroenterology and Nutrition* **6**: 84–88.

8

Endocrine changes in severe PEM

Introduction

Hormonal changes in severe malnutrition fall into two broad groups: those that reflect or determine short-term changes in metabolic pattern and those that influence the rate of growth. Although there is much overlap, insulin, growth hormone, glucagon and the corticosteroids fall broadly into the first group; thyroid hormones and the somatomedins into the second, together with a range of locally produced and locally acting polypeptide growth factors. Insulin plays a key role in anabolic reactions, often being permissive for the action of other hormones.

The net effects depend also on the amounts and activities of receptors in different tissues. In such a complex situation the account that follows is inevitably superficial; it can do little more than show that there are profound abnormalities, which may be interpreted in different ways, as distortions of metabolic pattern or as attempts at adaptation. One generalization can probably be made: that for growth to be restored the provision of food must be accompanied by an appropriate and co-ordinated response of the endocrine orchestra.

The changes in endocrine activity that have been found in severe PEM were reviewed in detail by Alleyne et al. (1977). Most of the results have been obtained in children in hospital; they are complemented by the unique prospective field studies of Whitehead and his colleagues in Uganda and The Gambia, which are of importance for understanding the development of PEM, and which have not received as much attention as they deserve.

It must also be remembered that all the measurements of hormones in malnourished children have been made on blood, but the blood level does not always reflect the activity of the hormone at its target site. This applies particularly to triiodothyronine (T_3) and somatomedin (SmC). Interpretation of plasma concentrations may also be affected by differences in the amount of binding protein, particularly with cortisol and T_3.

There are three questions of particular interest: (i) is the endocrine pattern different in kwashiorkor and marasmus? (ii) how are the changes in different hormones related? (iii) what information, if any, do they give us about mechanisms and pathogenesis? This last question is considered in Chapter 11.

Insulin and blood sugar

Many workers have described hypoglycaemia in children with PEM. Kerpel-Fronius and Kaiser (1967), writing about marasmus, give a vivid description of the clinical signs that should alert one to the danger. The commonest symptoms were 'deathly pallor' and apnoeic spells. Less common were hypothermia, rolling of the eyes and convulsions. The presence of symptoms was a sign of imminent death unless intravenous glucose was given immediately. Kerpel-Fronius showed a clear relationship between the fasting blood sugar and mortality but not with the degree of weight deficit (Table 8.1). The frequency of hypoglycaemia seems to vary from one region of the world to another; blood sugar concentrations below 2.2 mmol/l were found in 10 per cent of cases with severe PEM, mostly marasmic kwashiorkor, in Jamaica, compared with 24 per cent of children with kwashiorkor in Uganda. No consistent difference in blood sugar has been reported between kwashiorkor and marasmus.

Fasting plasma insulin levels are generally low in severe PEM, rising during recovery and peaking during the phase of rapid growth. In the five studies listed by Alleyne *et al.* (1977) there was no consistent difference between the fasting insulin levels in kwashiorkor and marasmus. During recovery glucagon followed the same pattern as insulin (Robinson and Seakins, 1982).

There is a subnormal insulin response to a glucose load (James and Coore, 1970; Hansen, 1975) or to stimulation with glucagon (Milner, 1971), which may persist for many months after recovery (James and Coore, 1970). Of interest is the finding by Pimstone *et al.* (1973) that the insulin response was significantly greater in children who received supplementary potassium than in those who were not supplemented.

As might be expected with a reduced insulin response, impaired glucose tolerance has been found in some studies, though not in all. The possibility of chromium deficiency aroused interest in the 1970s (see Alleyne *et al.*,

Table 8.1 Blood sugar and mortality rate in marasmus

	Mean blood glucose		Mortality (%)
	(mg/100 ml)	(mmol/l)	
'Dystrophy'	82	4.6	0
Marasmus, glucose > 50 mg/100 ml (> 2.8 mmol/l)	68	3.8	16.6
Marasmus, glucose < 50 mg/100 ml (< 2.8 mmol/l)	34	1.9	26.6
Marasmus with symptoms of hypoglycaemia	11	0.6	52

From Kerpel-Fronius and Kaiser (1967)

1977); in some cases, glucose tolerance was improved by the administration of small amounts of chromium (Chapter 9).

Insulin resistance may be a further factor contributing to glucose intolerance. The evidence has been summarized by Becker (1983). Possible causal factors are the raised concentrations of cortisol, growth hormone and free fatty acids that are characteristic in PEM. Recently Payne-Robinson *et al.* (1990) have shown reduced insulin binding by red cells of children with PEM, due to a reduction in the affinity of the binding sites rather than their number. This could perhaps result from the changes in the red cell membrane described in Chapter 10. It is not known whether there is reduced receptor affinity in other tissues. The binding of insulin by red cells increased rapidly with treatment.

The studies on clinic children in Uganda, where 'classical' kwashiorkor is the prevailing form of PEM, showed a beautiful parallelism between plasma concentrations of albumin and insulin (Whitehead *et al.*, 1973; Lunn *et al.*, 1973). In the light of recent work, summarized by Millward (1990), suggesting that protein is a more important stimulus for insulin production than carbohydrate, this relationship would make sense, if it is accepted that protein intake has anything to do with plasma albumin concentration (Chapter 11). In a later study on village children in The Gambia (Lunn *et al.*, 1979a), a remarkable correlation was found between plasma insulin concentration and rate of growth in length or height (Fig. 8.1). The parallel changes may, of

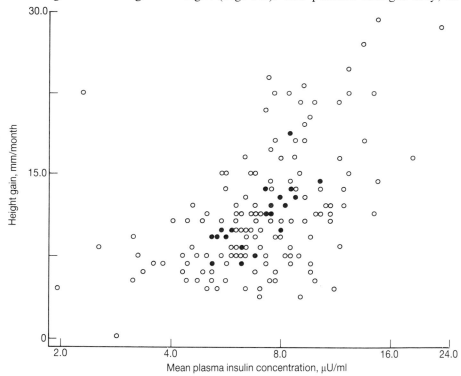

Fig. 8.1 Correlation between plasma insulin concentration and rate of growth in height in Gambian village children. Reproduced by permission from Lunn *et al.* (1979a). (●, two or more coincident points.)

course, be coincidental, unrelated effects of a single cause; however, there is a possible physiological explanation for the relationship, in that insulin stimulates the production of T_3 and SmC, which promote growth in muscle, cartilage and bone (Millward, 1990).

Insulin has an anabolic action on protein metabolism. It stimulates protein synthesis in the liver and in muscle and it appears to suppress protein breakdown (Pacy *et al.*, 1989). Low concentrations of insulin should therefore allow a greater liberation of amino acids from muscle, which would be available for protein synthesis in other tissues. This could be considered an adaptive change.

Glucocorticoids

Glucocorticoids are usually regarded as catabolic hormones. Their general action on protein metabolism is the opposite of that of insulin. In experiments on the rat glucocorticoids produced an increase in the synthesis of albumin, fibrinogen and transferrin in the liver (Jeejeebhoy *et al.*, 1973) and an increase in liver mass in animals on a low protein diet (Millward *et al.*, 1976). In muscle they inhibit protein synthesis; the mechanism has been discussed by Millward *et al.* (1983). The overall metabolic effect presumably depends, at least in part, on the balance between the two hormones insulin and cortisol. Thus the ratio of their levels in the plasma may be a useful index of metabolic state.

Glucocorticoid production, as judged by plasma concentrations, is increased in starvation and infection. From a teleological point of view this response should produce an increased supply of amino acids from muscle, which will provide on the one hand substrate for gluconeogenesis, on the other hand building blocks for protein synthesis in other more vital tissues, including that of acute phase proteins such as fibrinogen in the liver. This may be regarded as a favourable response in the short term; the end result is that described in Chapter 3 on body composition—a body in which muscle is much more depleted than the visceral tissues.

There is general agreement that plasma glucocorticoid levels, usually measured as cortisol, are raised in PEM. Becker (1983) discussed the very similar changes observed in anorexia nervosa and their relationship to the pituitary. Some authors have found that plasma cortisol was higher in marasmus than in kwashiorkor (Misra *et al.*, 1980) but reports in the literature are not consistent. In hospitalized children in Uganda there was a clear relationship between serum cortisol and both severity of infection on admission to hospital and degree of weight deficit (Fig. 8.2) (Lunn *et al.*, 1973).

In village studies in Uganda (Lunn *et al.*, 1973) cortisol levels rose as those of insulin and albumin fell. In individual children followed sequentially there was a reciprocal relationship between changes in cortisol and albumin. In The Gambia, where marasmus predominated, village children from the age of eight months tended to have higher cortisol and lower insulin levels than their counterparts in Uganda, where kwashiorkor was common (Whitehead *et al.*, 1977).

This exercise in what may be called hormonal epidemiology, comparing two different regions and sustained over several years, is unique and has not yet received the attention that it deserves.

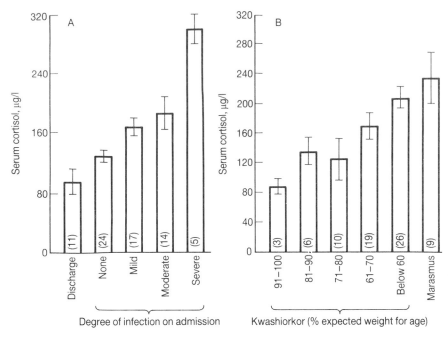

Fig. 8.2 Relationships between serum cortisol concentration and (A) degree of infection and (B) per cent of expected weight for age in children admitted to hospital with PEM in Uganda. Numbers of children in parentheses. Values are means with their standard errors. Reproduced by permission from Lunn *et al.* (1973).

Growth hormone

As Becker (1983) has pointed out, inadequate pituitary function was long thought to be the cause of growth failure in PEM, and it therefore came as a surprise when, with the availability of immunoassays, most authors reported high levels of growth hormone (GH) in malnourished children. Alleyne *et al.* (1977) tabulated the GH levels found in a number of studies in different countries. For the purpose of comparison between laboratories that may have differences in technique, in Table 8.2 the values found in the initial malnourished state are expressed as a ratio to the values in normal children or after recovery.

In both groups the GH concentrations are initially high, but on average the increase is almost three times greater in kwashiorkor than in marasmus. This is one of the rather rare cases in which there seems to be a fairly clear-cut distinction between the two syndromes. In kwashiorkor there was in most instances an adequate GH response to stimulation with arginine, whereas in marasmus this was less evident. One might speculate that the difference in GH levels between the two types of PEM arises from the probably greater duration of marasmus, leading to exhaustion of the pituitary. Mönckeberg *et al.* (1963) long ago described low plasma GH concentrations in nutritional dwarfs, infants who have hardly grown at all since birth but are of more or less normal weight for height, a clinical picture quite different from that of

Table 8.2 Elevation of fasting plasma growth hormone in children with PEM

	No. of studies	Ratio of initial: final concentration	
		Mean	Range
Kwashiorkor, weight for age > 60%	7	5.8	3.3–12
Marasmus, weight for age < 60%	4	2.1	0.5–3.6

Data from Alleyne *et al.* (1977)

marasmus, as the term is usually understood. Children with retarded growth as a result of psychosocial deprivation have low peak GH levels, which return to normal when the deprivation is corrected (Milner and King, 1985). By contrast, low birth-weight infants have high levels of GH (Becker, 1983) and in children with milder degrees of growth deficit plasma GH was inversely correlated with weight (Maung Maung Cho *et al.*, 1987).

In both marasmus and kwashiorkor a significant negative correlation has been found between plasma GH and albumin concentration (Pimstone *et al.*, 1968). Lunn *et al.* (1973) observed this also in Ugandan village children as hypoalbuminaemia developed. The relation cannot be causal, because with treatment GH levels return very rapidly to normal—in the series of Robinson and Seakins (1982) within seven days—long before albumin concentrations would have risen appreciably. Moreover, intravenous infusions of albumin had no effect on plasma GH (Hansen, 1975).

As a teleologist one seeks for a reason or function for the raised GH levels in malnutrition. A possible mechanism is that the rate of degradation of the hormone is decreased. It is degraded in the liver, whose function is more likely to be impaired in kwashiorkor than in marasmus (Chapter 5). This explanation remains a hypothesis, since the degradation rate of GH has not been measured in PEM. Another possibility is a process of negative feedback, by which low levels of somatomedin stimulate GH production. This would be a useful response when energy intake is low, because GH stimulates lipolysis and raises the concentration of circulating free fatty acids. It diminishes gluconeogenesis and so reduces the need for oxidation of amino acids.

Somatomedins

The somatomedins, also called insulin-like growth factors, are a group of polypeptide hormones which resemble insulin in structure and have insulin-like activity on protein and carbohydrate metabolism, as well as effects on growth. The physiology of the somatomedins and their behaviour in malnutrition and disease have been reviewed by Hall and Sara (1983) and Phillips and Unterman (1984). Root (1990) has summarized the effects of undernutrition on skeletal development and maturation. Daughady and Rotwein (1989) provide a review at the more molecular level.

Of this group of peptides, somatomedin-C (SmC) or insulin-like growth factor 1 (IGF-1) has the most direct effect on somatic growth. The circulating SmC in the plasma probably reflects synthesis in the liver under the influence of growth hormone (GH). Insulin promotes the production of SmC, perhaps by altering the binding potential of the hepatic GH receptors (Rappaport, 1988), while cortisol has an inhibitory effect (Unterman and Phillips, 1985).

Somatomedin-C is also synthesized locally in target tissues such as muscle and cartilage. Its activity in tissues is measured by the uptake of radioactive sulphate into proteoglycans of cartilage and connective tissues. Yahya *et al.* (1988) showed that in rats sulphate uptake into both muscle and bone was reduced to one-third of the initial rate after seven days on a low protein diet. However, the picture presented by the experimental work with protein deficient diets is not yet clear. First, large changes in the rate of tibial growth may occur with quite small changes in the concentration of SmC in the growth plate; secondly, and more important in the present context, the plasma SmC level does not reflect the concentration in the tissues. The data of Millward (1990) show that SmC concentrations in growth plate and skeletal muscle remained apparently unchanged over an almost ten-fold range of plasma SmC. Millward concluded: 'Changes in receptor number and sensitivity, associated with both stimulatory and inhibitory influences from other factors, mean that measurements of plasma hormone (SmC) concentrations provide at best a crude qualitative guide to their actual physiological role during growth'. A further problem in the interpretation of plasma levels is that the hormone is partially bound to carrier proteins.

In man all that we can measure is SmC in plasma, so the question is whether such measurements have any meaning or use. Plasma SmC is low at birth, gradually increases throughout childhood and rises sharply at puberty (Bala *et al.*, 1981; Hall and Sara, 1983). Table 8.3 shows plasma SmC in normal infants and children. There is clearly no direct relation between SmC concentration and the rate of growth—if anything the opposite. Bala concluded that possibly 'serum SM [somatomedin] concentrations may be reflecting the production of SM by various tissues, while tissue growth is primarily regulated by intracellular or local pericellular concentrations of SM'. The picture may be further complicated by the activity of somatomedin inhibitors.

In the light of these findings it is surprising that in practice plasma SmC levels reflect current nutritional state rather dramatically in both children and adults. Reductions in plasma SmC in PEM have been documented in a number of countries (Table 8.4). In most studies the initial levels were lower in kwashiorkor than marasmus, although in only one (Smith *et al.*, 1989) was the difference reported to be significant. As the table shows, in two studies there was a negative correlation with cortisol; in one only was there a positive correlation with insulin, although this relationship was shown very clearly by Millward (1990) in experiments with rats on a low protein diet.

Table 8.3   Effect of age on plasma somatomedin C (SmC) levels in normal children

Age (months)	SmC (U/ml)
4–6	0.175
7–12	0.288
13–18	0.289
19–24	0.598

Data of H. M. Payne-Robinson (personal communication)

Table 8.4 Changes in plasma somatomedin C in PEM

Reference	Country	Malnourished/recovered or malnourished/control (%)		Method
		Kwashiorkor	Marasmus	
Grant et al. (1973)	South Africa	50	–	Bioassay
Hintz et al. (1978)	Thailand		40	Bioassay
Mohan and Rao (1979)	India	63	89	Bioassay[1]
Smith et al. (1981)	Nigeria	22	10	Bioassay[2]
Soliman et al. (1986)	Egypt	34	35	RIA[a3]
Payne-Robinson et al. (1986)	Jamaica	46	65	RIA
Smith et al. (1989)	Nigeria*	56	70	RIA

* The actual values of SmC on admission were: oedematous 0.15 U/ml, marasmic 0.26 U/ml; $P < 0.05$
[a] Radioimmunoassay
Correlations: [1]positive with albumin; [2]negative with cortisol; [3] positive with albumin, insulin, but negative with cortisol, height deficit

A low plasma concentration of SmC is also seen in hospitalized adults with primary or secondary malnutrition and is coming to be regarded as a particularly sensitive indicator of nutritional state (Unterman *et al.*, 1985). In a study by Clemmons *et al.* (1985) the change of SmC during treatment was greater than that of other plasma proteins commonly used to monitor nutritional responses. In malnourished children the increase in SmC that occurred on a vegetable protein diet was regarded as good evidence that the treatment was effective (Smith *et al.*, 1989). In an elegant experiment on volunteers, Isley *et al.* (1983) tried to determine the relative importance of energy and protein in regulating the SmC concentrations. Their results (Fig. 8.3) show that after only five days of fasting SmC had fallen to about one-third of the initial level; energy appeared to be more effective than protein in restoring normal levels.

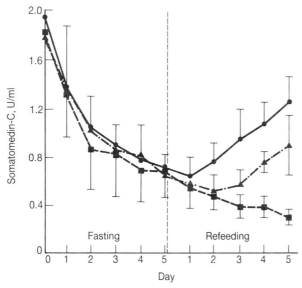

Fig. 8.3   Decrease of plasma somatomedin C in adult volunteers during a five-day fast and the effect of refeeding with different diets; ——●—— , normal diet; —·▲·—, low protein, isocaloric diet; ——■——, low protein, low energy diet. Reproduced by permission of the American Society for Clinical Investigation from Isley *et al.* (1983).

Knowledge of the somatomedins and their mode of action is expanding rapidly. The observations in malnourished children and adults cited above suggest that changes in SmC are reflecting the insulin-like activity rather than the growth-promoting effect of the hormone. It is not clear whether insulin is the prime mover, or whether SmC and insulin are operating synergistically. The scheme (Fig. 8.4) proposed by Rappaport (1988) postulated a relationship in series rather than in parallel, but it is likely that regulation differs in different tissues. In muscle it was insulin rather than SmC that was responsible for stimulating protein synthesis when protein-depleted rats were re-fed (Yahya *et al.*, 1988). More studies of this kind are needed which dissociate the effects of the two hormones.

Measurements made during recovery have indicated that the increase in plasma SmC is related more closely to the intake of energy than of protein

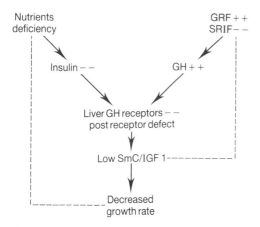

Fig. 8.4 Sequence of hormonal changes affecting growth that may occur as a result of malnutrition. Changes at the level of hepatic receptors for GH and inability to secrete adequate amounts of SmC play a central role. GH, growth hormone; GRF, growth hormone releasing factor; SRIF, somatostatin; SmC, somatomedin; IGF 1, plasma somatomedin. Reproduced by permission from Rappaport (1988).

(Fig. 8.3). If one believes in the 'protein deficiency' theory of kwashiorkor, it is then rather paradoxical that SmC levels should on the whole be lower in kwashiorkor than in marasmus.

The crucial question that remains is the relationship of these short-term nutritionally induced changes in SmC and other polypeptide factors to longer-term changes in growth and development. For example, there is evidence that SmC induces the development of oligodendrocytes in the brain (McMorris *et al.*, 1986), which are responsible for the synthesis of myelin. Is it possible that depression of SmC production plays a part in the impairment of mental development found in children who are stunted in linear growth (Chapter 19)?

Thyroid hormones

The last few years have seen important advances in our understanding of thyroid function in PEM, notably through the work of Ingenbleek and colleagues in Senegal (for review see Ingenbleek, 1986). Measurements of BMR, thyroidal iodine uptake and butanol-extractable iodine in the plasma had suggested that some degree of hypothyroidism is characteristic of PEM, but it is only more recently that sensitive radioimmunoassays have made possible accurate determination of bound and free hormone concentrations in blood.

Table 8.5 summarizes results from Senegal and Jamaica; the agreement is remarkable. The reduction in total T_4 is related to the low levels of the binding proteins. The changes in free T_4 (FT_4) are small. There are far greater decreases in both total and free T_3 and in the FT_3/FT_4 ratio, with an increase in reverse T_3 (rT_3), the inactive form of the hormone. T_3 is produced from T_4 by the enzyme 5'-monodeiodinase, The data suggest that the activity of this enzyme, which is a selenium-containing protein, is reduced and redirected towards the production of the inactive form rT_3. The iodinase activity has

Table 8.5 Thyroid hormone activity in children with PEM in Senegal and Jamaica in the malnourished state (M) and after recovery (R)

Thyroid hormone	Senegal[a]			Jamaica[b]		
	M	R	M/R, %	M	R	M/R, %
Total T_4, µg/dl	3.5	6.9	51	4.2	8.0	53
Free T_4, ng/dl	1.43	1.73	83	0.97	1.0	97
Total T_3, ng/dl	55	223	25	68	162	42
Free T_3, ng/dl	0.17	0.47	36	0.19	0.31	61
Free T_3/free T_4	0.12	0.27	44	0.20	0.31	64

[a] From Ingenbleek (1986); [b] From Robinson *et al.* (1985)

been shown to be affected by the carbohydrate content of the diet and by insulin.

In the Jamaican study at three stages of recovery the high energy feeding was interrupted for three days and the children returned to the maintenance diet which they had received initially. Thyroid hormone concentrations were measured at the beginning and end of each of these short periods. This made it possible to disentangle the short-term from the long-term effects of changes in food intake. Over these three-day periods on a low energy intake the FT_3/FT_4 ratio and the plasma insulin concentration both showed a significant fall. Thus the immediately preceding diet may have made some contribution to the low FT_3 levels found in PEM, but it is probably not the only factor, because both in Senegal and Jamaica it took two weeks of treatment before FT_3 reached the levels characteristic of recovery. It therefore becomes reasonable to regard the reduction in thyroid activity as an adaptation to malnutrition.

In hypothyroidism in the absence of malnutrition the concentration of thyroid-stimulating hormone (TSH) in plasma is increased, but the evidence summarized by Becker (1983) shows that in PEM, as in anorexia nervosa and secondary malnutrition, TSH levels are either normal or low. This implies some impairment of the feedback mechanism by which a low level of T_3 stimulates the production of TSH. The capacity of the pituitary to secrete TSH is maintained, since the thyroid-releasing hormone (TRH) evokes a normal or even increased production of TSH. It is therefore concluded that the major effect of malnutrition on thyroid function is at the peripheral level.

In hypothyroidism the rates of basal metabolism, whole-body protein turnover and ion pumping are all reduced. Experimentally, T_3 has a profound effect on muscle protein synthesis (Jepson *et al.*, 1988). Thyroidectomy caused a greater depression of protein synthesis in fast than in slow muscles (Brown and Millward, 1983). In hypothyroidism there appears to be a decrease in the proportion and size of fast muscle fibres, which use more energy per unit of force developed than the slow ones. There would therefore be an advantage in the selective preservation of slow fibres. All these phenomena taken together suggest that reduction in thyroid activity could be an important mechanism of adaptation to low energy intakes (Waterlow, 1986, 1990).

Such an adaptation, however, may possibly carry a serious cost. There is increasing evidence of impaired mental function in apparently normal children living in iodine-deficient areas (Hetzel, 1988). Iodine deficiency operates through reducing the production of thyroid hormones and their concentration in the brain. It would be logical to expect the same end result in children with PEM, even though the cause of the hypothyroidism may be different. At present this hypothesis is speculative. Wolter *et al.* (1979) reported that children who became hypothyroid between one and 12 months of age were usually not mentally retarded. Nevertheless, the possibility remains that depression of thyroid activity may play some part in the impairment of mental development of children with PEM (Chapter 19).

References

Alleyne, G. A. O., Hay, R. W. *et al.* (1977). *Protein-energy malnutrition*. Edward Arnold, London.

Bala, R. M., Lopatka, J. *et al.* (1981). Serum immunoreactive somatomedin levels in normal adults, pregnant women at term, children at various ages and children with constitutionally delayed growth. *Journal of Clinical Endocrinology and Metabolism* **52**: 508–512.

Becker, D. J. (1983). The endocrine responses to protein calorie malnutrition. *Annual Review of Nutrition* **3**: 187–212.

Brown, J. G., Millward, D. J. (1983). Dose response of protein turnover in rat skeletal muscle to triiodothyronin treatment. *Biochemica Biophysica Acta* **757**: 182–190.

Clemmons, D. R., Underwood, L. E. *et al.* (1985). Use of plasma somatomedin C/ insulin-like growth factor I. Measurements to monitor the response to nutritional repletion in malnourished patients. *American Journal of Clinical Nutrition* **41**: 191–198.

Daughady, W. H., Rotwein, P. (1989). Insulin-like growth factors I and II. Peptide, messenger ribonucleic acid and gene structures, serum and tissue concentrations. *Endocrine Reviews* **10**: 68–91.

Grant, D. B., Hambley, J. *et al.* (1973). Reduced sulphation factor in undernourished children. *Archives of Disease in Childhood* **48**: 596–600.

Hall, K., Sara, V. R. (1983). Growth and somatomedins. *Vitamins and Hormones* **40**: 175–233.

Hansen, J. D. L. (1975). Endocrines and malnutrition. In Olson, R. E. (ed) *Protein-calorie malnutrition*. Academic Press, New York, pp. 229–241.

Hetzel, B. S. (1988). *The prevention and control of iodine deficiency disorders*. Sub-committee on Nutrition: Nutrition Policy Discussion Paper No. 3. ACC/SCN, WHO, Geneva.

Hintz, R. L., Suskind, R. *et al.* (1978). Plasma somatomedin and growth hormone values in children with protein-calorie malnutrition. *Journal of Pediatrics* **92**: 153–156.

Ingenbleek, Y. (1986). Thyroid dysfunction in protein-calorie malnutrition. *Nutrition Reviews* **44**: 253–263.

Isley, W. L., Underwood, L. E., Clemmons, D. R. (1983). Dietary components that regulate serum somatomedin-C concentrations in humans. *Journal of Clinical Investigation* **71**: 175–182.

James, W. P. T., Coore, H. G. (1970). Persistent impairment of insulin secretion and glucose tolerance after malnutrition. *American Journal of Clinical Nutrition* **23**: 386–389.

Jeejeebhoy, K. N., Bruce-Robertson, A. *et al.* (1973). In *Protein turnover*. CIBA Foundation Symposium No. 9. Elsevier, Amsterdam, pp. 217–247.

Jepson, M. M., Bates, P. C., Millward, D. J. (1988). The role of insulin and thyroid hormones in the regulation of muscle growth and protein turnover in response to dietary protein in the rat. *British Journal of Nutrition* **59**: 397–415.

Kerpel-Fronius, E., Kaiser, E. (1967). Hypoglycaemia in infantile malnutrition. *Acta Paediatrica Scandinavica* Suppl. 172.

Lunn, P. G., Whitehead, R. G. *et al.* (1973). Progressive changes in serum cortisol, insulin and growth hormone concentrations and their relationship to the distorted amino acid pattern during the development of kwashiorkor. *British Journal of Nutrition* **29**: 399–422.

Lunn, P. G., Whitehead, R. G. *et al.* (1979a). The relationship between hormonal balance and growth in malnourished children and rats. *British Journal of Nutrition* **41**: 73–84.

Lunn, P. G., Whitehead, R. G., Coward, W. A. (1979b). Two pathways to kwashiorkor? *Transactions of the Royal Society of Tropical Medicine and Hygiene* **73**: 438–443.

McMorris, F. A., Smith, T. M. *et al.* (1986). Insulin-like growth factor I/somatomedin C: a potent inducer of oligodendrocyte development. *Proceedings of the National Academy of Sciences USA* **83**: 822–826.

Maung Maung Cho, Pyone Myint Han, Myo Thein (1987). Comparison of human growth hormone levels in children with satisfactory and unsatisfactory growth. *Human Nutrition:Clinical Nutrition* **41C**: 209–214.

Millward, D. J. (1990). The hormonal control of protein turnover. *Clinical Nutrition* **9**: 115–126.

Millward, D. J., Nnanyelugo, D. O. *et al.* (1976). Muscle and liver protein metabolism in rats treated with glucocorticoids. *Proceedings of the Nutrition Society* **35**: 47A.

Millward, D. J., Odedra, B., Bates, P. C. (1983). The role of insulin, corticosterone and other factors in the acute recovery of muscle protein synthesis on refeeding food-deprived rats. *Biochemical Journal* **216**: 583–587.

Milner, R. D. G. (1971). Metabolic and hormonal responses to glucose and glucagon in patients with infantile malnutrition. *Pediatric Research* **5**: 33–39.

Milner, R. D. G., King, J. M. (1986). Growth hormone. In Meadow, R. (ed) *Recent advances in paediatrics*, 8. Churchill Livingstone, London, pp. 33–49.

Misra, P. K., Agrawed, C. G. *et al.* (1980). Plasma cortisol, immunoreactive insulin and oral glucose tolerance in protein-calorie malnutrition. *Indian Pediatrics* **17**: 411–415.

Mohan, P. S., Jaya Rao, K. S. (1979). Plasma somatomedin activity in protein-calorie malnutrition. *Archives of Disease in Childhood* **54**: 62–64.

Mönckeberg, F., Donoso, G. *et al.* (1963). Human growth hormone in malnutrition. *Pediatrics* **31**: 58–64.

Pacy, P. J., Nair, K. S. *et al.* (1989). Failure of insulin infusion to stimulate fractional muscle protein synthesis in type 1 diabetic patients: anabolic effect of insulin and decreased proteolysis. *Diabetes* **38**: 618–624.

Payne-Robinson, H. M., Smith, I. F., Golden, M. H. N. (1986). Plasma somatomedin-C in Jamaican children recovering from severe malnutrition. *Clinical Research* **34**: 866A.

Payne-Robinson, H. M., Coore, H. G. *et al.* (1990). Changes in red cell insulin receptors during recovery from severe malnutrition. *European Journal of Clinical Nutrition* **44**: 803–812.

Phillips, L. S., Unterman, T. G. (1984). Somatomedin activity in disorders of nutrition and metabolism. *Clinics in Endocrinology and Metabolism* **13**: 145–189.

Pimstone, B. L., Barbazat, G. *et al.* (1968). Studies on growth-hormone secretion in protein-calorie malnutrition. *American Journal of Clinical Nutrition* **21**: 482–487.

Pimstone, B. L., Becker, B. *et al.* (1973). Insulin secretion in protein-calorie malnutrition. In Gardner, L. I., Amacher, P. (eds) *Endocrine aspects of malnutrition*. Kroc Foundation, Santa Ynez, California, pp. 289–302.

Rappaport, R. (1988). Endocrine control of growth. In Waterlow, J. C. (ed) *Linear growth retardation in less developed countries*. Nestlé, Vevey/Raven Press, New York, pp. 109–126.

Robinson, H. M. P., Seakins, A. (1982). Fasting pancreatic glucagon in Jamaican children during malnutrition and subsequent recovery. *Pediatric Research* **16**: 1011–1015.

Robinson, H. M. P., Betton, H., Jackson, A. A. (1985). Free and total triiodothyronine and thyroxine in malnourished Jamaican infants. *Human Nutrition: Clinical Nutrition* **39C**: 245–257.

Root, A. W. (1990). Effects of undernutrition on skeletal development, maturation and growth. In Simmons, D. J. (ed) *Nutrition and bone development*. Oxford University Press, pp. 115–130.

Smith, I. F., Latham, M. C. *et al.* (1981). Blood plasma levels of cortisol, insulin, growth hormone and somatomedin in children with marasmus, kwashiorkor and intermediate forms of protein-energy malnutrition. *Proceedings of the Society of Experimental and Biological Medicine* **167**: 607–611.

Smith, I. F. Taiwo, O., Payne-Robinson, H. M. (1989). Plasma somatomedin-C in Nigerian malnourished children fed a vegetable protein rehabilitation diet. *European Journal of Clinical Nutrition* **43**: 705–713.

Soliman, A. T., Hassan, A. H. I. *et al.* (1986). Serum insulin-like growth factors I and II concentrations and growth hormone and insulin responses to arginine infusion in children with protein-energy malnutrition before and after nutritional rehabilitation. *Pediatric Research* **20**: 1122–1130.

Unterman, T. G., Phillips, L. S. (1985). Glucocorticoid effects of somatomedins and somatomedin inhibitors. *Journal of Clinical Endocrinology and Metabolism* **61**: 618–626.

Unterman, T. G., Vasquez, R. M. *et al.* (1985). Nutrition and somatomedin. XIII. Usefulness of somatomedin-C in nutritional assessment. *American Journal of Medicine* **78**: 228–234.

Waterlow, J. C. (1986). Metabolic adaptation to low intakes of energy and protein. *Annual Review of Nutrition* **6**: 495–526.

Waterlow, J. C. (1990). Mechanisms of adaptation to low energy intakes. In Harrison, G. A., Waterlow, J. C. (eds) *Diet and disease in traditional and developing societies*. Cambridge University Press, pp. 5–23.

Whitehead, R. G., Coward, W. A., Lunn, P. G. (1973). Serum albumin concentration and the onset of kwashiorkor. *Lancet* **1**: 63–66.

Whitehead, R. G., Coward, W. A. *et al.* (1977). A comparison of the pathogenesis of protein-energy malnutrition in Uganda and The Gambia. *Transactions of the Royal Society of Tropical Medicine and Hygiene* **71**: 189–195.

Wolter, R., Noel, P. *et al.* (1979). Neuropsychological study in treated thyroid dysgenesis. *Acta Paediatrica Scandinavica* Suppl. **277**: 41–46.

Yahya, Z. A. H., Bates, P. C. *et al.* (1988). IgF-1 concentrations in protein deficient rat plasma and tissues in relation to protein and proteoglycan synthesis rates. *Biochemical Society Transactions* **16**: 624–625.

9

Trace elements

Introduction

In the last decade there has been a great upsurge of interest in trace element metabolism and deficiencies in man, no doubt in part because instruments for measuring these elements have become more widely available. The reviews of Golden (1982), Golden *et al.* (1985) and Prasad (1988) among many others provide general accounts. Cousins (1985) concentrates on the metabolism of zinc and copper. Casey and Walravens (1988) and Lönnerdal (1989) focus on infants. The trace elements that are known to be essential for man are zinc, copper, manganese, chromium, selenium, molybdenum and iodine. There are a further 11 referred to as 'ultratrace' elements where the evidence that they are essential is much more equivocal (Nielsen, 1988).

Most of the trace elements are essential constituents of all living tissues, but some of them have specific functions as well. Golden's distinction between specific deficiency with decreased tissue concentration (type I) and depletion with normal tissue concentration (type II) has already been referred to (Chapter 2). Of the trace elements, he puts copper (Cu), selenium (Se), manganese (Mn) and iodine (I) in the first category and zinc (Zn) in the second. All these elements, like iron, which can hardly be called a trace element, are components of enzymes. Some of them are also bound to specific proteins, either for storage or for transport or for both, e.g. Cu in caeruloplasmin and Cu and Zn in metallothionein.

Because all foodstuffs based on plant or animal cells contain trace elements in greater or lesser amounts, it has been difficult to establish the effects of deficiency of a specific element. An artificial situation which avoids this problem is that of total parenteral nutrition (TPN). Trace elements for which deficiencies have been established in patients on TPN include selenium, molybdenum (Rajagopalan, 1988) and chromium (Offenbacher and Pi-Sunyer, 1988). Infants and young children may be particularly at risk, because of their increased need for these elements during rapid growth.

Zinc

Effects of zinc deficiency

The prime example of severe zinc deficiency is the condition acrodermatitis enteropathica, caused by congenital impairment of the capacity to absorb Zn (Moynahan, 1974). The main clinical features, which it shares with severe PEM, are anorexia, stunted growth, severe skin lesions and intractable diarrhoea. The differential diagnosis may be difficult when the disease occurs in a region where PEM is common (James *et al.*, 1969).

In early studies in Egypt and South Africa on trace elements in PEM plasma Zn concentrations were found to be half those of recovered children or controls (Sandstead *et al.*, 1965; Hansen and Lehmann, 1969). Hansen reported that 'the only correlation we could find of serum Zn levels with specific symptoms or signs was a possible link with ulcerative skin lesions' and drew attention to the long-standing belief than Zn has an effect on wound-healing. He did, however, also find a correlation with serum albumin. This may be only an association, but a possible explanation could be that albumin acts as a carrier protein for the transport of zinc. Golden and Golden (1979) in Jamaica found low plasma Zn levels in oedematous PEM, but not in marasmus. There was no correlation with the degree of oedema nor, in contrast to Hansen, with plasma albumin concentration. Like Hansen, the Goldens observed a close association between low plasma Zn and ulcerative skin lesions, which responded rapidly to topical application of Zn salts (Golden *et al.*, 1980).

It seems that Zn is particularly important for cell multiplication in the epidermis and intestinal epithelium, which is not surprising since it is an essential component of enzymes involved in protein and RNA synthesis. This function of Zn probably contributes to the atrophy of the thymus and impairment of cell-mediated immunity that are characteristic of severe PEM (Fraker *et al.*, 1986) (Chapter 17). In an elegant experiment it was shown that when *Candida* antigen was injected intradermally in both arms of a child with PEM, and Zn applied topically to one arm only, there was a much larger reaction on the treated than on the other arm (Golden *et al.*, 1978). The general relationships of Zn deficiency to immune function have been reviewed by Keen and Gershwin (1990). It has also been found that Zn deficiency was associated with reduced activity of Na^+-K^+-ATPase in leucocytes (Patrick *et al.*, 1980).

Whereas these effects on skin, immune system and perhaps gut may be regarded as specific effects of deficiency, as defined in Chapter 2, a child with PEM is also Zn-depleted. Golden and Golden (1981*a*) showed that in children recovering from PEM and growing very rapidly, plasma Zn levels fell unless Zn supplements were given. Presumably this was because, in the absence of Zn stores, circulating Zn was being taken up into newly formed tissue. Figure 9.1 illustrates how weight gain may be limited by a diet containing an inadequate amount of available Zn. The limitation may be more serious than it seems from the weight curve because measurements of body composition showed that on a low Zn intake the tissue laid down contained an excess of fat. Growth in lean tissue cannot occur unless all the constituents of cells are

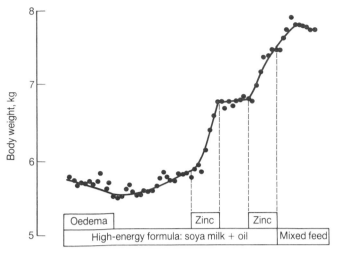

Fig. 9.1 Effect of a zinc supplement (2 mg Zn/kg/day as Zn acetate) on weight gain of a ten-month old child recovering from PEM on a soya-milk formula. Reproduced by permission from Golden and Golden (1981*b*).

provided. It has also been reported from Bangladesh that Zn supplements improved weight gain during the rehabilitation of children with PEM (Simmer *et al.*, 1988).

There is conflict of opinion about the importance of Zn deficiency among the many factors that contribute to the development of PEM. Sandstead (1975) considered that it was likely to be the rule rather than the exception, whereas Golden believes that 'in the hierarchy of deficiencies found in developing countries many other nutrients and energy are likely to become limiting before Zn' (Golden *et al.*, 1985).

The main effects of less severe Zn deficiency are loss of appetite and growth failure. In 1961 Prasad *et al.* described a syndrome of dwarfing with hypogonadism, mental apathy and skin changes in older children and adolescents in the Middle East, which they claimed to be the result of Zn deficiency, but the results of trials with Zn supplements were rather equivocal (Golden and Golden, 1985*a*). Hambidge's group in Colorado have produced evidence of Zn deficiency even in the United States. Zinc supplements given for a year to the children of poor Mexican immigrants resulted in a significant increase in height growth compared with controls (Walravens *et al.*, 1983). The supplemented children also had better appetites and larger food intakes. These findings clearly have a bearing on the cause of stunting in Third World children (Chapter 13).

There is much discussion at the present time about the prevalence of marginal Zn deficiency. The outcome must depend on better methods of diagnosis.

Diagnosis of zinc deficiency

Golden (1988), on the basis of extensive experience in Jamaica, considers that in established PEM the plasma Zn concentration is probably the best available indicator of Zn status, because it reflects the adequacy of supply in relation to demand. However, this measure is evidently not sensitive in marginal deficiency states. Great sensitivity has been claimed for the concentration of Zn in leucocytes, although it is much more difficult to measure. Thus Meadows *et al.* (1981) found a close correlation between the Zn concentration in maternal leucocytes and in muscle taken at Caesarean section. These concentrations were significantly lower in mothers of small-for-dates babies than in controls, whereas there was no difference in maternal plasma Zn levels. Golden (1988), however, argues that as with protein, a true deficit in tissue Zn, including that in leucocytes, can only be established when it is related to DNA (Chapter 2).

Hopes that the Zn content of hair would be useful for diagnosis at the community level have not been realized, because the values cover a very wide range (Dorea and Paine, 1985). Recently it has been suggested that a useful diagnostic measure would be the red cell content of the protein metallothionein, which contains both Zn and Cu. In experimental subjects on low Zn intakes there was a substantial fall in red cell metallothionein within eight days and a several-fold increase with Zn supplements (Grider *et al.*, 1990). Unfortunately from the diagnostic point of view, the results may be influenced by the presence of infections, since the cytokines interleukin-1 and -6 that are produced in response to infection stimulate the synthesis of metallothionein (Cousins and Leinart, 1988; Shroeder and Cousins, 1990).

Causes of zinc deficiency

Most authors have found that the Zn content of breast milk falls as lactation progresses, the concentration at six months being about half that at one month (Vuori and Kuitunen, 1979; Krebs *et al.*, 1985; Lönnerdal, 1989). The values found by Lehti (1990) in Amazonia are quite close to those of Vuori in Finland. On the other hand Bates and Tsuchiya (1990) found that at comparable stages of lactation the Zn concentration in the milk of Gambian women was twice as high as in that of mothers in Cambridge, UK.

Zinc intake becomes low at a time when there is still a considerable demand for growth. Weaning, therefore, is a critical period. The Zn in breast milk is particularly well absorbed, but in the foods given at weaning both the content and the bio-availability of Zn are likely to be low. Phytate and fibre in mainly vegetable diets can impair the absorption of Zn, although their effect seems to be quite variable (Solomons, 1982; Fairweather-Tait, 1988). Iron and copper may also inhibit Zn absorption.

Some balance studies have been made of Zn absorption in children recovering from PEM (B. Golden and M. Golden, unpublished). To obtain net absorption from the food, endogenously secreted Zn was measured with the stable isotope ^{70}Zn. Control children absorbed about 15 per cent of their Zn intake, children with PEM much less, particularly those with oedema. Hypoalbuminaemia has been found to reduce Zn absorption (Cousins, 1985).

Infections may also contribute to Zn deficiency, because it has long been known that the loss of nitrogen from the body is accompanied by a loss of Zn, supposed to be derived from muscle. The plasma Zn concentration falls as part of the acute phase response (Chapter 17), and it has been suggested that this reflects the increased synthesis of metallothionein mentioned above

(Cousins, 1985). Diarrhoea probably also causes losses of Zn, although Golden and Golden (1985b) were not able to substantiate this. In a controlled trial in Bangladesh Behrens *et al.* (1990) showed that children with diarrhoea who received a supplement of 15 mg Zn acetate per day had significantly greater gains in height and weight in the following nine weeks than unsupplemented children.

For all these reasons children with PEM are very likely to be deficient in Zn, and it is essential that during treatment the intake should be adequate to match the demands of rapid growth (Chapter 12).

Copper

As long ago as 1964 Cordano *et al.*, working in Peru, reported that children recovering from malnutrition on a milk-based diet low in Cu developed an anaemia which was not responsive to iron, with low plasma levels of Cu and of the Cu-containing protein caeruloplasmin. In some children there was osteoporosis and pathological fractures resembling those of scurvy, which responded to Cu supplements. These skeletal lesions, which as far as we know have not been described elsewhere, could be explained by the fact that Cu is essential for the formation of cross-linkages in collagen and elastin (O'Dell, 1981; Danks, 1988).

The group in Peru considered that about one-third of their children with PEM were deficient in Cu. This is to be expected, since the causes are much the same as those of Zn deficiency. In fact, the position could be worse for Cu. Both Zn and iron inhibit the absorption of Cu (Bremner and Mills, 1981), and although this inhibition is reciprocal, if there is competition for binding sites on the enterocyte Cu is likely to come off badly, since its concentration in foods is much lower.

Hansen and Lehmann (1969) found low plasma Cu levels in PEM, the values in marasmus being about 50 per cent higher than in kwashiorkor, but still well below control levels. They pointed out that the concentrations of Cu were much more variable than those of Zn, and they could not establish a relationship between plasma Cu and any of the features of PEM except perhaps the skin lesions. Although they had demonstrated a reduced Cu content in the liver in PEM, other tissues had not been examined, and Hansen and Lehmann concluded 'should future work show that there is in fact significantly less copper in the tissues of cases of PEM we are still left wondering whether this has any relation to the clinical state of the patient'.

There has only been a modest advance in knowledge since then. Golden (1982) has stated that their experience in Jamaica supported the findings in Peru. Plasma concentrations of Cu were reduced in children with oedematous malnutrition but not in those with marasmus (Golden and Golden, 1984). However, there is still a problem in assessing how far these changes really reflect Cu status. In plasma 90 to 95 per cent of Cu is in the bound form as caeruloplasmin. This protein is one of the acute phase proteins secreted by the liver in response to infection or stress (Chapter 17) so that the plasma concentration of Cu increases. Metallothionein, another acute phase protein, contains Cu as well as Zn (Bremner and Beattie, 1990). In the case of both these proteins, infection masks the effects of deficiency.

Another approach to the problem of assessment is to measure the activity in erythrocytes of the Cu-containing enzyme superoxide-dismutase (SOD), which has a role in the scavenging of free radicals (Chapter 10). Bennett *et al.* (1985) found that nearly 50 per cent of children with PEM had SOD levels on admission below the lower limit of Jamaican controls. In children who were given supplementary Cu during recovery, there was no increase in erythrocyte SOD from the initial values, and in unsupplemented children there was a fall. In a study in Chile children who had recovered from PEM still had low plasma concentrations of Cu, caeruloplasmin and SOD, which were restored to normal by Cu supplements (Uauy *et al.*, 1985). In these children SOD correlated well with plasma Cu.

The extent and functional significance of Cu deficiency in PEM are still not very clear. However, it can be concluded that, as with Zn, during rapid growth enough Cu must be available for the formation of new tissue. Since milk, which is the basis of most feeding regimes, is low in Cu a supplement should be given as routine during this phase of treatment.

Selenium

Selenium deficiency has long been recognized in cattle and sheep grazing on pastures where the soil is deficient in Se, but it was not until the late 1970s that deficiency of this trace element was identified as the cause of disease in man: a fatal cardiomyopathy called Keshan disease, which was common in south-west China. The results of Chen *et al.* (1980), summarized by Golden (1982), on the reduction in mortality by selenium supplements, are truly impressive. Many workers now consider that milder degrees of Se deficiency may be quite common. For example, Pearson *et al.* (1990), on the basis of measurements of Se in plasma and of glutathione peroxidase (GPX), a selenium-containing enzyme, in platelets, argue that Se deficiency is widespread in north-western England. Low levels of plasma Se have also been recorded in other parts of Europe (Fernandez-Banares *et al.*, 1990). Since GPX is an important scavenger of free radicals (Chapter 10) it seems a reasonable proposition that deficiency of this enzyme may contribute to the pathogenesis of many disease states. Thus Golden (1982) wrote: 'over the past two decades we have reached the stage with selenium that iodine enjoyed in the 1920s . . . the present evidence strongly suggests that selenium is a trace element which will have a definite role in clinical medicine'. It is all the more likely to have a role in PEM, in which there is a deficiency of most nutrients.

In 1967 Burk *et al.* in Guatemala demonstrated low levels of selenium in whole blood and increased uptake of Se into red cells in children with PEM. In Thailand Se concentrations were greatly reduced in plasma and normal or high in red cells. In Zaïre Fondu *et al.* (1978) also reported low Se in plasma but not in erythrocytes in marasmic kwashiorkor. In Jamaica Murphy *et al.* (1988) found reduced concentrations of erythrocyte GPX in malnourished children, but plasma GPX and Se were low only in those with oedema. Selenium supplements were necessary to restore the levels to normal. Mathias and Jackson (1982) reported on a child with increased red cell fragility and a low plasma vitamin E who showed dramatic improvement when given small doses of Se.

In a group of 26 children in Jamaica with low Se status, 11 developed cardiac failure and four died (Golden and Golden, 1984). It was not reported whether the pathology in those cases had any relation to that of Keshan disease. Although it is not possible to be certain about cause and effect, a fatality rate of 15 per cent indicates that a low Se status carries a bad prognosis. Since the measurements are difficult, it may be well to give Se supplements as a routine in the early stages of treatment (Chapter 12).

In this section only three trace elements have been discussed, for which there is good evidence of deficiency in PEM: zinc, copper and selenium. This is not to imply that they are the only ones of importance. For example, animal experiments have shown that deficiency of chromium led to a decrease in glucose tolerance. In Jordan a clear correlation was found between glucose tolerance and the chromium content of drinking water (Hopkins *et al.*, 1968). Gürson and Saner (1971), following up this observation, found that in nine out of 14 severely marasmic children a single dose of $CrCl_3$ produced a significant increase in glucose removal rate, from 1.5 to 5.0 per cent per minute. However, other such studies have given inconclusive or negative results. In the words of Offenbacher and Pi-Sunyer (1988): 'a clinical measure of Cr status has eluded investigators'.

The possible effects of vanadium deficiency in PEM have been discussed by Golden and Golden (1981*b*). They summarized evidence that vanadium may control the activity of the sodium pump, and suggested that deficiency of this element could explain the retention of salt and water in nutritional oedema (Chapter 11). Low plasma concentrations of vanadium have indeed been recorded in children with kwashiorkor (Burger and Hogewind, 1974).

Conclusion

Golden *et al.* (1985) have said: '. . . we must never lose sight of the fact that these substances [trace elements] fit into a much larger and more complex situation. . . . There is evidence for deranged metabolism of almost all the trace elements in malnourished individuals'. In a multifactorial situation it is difficult to disentangle specific effects of specific deficiencies, but to attempt to do so is worthwhile if we are to get a better understanding of the metabolic changes in PEM and of the biological function of individual micronutrients.

References

Bates, C. J., Tsuchiya, H. (1990). Zinc in breast milk during prolonged lactation: comparison between the UK and The Gambia. *European Journal of Clinical Nutrition* **44**: 61–69.
Behrens, R. H., Tomkins, A. M., Roy, S. K. (1990). Zinc supplementation during diarrhoea: a fortification against malnutrition? *Lancet* **2**: 442–443.
Bennett, F. I., Golden, M. H. N. *et al.* (1985). Red cell superoxide dismutase as a measure of copper status in man. In Mills, C. F., Bremner, I., Chesters, J. K. (eds) *Trace element metabolism in man and animals. 5.* Commonwealth Agricultural Bureaux, Aberdeen, pp. 578–581.

Bremner, I., Beattie, J. H. (1990). Metallothionein and the trace minerals. *Annual Review of Nutrition* **10:** 63–83.

Bremner, I., Mills, C. F. (1981). Absorption, transport and tissue storage of essential trace elements. *Philosophical Transactions of the Royal Society of London B* **294:** 75–90.

Burger, F. J., Hogewind, Z. A. (1974). Changes in trace elements in kwashiorkor. *South African Medical Journal* **48:** 502–504.

Burk, R. F., Pearson, W. N. *et al.* (1967). Blood selenium levels and in vitro red blood cell uptake of ^{75}Se in kwashiorkor. *American Journal of Clinical Nutrition* **20:** 723–733.

Casey, C. E., Walravens, P. A. (1988). Trace elements. In Tsang, R. C., Nichols, B. L. (eds) *Nutrition during infancy.* Hanley and Belfus, Philadelphia, pp. 190–215.

Chen, X., Yang, G. *et al.* (1980). Studies on the relations of selenium and Keshan disease. *Biological Trace Element Research* **2:** 91–107.

Cordano, A., Baertl, J. M., Graham, G. G. (1964). Copper deficiency in infancy. *Pediatrics* **34:** 324–336.

Cousins, R. J. (1985). Absorption, transport and hepatic metabolism of copper and zinc: special reference to metallothionein and caeruloplasmin. *Physiological Reviews* **65:** 238–309.

Cousins, J., Leinart, A. S. (1988). Tissue-specific regulation of zinc metabolism and metallothionein genes by interleukin 1. *FASEB Journal* **2:** 2884–2890.

Danks, D. M. (1988). Copper deficiency in humans. *Annual Review of Nutrition* **8:** 235–257.

Dorea, J. G., Paine, P. A. (1985). Hair zinc in children: its uses, limitations and relationship to plasma zinc and anthropometry. *Human Nutrition: Clinical Nutrition* **39C:** 389–398.

Fairweather-Tait, S. J. (1988). Zinc in human nutrition. *Nutrition Research Reviews* **1:** 23–38.

Fernandez-Banares, F., Dolz, C. *et al.* (1990). Low serum selenium concentration in a healthy population in Catalunya: a preliminary report. *European Journal of Clinical Nutrition* **44:** 225–230.

Fondu, P., Hariga-Muller, C. *et al.* (1978). Protein-energy malnutrition and anemia in Kivu. *American Journal of Clinical Nutrition* **30:** 40–50.

Fraker, P. J., Gershwin, M. E. *et al.* (1986). Interrelationships between zinc and immune function. *Federation Proceedings* **45:** 1474–1479.

Golden, M. H. N. (1982). Trace elements in human nutrition. *Human Nutrition: Clinical Nutrition* **36C:** 185–202.

Golden, M. H. N. (1988). The role of individual nutrient deficiencies in growth retardation of children as exemplified by zinc and protein. In Waterlow, J. C. (ed) *Linear growth retardation in less developed countries.* Nestlé Nutrition, Vevey; Raven Press, New York, pp. 143–164.

Golden, B. E., Golden, M. H. N. (1979). Plasma zinc and the clinical features of malnutrition. *American Journal of Clinical Nutrition* **32:** 2490–2494.

Golden, B. E., Golden, M. H. N. (1981*a*). Plasma zinc, rate of weight gain and the energy cost of tissue deposition in children recovering from severe malnutrition on a cow's milk or soya protein based diet. *American Journal of Clinical Nutrition* **34:** 892–899.

Golden, M. H. N., Golden, B. E. (1981*b*). Trace elements: potential importance in human nutrition, with particular reference to zinc and vanadium. *British Medical Bulletin* **37:** 31–36.

Golden, B. E., Golden, M. H. N. (1984). New aspects of trace element metabolism; particularly zinc. In Fernandez, J., Buersma, R. (eds) *Nutrition a universal problem: the Jonxis lectures.* Foundation for Clinical Higher Education, Netherlands Antilles, pp. 69–73.

Golden, M. H. N., Golden, B. E. (1985*a*). Problems with the recognition of human zinc responsive conditions. In Mills, C. F., Bremner, I., Chesters, J. K. (eds) *Trace element metabolism in man and animals, 5.* Commonwealth Agricultural Bureaux, Aberdeen, pp. 933–938.

Golden, B. E., Golden, M. H. N. (1985*b*). Zinc, sodium and potassium losses in the diarrhoeas of malnutrition and zinc deficiency. In Mills, C. F., Bremner, I., Chesters, J. K. (eds) *Trace elements in man and animals, 5.* Commonwealth Agricultural Bureaux, Farnham Royal, UK, pp. 228–232.

Golden, M. H. N., Golden, B. E., Jackson, A. A. (1980). Skin breakdown in kwashiorkor responds to zinc. *Lancet* **1:** 1256.

Golden, M. H. N., Golden, B. E., Bennett, F. I. (1985). Relationship of trace element deficiencies to malnutrition. In Chandra, R. K. (ed) *Trace elements in nutrition of children.* Raven Press, New York, pp. 185–207.

Golden, M. H. N., Golden, B. E. *et al.* (1978). Zinc and immunocompetence in protein-energy malnutrition. *Lancet* **1:** 1226–1228.

Grider, A., Bailey, L. B., Cousins, R. J. (1990). Erythrocyte metallothionein as an index of zinc status in humans. *Proceedings of the National Academy of Sciences USA* **87:** 1259–1262.

Gürson, C. T., Saner, G. (1971). Effect of chromium on glucose utilization in marasmic PCM. *American Journal of Clinical Nutrition* **24:** 1313–1319.

Hansen, J. D. L., Lehmann, B. H. (1969). Serum zinc and copper concentrations in children with protein-calorie malnutrition. *South African Medical Journal* **43:** 1248–1251.

Hopkins, L. L., Ransome-Kuti, O., Majaj, A. S. (1968). Improvement of impaired carbohydrate metabolism by chromium (III) in malnourished infants. *American Journal of Clinical Nutrition* **21:** 203–211.

James, W. P. T., Ragbeer, M. M. S., Walshe, M. M. (1969). Acrodermatitis enteropathica. *West Indian Medical Journal* **18:** 17–24.

Keen, C. L., Gershwin, E. G. (1990). Zinc deficiency and immune function. *Annual Review of Nutrition* **10:** 415–432.

Krebs, N. F., Hambidge, K. M. *et al.* (1985). The effects of a dietary zinc supplement during lactation on longitudinal changes in maternal zinc status and milk zinc concentrations. *American Journal of Clinical Nutrition* **41:** 560–570.

Lehti, K. K. (1990). Breast milk folic acid and zinc concentrations of lactating, low socio-economic, Amazonian women and the effect of age and parity on the same two nutrients. *European Journal of Clinical Nutrition* **44:** 675–680.

Levine, R. J., Olson, R. E. (1970). Blood selenium in Thai children with protein-calorie malnutrition. *Proceedings of the Society of Experimental Biological Medicine* **134:** 1030–1034.

Lönnerdal, B. (1989). Trace element nutrition in infants. *Annual Review of Nutrition* **9:** 109–125.

Mathias, P. M., Jackson, A. A. (1982). Selenium deficiency in kwashiorkor. *Lancet* **1:** 1312–1313.

Meadows, N. J., Ruse, W. *et al.* (1981). Zinc and small babies. *Lancet* **2:** 1135–1137.

Moynahan, F. J. (1974). Acrodermatitis enteropathica: a lethal inherited human zinc deficiency disorder. *Lancet* **2:** 399–400.

Murphy, C., Golden, B. *et al.* (1988). Selenium status during recovery from malnutrition: effect of selenium supplementation. In Hurley L S., Keen, C. L. *et al.* (eds) *Trace element metabolism in animals and man.* Vol. 6. Plenum, New York, pp. 11–12.

Neilsen, F. H. (1988). Possible future implications of ultratrace elements in human health and disease. In Prasad, A. S. (ed) *Essential and toxic trace elements in nutrition and disease.* Alan Liss, New York, pp. 277–292.

O'Dell, B. L. (1981). Roles for iron and copper in connective tissue biosynthesis. *Philosphical Transactions of the Royal Society London B* **294:** 91–104.

Offenbacher, E. G., Pi-Sunyer, F. X. (1988). Chromium in human nutrition. *Annual Review of Nutrition* **8**: 543–563.

Patrick, J., Golden, B. E., Golden, M. H. N. (1980). Leucocyte sodium transport and dietary zinc in protein energy malnutrition. *American Journal of Clinical Nutrition* **33**: 617–620.

Pearson, D. J., Day, J. P. *et al.* (1990). Human selenium status and glutathione peroxidase activity in north-west England. *European Journal of Clinical Nutrition* **44**: 277–284.

Prasad, A. S. (ed). *Essential and toxic trace elements in human health and disease.* Alan Liss, New York.

Prasad, A. S., Halstead, J. A., Nadimi, M. (1961). Syndrome of iron deficiency anaemia, hepatosplenomegaly, hypogonadism, dwarfing and geophagia. *American Journal of Medicine* **31**: 532–546.

Rajagopalan, K. V. (1988). Molybdenum: an essential trace element in human nutrition. *Annual Review of Nutrition* **8**: 401–427.

Sandstead, H. H. (1975). Mineral metabolism in protein malnutrition. In Olson, R. E. (ed) *Protein-calorie malnutrition.* Academic Press, New York, pp. 201–220.

Sandstead, H. H., Shukry, A. S. *et al.* (1965). Kwashiorkor in Egypt. I. Clinical and biochemical studies, with special reference to plasma zinc and serum lactic dehydrogenase. *American Journal of Clinical Nutrition* **17**: 15–26.

Schroeder, J. J., Cousins, R. J. (1990). Interleukin 6 regulates metallothionein gene expression and zinc metabolism in hepatocyte monolayer cultures. *Proceedings of the National Academy of Sciences USA* **87**: 3137–3141.

Simmer, K., Khanum, S. *et al.* (1988). Nutritional rehabilitation in Bangladesh—the importance of zinc. *American Journal of Clinical Nutrition* **47**: 1036–1040.

Solomons, N. W. (1982). Biological availability of zinc in humans. *American Journal of Clinical Nutrition* **35**: 1048–1075.

Uauy, R., Castillo-Duran, C. *et al.* (1985). Red cell superoxide dismutase as an index of human copper nutrition. *Journal of Nutrition* **115**: 1650–1655.

Vuori, E., Kuitunen, P. (1979). The concentrations of copper and zinc in human milk. *Acta Paediatrica Scandinavica* **68**: 33–37.

Walravens, P. A., Krebs, N. F., Hambidge, K. M. (1983). Linear growth of low income pre-school children receiving a zinc supplement. *American Journal of Clinical Nutrition* **38**: 195–201.

10

Cell membranes and free radicals

Changes in cell membranes

It was suggested in an earlier chapter that hyponatraemia might be the result of what has been called the 'sick cell syndrome', and that this in turn might be caused by leakiness of the cell membrane. Here we examine the evidence for leakiness and the concept of damage by free radicals as a cause of it.

There is indeed evidence that in PEM alterations occur in the structure and functioning of cell membranes. Most of it is derived from studies on red blood cells, whose membranes are not necessarily representative of those of other cells. The earliest observations came from South Africa (Lanzowsky et al., 1967) and Uganda (Coward, 1971). Later studies were those of Brown and co-workers (1978) in Thailand and Fondu et al. (1978) in Zaïre. Both groups reported that in PEM the red cells were more than normally resistant to osmotic stress, but had a shortened life-span. They also found an increase in the phospholipid and cholesterol content of the membranes (Fondu et al., 1980). The higher cholesterol content would have the effect of increasing the rigidity or decreasing the fluidity of the membrane and possibly of altering its permeability (Claret et al., 1978). Divalent cations also affect the characteristics of the membrane; Ca^{++} makes it more rigid (Kaplay, 1984) and Mg^{++} deficiency, which is not uncommon in PEM (Chapter 4), makes it more fluid (Heaton et al., 1988).

These findings on structural changes naturally directed attention to changes in function. Kaplay (1978) and Fondu et al. (1979) reported an increase in activity in the ouabain-sensitive Na^+-K^+-ATPase (the 'sodium pump') of isolated red cell membranes from children with PEM, without any increase in intracellular Na^+. In a very interesting and comprehensive review in 1984 Kaplay suggested that increases in the activity of the pump and the number of pump sites were a mechanism to compensate for increased permeability to Na^+. Willis and Golden (1988) confirmed that both in kwashiorkor and in marasmus the membrane was 'leaky', with increased passive permeability to both K^+ (efflux) and Na^+ (influx). However, in their patients pump activity was increased only in kwashiorkor and not in marasmus. They made the important observation that in normal children the pump-rate is affected by age, being slower in younger children, so that the absence of a rise in marasmus might be regarded as reversion to an earlier stage of development.

The erythrocyte is a very specialized cell. It was therefore satisfactory that these findings agreed well with the studies of Patrick on a physiologically much more representative tissue, the leucocytes of children with PEM. Patrick and Golden (1977) reported that in kwashiorkor the leucocytes contained an excess of Na^+, with an increased activity of the sodium pump responsible for active transport of Na^+ out of the cells. This effect was not found in marasmic children. In a later study on recovering children Patrick *et al.* (1980) found that supplements of zinc stimulated the sodium pump. They concluded that there are at least two defects of Na^+ transport in PEM: increased passive permeability (leakiness) in kwashiorkor and decreased active transport of Na^+ in marasmus. A most interesting further observation was that in some children who died unexpectedly, with tachycardia, tachypnoea and watery diarrhoea, after they had started treatment on a high energy diet, leucocyte Na^+ was actually reduced and the activity of the sodium pump greatly increased, suggesting an over-compensation (Patrick, 1977). When these conditions were observed in subsequent cases, treatment with frusemide and digoxin caused dramatic improvement, with restoration of leucocyte Na^+ concentration and pump activity to normal levels.

These results taken together lead to the conclusion that in preparations as diverse as intact red cells (Fondu, Willis), isolated red cell membranes (Kaplay) and intact leucocytes (Patrick), children with kwashiorkor show increased sodium pump activity, perhaps as a compensation for a rise in passive permeability or leakiness. Secondly, although, as one might expect, there is a good deal of variability in the results, in all the studies the changes seem to be more marked in kwashiorkor than in marasmus; in other words, they seem to be related in some way to the presence of oedema. This conclusion clearly may be an important clue to the pathogenesis of oedema, discussed in the next chapter.

One might speculate that with further membrane damage a point comes where the compensation breaks down, leading to a rise in intracellular sodium, a loss of potassium and a truly sick cell. Moreover, in addition to the sodium pump there is a calcium pump, which maintains a 10 000-fold concentration gradient of free Ca^{++} between the outside and the inside of the cell. An accumulation of Ca^{++} at intracellular sites has been implicated in the mechanism of several types of cell damage (Jackson, 1990). Therefore the integrity of the cell membrane and of the calcium pump is of crucial importance for the viability of the cell. Both the sodium and the calcium pumps are driven by ATP and therefore require an energy supply. It used to be thought that about 50 per cent of basal oxygen consumption is used for maintaining these ion pumps, but that is now considered to be much too high (Chinet, 1989). Nevertheless, if the argument in Chapter 6 is correct, reduction in the metabolic rate of vital tissues in PEM could represent impairment of pump activity just at a time when an increase is demanded to compensate for leakiness of cell membranes. In the next section we consider the possibility that leakiness results from damage by free radicals.

Free radicals in the pathogenesis of kwashiorkor

Free radicals are defined as molecules or molecular fragments containing a single unpaired electron, which makes them highly reactive, frequently with toxic effects. In chemical formulae the presence of this unpaired electron is denoted by a dot, as in the hydroxyl free radical OH$^\bullet$. The book by Halliwell and Gutteridge (1985) gives a general account of the chemistry and biology of free radicals.

Golden's hypothesis is that kwashiorkor results from an imbalance between the production of toxic radicals and their safe disposal (Golden, 1985; Golden and Ramdath, 1987; Golden *et al.*, 1991). This hypothesis is a break from the conventional view that marasmus and kwashiorkor represent the ends of a continuous spectrum. Instead it postulates that the two conditions are causally distinct; in both there is a background of energy and protein deficiency; kwashiorkor is precipitated by a variety of environmental insults, termed by Golden 'noxae', which increase the production of free radicals. At the same time the child's protective mechanisms are compromised by a whole range of dietary deficiencies or depletions. The important noxae are infections, which are well-known to precipitate the onset of kwashiorkor, and particular emphasis is laid on bacterial overgrowth in the bowel which, in Golden's words, constitutes a 'biochemical powerhouse', capable of producing numerous toxic products. Other possible noxae are exogenous toxins, such as aflatoxin and its metabolites. In children in the Sudan these substances were found somewhat more often, and in greater concentration, in serum and urine in PEM than in controls (Coulter *et al.*, 1986).

Free radicals are nowadays implicated in many disease processes (Halliwell and Gutteridge, 1985; Slater *et al.*, 1987). In the present context perhaps the most important effects are those on the lipids of cell membranes, since free radicals acting on polyunsaturated fatty acids can start a chain reaction of lipid peroxidation (Halliwell, 1987).

Free radicals are not always and in all situations harmful. They are produced in many normal metabolic reactions, e.g. those involving oxygenases and dehydrogenases. The free radical superoxide ($O_2^{\bullet -}$) is produced by neutrophils when they are activated by bacteria and probably has an important bactericidal action. It has been suggested that free radical activity may be part of the body's defence mechanism against the proliferation of cancer cells (Dormandy, 1988).

Radicals vary in their activity and one can be transformed into another. For example, the relatively unreactive superoxide radical $O_2^{\bullet -}$ can be converted into the much more reactive and toxic species OH$^\bullet$ under the catalytic influence of iron. The chemistry of the reactions that are likely to be important in PEM has been described in detail by Slater *et al.* (1987) and Golden and Ramdath (1987).

Even though some of the reactions may be beneficial components of normal metabolism, the problem for the body is to prevent them from getting out of hand. There are two kinds of protective mechanisms; one is prevention of the formation of toxic radicals, particularly OH$^\bullet$; the other is disposal or scavenging of them once they have been formed. In both mechanisms trace metals and the tripeptide glutathione (GSH) play an important part. Caeruloplasmin and transferrin, by mopping up free iron and converting the highly toxic Fe^{2+} into the less toxic Fe^{3+}, are major preventive antioxidants (Thurnham, 1990).

Increased production of free radicals

The role of iron

Iron repletion has an adverse effect on the course of some infections (Murray *et al.*, 1978). The subject has been reviewed by Oppenheimer and Hendrickse (1983). There seem to be two mechanisms: iron promotes bacterial growth and it also plays a very important role in promoting free radical formation. It was observed long ago that children dying of PEM had abnormally large amounts of Fe in the liver (Waterlow, 1948). At the time this was attributed to decreased uptake into haemoglobin because protein and other factors were limiting. It has also long been recognized that plasma transferrin levels are low in PEM (Chapter 7). Since plasma Fe concentrations are normal, it follows that transferrin saturation is increased and the capacity to deal with an iron overload reduced. Ramdath and Golden (1989) have shown that transferrin saturation of more than 90 per cent was much commoner in kwashiorkor than marasmus and was associated with a high mortality.

Ferritin is iron conjugated with a protein, and its synthesis is stimulated by iron salts (Drysdale and Munro, 1966). The serum ferritin concentration is usually considered to be a measure of Fe stores, but it is increased in infections. Several workers have found that in PEM serum ferritin levels are higher than normal; in Jamaica they were higher in kwashiorkor than marasmus, though with a good deal of overlap. High levels were a bad prognostic sign (Fig. 10.1): 14 out of 24 children with levels above 250 µg/ml died (Ramdath and Golden, 1989). These authors also showed that in response to the iron-chelator, desferrioxamine, children with kwashiorkor had a much greater excretion of Fe in the urine than those with marasmus. These findings, summarized in Table 10.1, point to iron overload as an important feature of PEM, more severe in kwashiorkor than marasmus and carrying a serious risk of death. It is therefore not surprising that mortality was increased when children were treated with ferrous sulphate at an early stage after admission to hospital (Smith *et al.*, 1989). What is not clear is where the iron overload comes from; perhaps the original explanation of it—a block in haemoglobin synthesis—

Table 10.1   Iron status of children with PEM

	Control	Marasmus	Marasmic kwashiorkor	Kwashiorkor
Iron-binding capacity, µg/l	358	250	116	124
Transferrin saturation, %	~ 30	45	55	68[a]
Plasma ferritin, µg/l	–	82	300	329
Urinary iron after desferrioxamine, µg/24 hours	–	367	708	987

[a] Recalculated from Ramdath and Golden (1989), Fig. 3.
From Ramdath and Golden (1989), Golden *et al.* (1990)

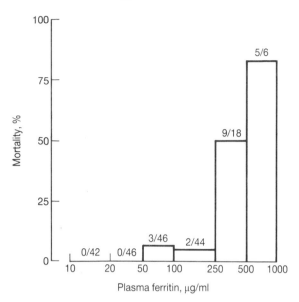

Fig. 10.1 Plasma ferritin concentrations and mortality in Jamaican children with PEM. Reproduced by permission from Ramdath and Golden (1989).

was correct. In the very interesting case of rhesus haemolytic disease, where there is an obvious source of iron overload, increased ferritin levels have been found, compared with controls, together with increased concentrations of lipid-peroxidation products in the plasma (Berger *et al.*, 1990).

Deficiency of protective dietary factors

Three vitamins, A (or rather its precursor, β-carotene), C and E, together with essential (polyunsaturated) fatty acids help to protect against free radical attack in virtue of their chemical function as antioxidants. In some parts of the world vitamin A deficiency is frequently associated with PEM. Since Third World diets in general contain very little preformed vitamin A, the basic deficiency must be of β-carotene. McLaren and Shirajian (1969) showed that children with kwashiorkor had lower plasma carotene levels than those with marasmus. This could be because in kwashiorkor there is greater destruction of carotene by free radicals, rather than a difference in intake (Golden and Ramdath, 1987).

Plasma vitamin E concentrations have also been found to be low in children with severe PEM (McLaren and Shirajian, 1969; Mathias, 1983). In the series reported by Golden and Ramdath (1987) plasma vitamin E was below the accepted normal level in 25 out of 29 children with oedema and in 11 out of 22 with marasmus. The distinction is therefore suggestive but not absolute. It is interesting in this connection that in experiments *in vitro* vitamin E deficiency was associated with an increased uptake of water and sodium by liver slices (McLean, 1963).

Clinical signs of scurvy have not been described in kwashiorkor and we know of no investigations of vitamin C status. Recently reported outbreaks of scurvy in refugee camps might provide an opportunity for further studies on this subject.

Naismith (1973) found biochemical evidence of essential fatty acid deficiency in children with kwashiorkor in Nigeria, and James (1977) pointed out that kwashiorkor presents many of the factors found in essential fatty acid deficiency in animals: skin rashes and dyspigmentation; thin hair; fatty liver; gut lesions; increased capillary permeability and enhanced susceptibility to infection. A decrease in the n-6 fatty acids of the red cell phospholipids has been reported, down to one-third of the control level, in grade III malnutrition (Marín *et al.*, 1991). Nevertheless, children can make a full recovery on a diet with the main source of fat as coconut oil, which has a very low content of essential fatty acids.

Golden and Ramdath (1987) also suggested that zinc might have a protective effect, acting in the form of zinc-metallothionein as a free radical sink. Plasma zinc concentrations were consistently low in oedematous PEM, whereas in marasmus the results were more variable (Chapter 9).

Mechanisms for scavenging free radicals

The role of glutathione and of trace metals

There are several reactions which are of particular importance in protection against free radicals and in all of them the tripeptide glutathione (cysteine-glutamic acid-glycine) plays a central role. It therefore provided strong support for the free radical theory when Jackson (1986) demonstrated that the glutathione content of red cells was greatly reduced in kwashiorkor but not in marasmus (Fig. 10.2). These observations were confirmed and extended by Golden and Ramdath (1987). It has also been shown that reduction *in vitro* of red cell glutathione reproduces the defects of cellular sodium transport in oedematous malnutrition (Forrester *et al.*, 1990).

Glutathione normally exists mainly in the reduced form GSH; free radicals and their products are oxidizing agents, which react with GSH to produce oxidized glutathione, GSSG. The following reactions are an example of such a sequence:

$$(1) \quad 2O_2^{\cdot -} + 2H^+ \xrightarrow[-O_2]{\text{SOD}} H_2O_2 + O_2$$

(superoxide radical)   (hydrogen peroxide)

$$(2) \quad H_2O_2 + 2GSH \xrightarrow{\text{GPX}} GSSG + 2H_2O$$

$$(3) \quad GSSG + 2NADPH \xrightarrow{\text{EGR}} 2GSH + 2NADP$$

The following account of these reactions in PEM is based on the work of Golden and Ramdath (1987) and Golden *et al.* (1991). Reaction (1) is catalysed by the enzyme superoxide dismutase (SOD), which may therefore be

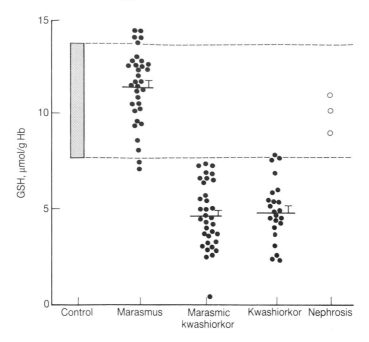

Fig. 10.2 Reduced glutathione (GSH) content of erythrocytes in Jamaican control children and in children with PEM. Data from Golden and Ramdath (1987).

regarded as a 'protective' enzyme. A reduced activity of this enzyme in red cells was found in 25 per cent of cases of kwashiorkor. The red cell enzyme is a metalloprotein in which the metal is copper. In mitochondria, where there is a much more active oxidizing environment, the metal is manganese. In view of the evidence for deficiency of trace metals in PEM (Chapter 9) the activity of the mitochondria as well as of the red cell superoxide dismutase might be compromised.

Reaction (2) is catalysed by the selenium-containing enzyme glutathione peroxidase (GPX). The activity of GPX in erythrocytes is often reduced in severe PEM, to a greater extent in oedematous than in non-oedematous cases. It will be recalled that selenium is another trace element that is deficient in PEM. Supplements of selenium produced a large increase in GPX activity.

The regeneration of GSH by reaction (3) is catalysed by erythrocyte gluta-thione reductase (EGR), for which riboflavin is an essential co-factor. Although Golden and co-workers did not find any reduction in this enzyme in PEM, its activity would presumably be limited if there was a concomitant riboflavin deficiency. In the old days clinical signs of this deficiency (cheilosis and angular stomatitis) were quite often seen in kwashiorkor (Waterlow, 1948). In reaction (3) reduction of GSSG occurs at the expense of oxidation of NADPH. This could be a limiting factor: erythrocyte NADPH was very low in kwashiorkor and marasmic kwashiorkor but not in marasmus.

A further pathway for removal of the peroxides generated by free radicals is by direct conjugation with GSH, catalysed by the enzyme glutathione-S-transferase (GST). The conjugates are then broken down to sulphur-containing mercapturic acids, which are excreted. Figure 10.3 shows that mercapturic acid excretion was very much higher in PEM than in control children and did not return to normal levels on recovery. Whereas in the sequence of reactions (1) to (3) GSH is regenerated, the direct conjugation catalysed by GST leads to a net consumption of glutathione. This could be an important cause of the reduction in glutathione which, in the light of the preceding discussion, is perhaps the mose sensitive indicator of free radical stress and failure of the protective mechanisms. However, Jackson (1990) has also suggested that the synthesis of glutathione may be impaired, because of a shortage of the semi-essential amino acids glycine and cysteine (Chapter 6).

Table 10.2 summarizes factors in the free radical story in which Golden

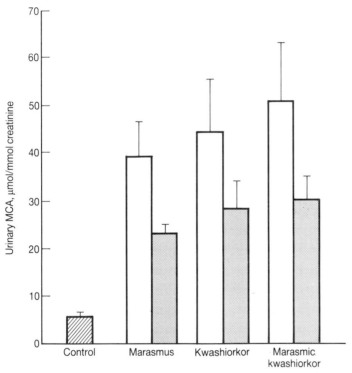

Fig. 10.3 Urinary mercapturic acid (MCA) output in Jamaican control children and in children with PEM; ⬜, on admission; ▩, on discharge. Reproduced by permission from Golden *et al.* (1991).

Table 10.2 Summary of differences between kwashiorkor and marasmus in factors that protect against free radicals

A. *Large difference with little or no overlap*
  Decrease in red cell GSH concentration (Fig. 10.2)
  Decrease in red cell NADPH concentration
B. *Moderate difference, with considerable overlap*
  Plasma vitamin E concentration
  Red cell GPX activity
  Urinary mercapturic acid output (Fig. 10.3)

and co-workers have demonstrated a difference between kwashiorkor and marasmus. Most of their studies have been made on red blood cells and it remains to be determined whether the same effects are found in other tissues. As mentioned earlier, it has indeed been found that membrane changes in red cells are reproduced also in leucocytes. Whether the specific characteristics of kwashiorkor such as oedema and fatty liver can be explained by free radical damage is considered in the next chapter.

References

Berger, H. M., Lindeman, J. H. N. *et al.* (1990). Iron overload, free radical damage and rhesus haemolytic disease. *Lancet* **335**: 933–936.
Brown, K. H., Suskind, R. M. *et al.* (1978). Changes in the red blood cell membrane in protein-calorie malnutrition. *American Journal of Clinical Nutrition* **31**: 574–578.
Chinet, A. E. (1989). Energy cost of ionic homeostasis in mammalian skeletal muscle. In Wieser, W., Gnäger, E. (eds) *Energy transformations in cells and organisms.* Thieme Verlag, Frankfurt, pp. 58–65.
Claret, M., Garay, R., Giraud, F. (1978). The effect of membrane cholesterol in the sodium pump in red blood cells. *Journal of Physiology* **274**: 247–263.
Coulter, J. B. S., Hendrickse, R. G. *et al.* (1986). Aflatoxins and kwashiorkor: clinical studies in Sudanese children. *Transactions of the Royal Society of Tropical Medicine and Hygiene* **80**: 945–951.
Coward, W. A. (1971). The erythrocyte membrane in kwashiorkor. *British Journal of Nutrition* **25**: 145–151.
Dormandy, T. L. (1988). In praise of peroxidation. *Lancet* **2**: 1126–1128.
Drysdale, J. W., Munro, H. N. (1966). Regulation of synthesis and turnover of ferritin in rat liver. *Journal of Biological Chemistry* **241**: 3630–3637.
Fondu, P., Hariga-Muller, C. *et al.* (1978). Protein-energy malnutrition and anemia in Kivu. *American Journal of Clinical Nutrition* **31**: 46–56.
Fondu, P., Mandelbaum, I. N., Vis, H. L. (1979). The erythrocyte membrane in protein energy malnutrition. *American Journal of Clinical Nutrition* **31**: 717–719.
Fondu, P., Mozes, N. *et al.* (1980). The erythrocyte membrane disturbances in protein-energy malnutrition. *British Journal of Haematology* **44**: 605–613.
Forrester, T., Golden, M. *et al.* (1990). Reduction *in vitro* of red cell glutathione reproduces defects of cellular sodium transport seen in oedematous malnutrition. *European Journal of Clinical Nutrition* **44**: 363–370.
Golden, M. H. N. (1985). The consequences of protein deficiency in man and its relationship to the features of kwashiorkor. In Blaxter, K. L., Waterlow, J. C. (eds) *Nutritional adaptation in man.* John Libbey, London, pp. 169–188.
Golden, M. H. N., Ramdath, D. (1987). Free radicals in the pathogenesis of kwashiorkor. *Proceedings of the Nutrition Society* **46**: 53–68.
Golden, M. H. N., Ramdath, D. D., Golden, B. E. (1991). Free radicals and malnutrition. In Dreosti, I. E. (ed) *Trace elements, micronutrients and free radicals.* Humana Press, Clifton, New Jersey, in the press.
Halliwell, B. (1987). Free radicals and metals ions in health and disease. *Proceedings of the Nutrition Society* **46**: 13–26.
Halliwell, B., Gutteridge, J. M. C. (1985). *Free radicals in biology and medicine.* Clarendon Press, Oxford.
Heaton, F. W., Tongyai, S., Rayssiguier, Y. (1988). Increased fluidity of the erythrocyte membrane in magnesium deficiency. *Proceedings of the Nutrition Society* **47**: 162A.
Jackson, A. A. (1986). Blood glutathione in severe malnutrition in childhood. *Transactions of the Royal Society of Tropical Medicine and Hygiene* **80**: 911–913.

Jackson, M. J. (1990). Intracellular calcium, cell injury and relationships to free radicals and fatty acid metabolism. *Proceedings of the Nutrition Society* **49:** 77–81.

James, W. P. T. (1977). Kwashiorkor and marasmus: old concepts and new developments. *Proceedings of the Royal Society of Medicine* **70:** 611–615.

Kaplay, S. S. (1978). Erythrocyte membrane Na^+, K^+-activated adenosine-triphosphatase in protein-calorie malnutrition. *American Journal of Clinical Nutrition* **31:** 579–584.

Kaplay, S. S. (1984). Na^+ 'pump' and cell energetics in protein-energy malnutrition. *Nutrition Research* **4:** 935–948.

Lanzowsky, P., McKenzie, D. *et al.* (1967). Erythrocyte abnormality induced by protein malnutrition. II. 51-Chromium labelled erythrocyte studies. *British Journal of Haematology* **13:** 639–649.

McLaren, D. S., Shirajian, E. (1969). Short-term prognosis in protein-calorie malnutrition. *American Journal of Clinical Nutrition* **22:** 863–870.

McLean, A. E. M. (1963). Vitamin E deficiency and ion transport in rat liver slices. *Biochemical Journal* **87:** 164–167.

Marín, M. C., De Thomas, M. E. *et al.* (1991). Interrelationship between protein-energy malnutrition and essential fatty acid deficiency in nursing infants. *American Journal of Clinical Nutrition* **53:** 466–468.

Mathias, P. M. (1983). Vitamin status of children during recovery from severe malnutrition. *Proceedings of the Nutrition Society* **41:** 143A.

Murray, M. J., Murray, A. B. *et al.* (1978). The adverse effect of iron repletion on the course of certain infections. *British Medical Journal* **2:** 1113–1115.

Naismith, D. J. (1973). Kwashiorkor in western Nigeria: a study of traditional weaning foods, with particular reference to energy and linoleic acid. *British Journal of Nutrition* **30:** 567–576.

Oppenheimer, S., Hendrickse, R. (1983). The clinical effects of iron deficiency and iron supplementation. *Nutrition Abstracts and Reviews* (A) **53:** 585–598.

Patrick, J. (1977). Death during recovery from severe malnutrition and its possible relationship to sodium pump activity in leucocytes. *British Medical Journal* **1:** 1051–1054.

Patrick, J., Golden, M. H. N. (1977). Leucocyte electrolytes and sodium transport in protein energy malnutrition. *American Journal of Clinical Nutrition* **30:** 1478–1481.

Patrick, J., Golden, B. E., Golden, M. H. N. (1980). Leucocyte sodium transport and dietary zinc in protein energy malnutrition. *American Journal of Clinical Nutrition* **33:** 617–620.

Ramdath, D. D., Golden, M. H. N. (1989). Non-haematological aspects of iron nutrition. *Nutrition Research Reviews* **2:** 29–50.

Slater, T. F., Cheeseman, K. H. *et al.* (1987). Free radical mechanisms in relation to tissue injury. *Proceedings of the Nutrition Society* **46:** 1–12.

Smith, I. F., Taiwo, O., Golden, M. H. N. (1989). Plant protein rehabilitation diets and iron supplementation of the protein-energy malnourished child. *European Journal of Clinical Nutrition* **43:** 763–768.

Thurnham, D. I. (1990). Antioxidants and prooxidants in malnourished populations. *Proceedings of the Nutrition Society* **49:** 247–259.

Waterlow, J. C. (1948). *Fatty liver disease in infants in the British West Indies.* Medical Research Council Special Report Series No. 263. HM Stationery Office, London.

Willis, J. S., Golden, M. H. N. (1988). Active and passive transport of sodium and potassium ions in erythrocytes of severely malnourished Jamaican children. *European Journal of Clinical Nutrition* **42:** 635–646.

11

Causes of oedema and its relation to kwashiorkor

Causes of oedema

Few aspects of PEM have aroused as much discussion as the pathogenesis of oedema. The question is more than academic, because of the key role of oedema in the diagnosis of kwashiorkor (Chapter 1) and the clues that it may give to the dietary background.

Oedema is the clinical manifestation of expansion of the extracellular fluid volume. Whether or not there is an increase in intracellular water is an entirely different question (Chapter 3). In general medicine there is still much discussion and disagreement about the mechanisms by which the body controls its extracellular volume (e.g. Simpson, 1988). Are there volume receptors? Or is it the total sodium content that is controlled? Or is there really no control, but only passive extravasation of fluid into flaccid and wasted subcutaneous tissues? Because the oedema of PEM is usually readily reversible, a better understanding of its pathogenesis might have wider implications than in the particular context of malnutrition.

Hypoalbuminaemia

The longest standing candidate to be regarded as the cause of oedema is hypoalbuminaemia, and this is one of the most striking biochemical changes which differentiate kwashiorkor from marasmus. Starling's classical theory linked oedema to hypoalbuminaemia through a reduction in colloid osmotic pressure of the plasma (COP). Fibrinogen contributes less than 1 per cent to the COP of plasma (Guyton, 1981), so that from this point of view serum and plasma are equivalent. Coward (1975) showed that children in Uganda with low serum albumin concentrations did indeed have a decrease in serum COP, which was roughly, but not linearly, related to the degree of oedema. Guyton (1981) has described in detail the forces controlling the transfer of fluid from the capillaries to the interstitial space. According to his analysis, the interstitial space is normally at negative pressure; the moment that this pressure rises to equal that of the atmosphere, either from a decrease in serum COP or through haemodynamic changes, there is an enormous increase in outflow of fluid from the capillaries to the interstitial space (Fig. 11.1). Thus, there is a threshold effect in the formation of oedema and a strict concordance between a reduction in albumin concentration and degree of oedema is not to be expected. The demonstration in prospective studies on children in Uganda that a fall in plasma albumin preceded the development of oedema is entirely consistent with the Starling theory (Frood *et al.*, 1971; Whitehead *et al.*, 1973).

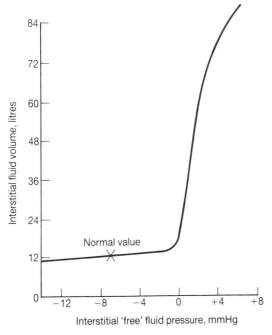

Fig. 11.1   Relation between interstitial fluid volume and interstitial fluid pressure. Reproduced by permission from Guyton (1981).

Many authors have commented on the overlap in serum albumin levels between oedematous and non-oedematous cases, ranging from Montgomery (1963) in his studies on PEM in Jamaica, to Gounelle (1962), who was investigating famine oedema in adults in France during World War II. Nevertheless, Gounelle stated that the lower the plasma albumin, the greater the degree of oedema. The classical studies of Weech and co-workers (1939) on dogs fed a low protein diet give an excellent example of the overlap (Fig. 11.2) (Weech *et al.*, 1933; Weech, 1939). The important point here is that although when plasma albumin levels were below 2 g/dl quite a large proportion of the dogs did not have oedema, there were few examples of the opposite inconsistency: only three out of 50 dogs were oedematous with an albumin level above 2 g/dl. This suggests that hypoalbuminaemia may be a necessary but not a sufficient cause and that some other factor may be needed, at least in some cases, for oedema to appear. One such factor is the availability of water and sodium; thus oedema can be produced in a child with marasmus

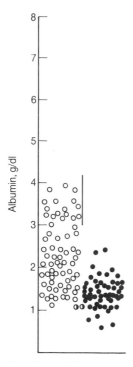

Fig. 11.2 Relation between plasma albumin concentration and oedema in dogs on a low protein diet; ○ , no oedema; ● , oedema present. Reproduced by permission from Weech (1939).

by excessive infusion of saline. Another factor is increased capillary permeability as a result of infection. Not only is there greater extravasation of fluid, but also an increase in the transcapillary escape of albumin (Fleck *et al.*, 1985), raising the COP in the interstitial space and promoting the accumulation of fluid there. Normally the protein content of the oedema fluid is very low (Tripathi *et al.*, 1983).

The problem of hunger oedema or famine oedema in adults is interesting and relevant. There is a general impression that this condition is not associated with hypoalbuminaemia, but the facts do not bear that out. Since measurements of plasma albumin have only been made in the last 60 years or so, the greater part of McCance's (1951) superb historical account of famine oedema, going back to the book of Deuteronomy, can neither confirm nor refute the relationship under discussion. It is true that McCance himself, working in Germany, did not find hypoalbuminaemia in adults with hunger oedema, nor did Sinclair (1948) in The Netherlands. However, Beattie *et al.* (1948), also working in Holland, recorded low plasma albumin in some but by no means all their subjects with oedema. Gounelle's findings in France have already been mentioned.

Thus the results from post-war Europe are contradictory; those from developing countries are more consistent. During the Japanese war in China Weech and Ling (1931) recorded that when the serum albumin level fell below 2.5 g/dl, oedema was invariably present. Kurnick (1948), also working in China, did not measure albumin, but noted that total serum protein levels were invariably low in subjects with oedema, sometimes falling below 2.5 g/dl. In the Bihar famine in India in 1966 plasma albumin concentrations in oedematous adults were even lower than in children (average 1.5 *versus* 2.65 g/dl) (Ramalingaswami *et al.*, 1971), and in an earlier famine values as low as 1.0 g/dl were found (Bose *et al.*, 1946). Gopalan *et al.* (1952) reported hypoalbuminaemia in their adult patients with nutritional oedema in South India. Trowell *et al.* (1954) described adult kwashiorkor in Uganda. His illustration shows oedema of the legs, severe wasting and changes in skin and hair. The average serum albumin level in these patients was 2.09 g/dl (Trowell and Muwazi, 1945).

The difference between nutritional oedema in adults and children is that in adults effusions in the serous cavities and ascites have been described. In our experience these effects are not found in PEM. In Jamaica when ascites was present it turned out to be due to the condition called veno-occlusive disease of the liver, caused by Senecio poisoning (Bras and Hill, 1956; Rhodes, 1957).

My conclusion is that there are some differences, but they are not fundamental, between nutritional oedema in adults and in children. There are also differences between the findings in Europe on the one hand and Asia and Africa on the other, in the extent to which oedema is accompanied by hypoalbuminaemia. This may be because in the Third World countries the shortage of food was of longer standing.

The experimental production of hypoalbuminaemia, sometimes with oedema, in animals on low protein diets has been cited earlier (Chapter 6). Almost in the category of an experiment is iatrogenic oedema appearing in children with milk allergy who were fed a low protein diet (Sinatra and Merritt, 1981). There is therefore a reasonably consistent body of evidence in children, adults and experimental animals of a strong, though not invariable, association between nutritional oedema and hypoalbuminaemia.

Criticism of the theory is based largely on the point already made, that hypoalbuminaemia may occur without oedema. The classical example is congenital analbuminaemia, in which oedema, if present at all, is minimal (Bearn and Litwin, 1978; Joles *et al.*, 1989). Much stress has been laid on the lack of correlation between oedema and albumin level in the response to treatment. Hansen (1956) found that the oedema of kwashiorkor could disappear completely on a protein-free diet containing only glucose and a salt mixture which included potassium. Golden *et al.* (1980*a*) observed that on treatment oedema disappeared without any increase in plasma albumin concentration. In a later study (Golden, 1982) they examined the rate of disappearance of oedema in children fed a number of different diets that had been used in Jamaica over the years and showed that the rate of loss was significantly related to the energy intake and not at all to the protein intake.

Although historically the therapeutic test has played an important role in the diagnosis of nutritional deficiencies, one could argue, with Fiorotto and Nichols (1982), that when a condition responds to a particular agent, it does not necessarily follow that the condition was caused by deficiency of that agent. As a historical aside, I recall a meeting in Uganda, when Brock was presenting his findings on the 'initiation of cure' of kwashiorkor, as judged by loss of oedema, with a mixture of amino acids alone (Brock *et al.*, 1955); the late Joseph Gillman of Johannesburg responded: 'When you cure a head-ache with aspirin, do you say that the cause was aspirin deficiency?'

Other causes of water and salt retention

The hypoalbuminaemic theory of oedema implies that there is a pre-renal diversion of fluid from the capillary bed to the extracellular space. This would fit in with Alleyne's finding of reduced glomerular filtration rate and renal plasma flow (Chapter 5). However, if the primary defect is inability of the kidney to control the extracellular fluid volume and body sodium content, this could lead to secondary hypoalbuminaemia through dilution. Mukherjee *et al.* (1954) described a group of critically ill adult patients in Calcutta with nutritional oedema and a mean plasma albumin concentration of 1.7 g/dl. They concluded that if hypoalbuminaemia has any role in the cause of oedema, it is not because of disturbance of the Starling equilibrium, but because the colloid osmotic pressure in the renal cortex is one of the factors conditioning salt and water excretion by the kidney. This dilutional theory of hypoalbuminaemia would suggest that the intravascular albumin mass is unchanged; in fact the evidence is that in spite of compensatory changes it is often reduced (Chapter 6).

Potassium deficiency is undoubtedly very important in promoting water and salt retention (Chapter 4). Walter *et al.* (1988) described the evidence as 'compelling', although the precise mechanism of the effect is not fully understood. Golden (1982), on the basis of his observations on the effect of energy intake in reducing oedema, put forward the interesting idea that oedema might be a result of energy deficiency, energy being needed to fuel the sodium pump and allow restoration of intracellular K^+ deficits.

The difficulty in allotting a primary role to potassium deficiency is our inability so far to show that children with kwashiorkor are more severely K deficient than those with marasmus. To do this, as discussed in Chapter 4, it would be necessary to demonstrate a greater reduction in K content in relation to active cell mass. An alternative would be to find out by balance measurements whether the ratio of K to N retained was consistently greater in kwashiorkor than in marasmus. Such studies have not to our knowledge been done. Moreover, although Alleyne (1966) showed that children with PEM have an impaired capacity to excrete a sodium load, which is a characteristic effect of K deficiency, there was no difference between those with and without oedema. Mönckeberg (1988) showed the same effect in marasmic children.

Alleyne's concept of the pathogenesis of oedema in PEM is shown in Fig. 11.3 (Klahr and Alleyne, 1973). What this diagram depicts is more in the nature of a mechanism than a cause. The initial trigger is supposed to be a decrease in plasma volume, which is put with a question-mark, because the literature on this is somewhat conflicting (Chapter 5). No evidence has been produced of increased aldosterone activity in children with oedematous PEM, although, paradoxically, Migeon *et al.* (1973) reported a great increase in the rate of aldosterone production in children with marasmus, but not in those with kwashiorkor, the opposite of what one might expect.

Renin is another hormone that may be involved in the production of oedema. It has been shown experimentally that chronic K deficiency produces

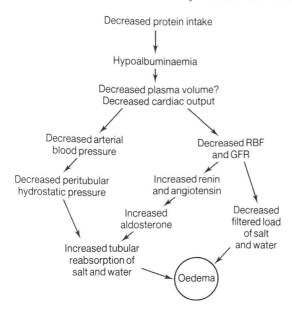

Fig. 11.3 Possible mechanisms for the development of oedema in malnourished subjects. RBF, renal blood flow; GFR, glomerular filtration rate. Reproduced by permission from Klahr and Alleyne (1973).

an increase in plasma renin activity with retention of Na (Abbrecht and Vandar, 1970). In a study on children with marasmic kwashiorkor in Bolivia Godard *et al.* (1986) found marked increases in plasma renin activity. High renin levels had earlier been found in children with PEM who died (Kritzinger *et al.*, 1972). Although Godard did not comment on it, in their series there was a striking inverse correlation between plasma renin activity and serum Na concentration. A similar inverse correlation was found between plasma renin and urinary Na excretion (Fig. 11.4). These two relationships suggest that renin must promote a disproportionate reabsorption of water, which would be a mechanism underlying the production of hyponatraemia (Chapter 4). This explanation, however, does not tally with the fact that in PEM the urine is typically hypotonic.

Many years ago it was suggested that oedema in PEM might be the result of increased antidiuretic hormone (ADH) activity. Gopalan (1950) reported that the urine of adult patients with nutritional oedema contained a substance that had antidiuretic activity in rats. Later it was found that ferritin stimulates ADH production by the posterior pituitary, and Srikantia and Gopalan (1959) showed that in monkeys on a low protein diet ferritin appeared in the serum after a few weeks and disappeared when the animals were restored to a normal diet. Srikantia and Mohanham (1970) subsequently reported that in children with PEM the level of circulating ADH differentiated between those with and without oedema. The hypothesis proposed was that ferritin is discharged into the circulation as a result of liver damage. These early observations gain added interest from the demonstration by Ramdath and Golden (1989) of higher serum ferritin levels in kwashiorkor and marasmic kwashiorkor than in marasmus (Chapter 10). Again, however, if increased ADH

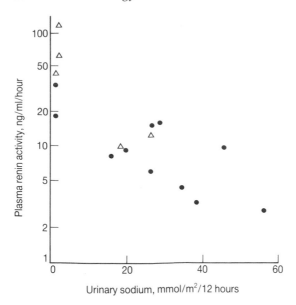

Fig. 11.4   Relation of plasma renin activity (log scale) to urinary sodium excretion in children with marasmic kwashiorkor; △ , on admission; • , after 3–4 days on an equilibration diet. Reproduced by permission from Godard *et al.* (1986).

production is a factor, one would expect a more concentrated urine in oedematous cases. This has not to our knowledge been reported.

There seems, therefore, to be no clear consensus about the role of the kidney or of salt-retaining hormones in the production of oedema in PEM. No proposed mechanism fits all the facts. Patrick (1979), in an excellent discussion of the control of water and sodium balance in PEM, concluded that 'either the signals from the "volume receptors" are inhibited or the kidney cannot regulate the rate of Na⁺ reabsorption from the nephron in response to ECF expansion because of an intrinsic defect'. However, Alleyne, who made the pioneer studies on kidney function in PEM, did not believe that renal impairment could be the primary cause of oedema (Klahr and Alleyne, 1973).

Damage to cell membranes

We have already discussed (Chapter 10) the evidence for leakiness of cell membranes in PEM, possibly caused by the damaging effects of free radicals. If a reduction in red cell glutathione content is a measure of free radical stress, then the stress does seem to be greater in oedematous than in non-oedematous cases (Jackson, 1986*b*; Golden and Ramdath, 1987). The question then is, how does leakiness of cells lead to oedema? One explanation proposed is that the cells of the renal tubule allow more Na⁺ to enter, which is then discharged into the circulation. To maintain tonicity water must enter with Na⁺. Such an effect must be specifically located in the distal tubule, since Klahr and Alleyne (1973) showed that in PEM reabsorption of Na⁺ in the proximal tubule is actually reduced. They therefore speculated that reabsorption must be increased distally. It is a little difficult, though not impossible, to visualize that a generalized stress—the toxic effect of free radicals—should operate so selectively.

Another possible mechanism for the production of oedema is that damage to the capillary endothelial cells could lead to increased leakage of albumin, as has been shown to occur in infections (Fleck *et al.*, 1985). At the same time the response to acute inflammation, which plays a prominent part in the free radical theory, involves diversion of export protein synthesis in the liver from albumin to acute phase proteins (Chapter 6). At this point the two theories, that of free radical damage and that of dietary protein deficiency, converge in providing an explanation for hypoalbuminaemia.

Conclusion

It is evident from this description that the factors which could promote the development of oedema are numerous, complex and interrelated. Most of those who have considered the subject have concluded that there is no single cause. Waterlow and Alleyne (1971), reviewing the evidence available up to that time, said 'hypoproteinaemia is a modifying factor and not the basic cause of the water and salt retention'. Similarly, Patrick (1979) concluded that 'provided the scene is set with a low albumin, any stimulus to sodium retention such as potassium depletion or inadequately treated acidosis may all lead to oedema'. In a more recent paper (Waterlow, 1984) I tentatively ranked hypoalbuminaemia as the number one cause and potassium deficiency as the number two, and I maintain that opinion.

Perhaps, however, a different approach may be more productive: that, from the point of view of pathogenesis, oedema in PEM is not a single entity. Clinically there is a great difference between 'classical' kwashiorkor and marasmic kwashiorkor. The former has only moderate deficits in weight and height, with relatively well preserved body fat. Plasma albumin may be very low and oedema generalized and gross, but the child responds quite easily to treatment. Admittedly Hay *et al.* (1975) and Vis (1985) found a close relationship between albumin concentration and mortality, but Vis's cases were mainly marasmic kwashiorkor. The fact remains that Gürson *et al.* (1976) quote no less than five authors in whose experience oedema did not carry a bad prognosis. In such cases, I suggest that hypoalbuminaemia is indeed the most important cause of oedema.

By contrast, the child with marasmic kwashiorkor, like the adult cases of famine oedema described in India, is grossly wasted and severely ill. In both, a history of prolonged dysentery and diarrhoea, perhaps leading to potassium deficiency, is characteristic. In Britain at the turn of the century Thomson (1908) and Still (1909) in their textbooks of paediatrics mentioned oedema occurring in marasmic children with a history of frequent attacks of diarrhoea, and the same pattern was described by the older German paediatricians. The fairly common finding of hyponatraemia in marasmic kwashiorkor is perhaps a sign of the generalized impairment of cellular composition and function described as the 'sick cell syndrome' (Chapter 4). It is here that damage by free radicals may be important. I suggest that in these cases factors other than hypoalbuminaemia, particularly potassium deficiency, play a dominant role in the production of oedema.

The cause of oedema is important and has been discussed at some length, because it has practical implications which will now be considered.

Aetiology of kwashiorkor

This phrase is shorthand for 'the causal factors determining the pathological changes characteristic of kwashiorkor'. We are concerned here with factors operating at the level of metabolism and nutrition rather than at the social and family level. Reviews of current thinking have been published by Golden (1985) and Jackson (1986*a*, 1990).

Although the presence of oedema has been accepted as essential for the diagnosis of kwashiorkor, in fact kwashiorkor is more than oedematous malnutrition. Any theory of cause, to be satisfactory, must also explain the other characteristic features of the syndrome, particularly fatty liver and skin lesions.

Why do some children develop kwashiorkor and others marasmus? The differences in clinical picture and pathology are complemented by differences in natural history and epidemiology (Fig. 11.5). However, in none of these characteristics are the syndromes clear-cut and distinct. There are always intermediate forms, blurring of distinctions, and overlap in almost every measurable characteristic. Nevertheless, the extremes are different and we need to know why.

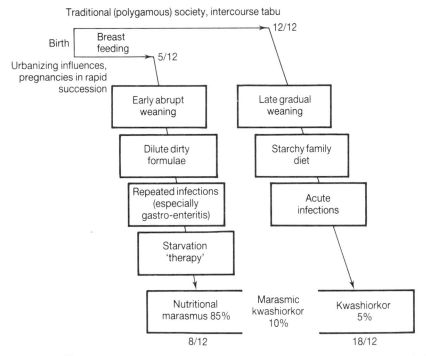

Fig. 11.5 Flow diagram illustrating the routes of evolution of marasmus and kwashiorkor. Reproduced by permission from McLaren (1966).

There are two principal theories: the classical theory of protein deficiency and the new theory of 'noxae' and free radical damage, of which the chief proponent and originator was Golden. The two theories emphasize, although not exclusively, different aspects of the environment: on the one hand the nutrients, on the other the stresses. Genetic differences in response are, of course, common to both. There are also some differences in the implications, which is why this whole question is more than academic. The protein deficiency theory has implications for nutrition policy but little impact on the treatment of established PEM. The free radical theory, described by Golden as 'holistic', brings together many features of the environment, but because none is singled out it provides no pointer to specific preventive action. On the other hand, its analysis of pathological processes has implications for treatment.

The classical theory of protein deficiency

The theory is called classical because it had its origin in Cicely Williams' observation that kwashiorkor developed in children weaned onto starchy paps, and was cured by milk. Dean and Whitehead, writing in 1964, said: 'Our experience has convinced us that the chief cause of kwashiorkor in Uganda is lack of protein in the diet'. Two points are important about this statement. First, protein deficiency in this context refers to the diet—one in which protein is inadequate or limiting in relation to energy (Chapter 2). The second point relates to the words 'chief cause'. It has always been recognized that kwashiorkor is multifactorial. If an inadequate protein intake does play a major role, it is likely to be accompanied by deficiencies of other nutrients associated with protein in foods, such as trace elements and vitamins of the B complex.

The protein deficiency theory relies on a causal chain with three links (Waterlow, 1984; Jackson, 1990). Starting with the agreed point that oedema is the prime feature of kwashiorkor, the links are as follows.

A. First link   Oedema is caused by hypoalbuminaemia. The discussion in the preceding section concluded that hypoalbuminaemia is probably a necessary condition, but not always a sufficient one. The theory can easily accommodate a role for potassium deficiency in the production of oedema, because potassium is associated with protein in foods. For the same reason it is compatible with the hypothesis that the skin lesions are caused by deficiency of zinc.

B. Second link   Hypoalbuminaemia is caused by an inadequate amino acid supply, which depresses albumin synthesis in the liver. For this there is strong experimental evidence (Chapter 6). The depression of synthesis may be reinforced by infections. The theory is strengthened by the association of fatty liver with oedema, if one accepts that the most probable cause of the fatty infiltration is depression of apolipoprotein synthesis, *pari passu* with that of albumin (Chapter 5). Experimental studies provided a convincing explanation of why a large deficit in energy intake, which we assume to be characteristic of marasmus, tends to inhibit the appearance of hypoalbuminaemia and fatty liver. These animal investigations have received some support from observations in the field (Whitehead *et al.*, 1977).

C. Third link   Children who develop kwashiorkor have had a protein-deficient diet, by which is meant a low concentration of protein in relation to energy. This is the weakest link in the chain and the one that has attracted the most serious criticism. There are, however, features in the natural history and epidemiology of kwashiorkor that provide some support for the hypothesis. Kwashiorkor is seldom seen in the first year of life; it usually presents in the second year or later, when the child is fully weaned, or at the best partially breast-fed, and may well have a low intake of protein (Chapter 16). Up to this point growth has been relatively good, as shown by the almost universal finding, wherever such measurements have been made, that children with kwashiorkor are less retarded in length than those with marasmus (Chapter 1, Fig. 1.1). Then something happens which precipitates the onset, often an infection, particularly measles. A further depression of albumin synthesis and increased leakiness of capillaries lead to the appearance of oedema in a child whose albumin status was already marginal.

There is also some epidemiological evidence, inconclusive but nevertheless relevant. As pointed out in Chapter 1, there do not exist any statistics for the real prevalence of kwashiorkor, only clinical data on hospital admissions, which do no more than give an indication of regions where it is relatively common or where it is seldom seen. It may be noted in passing that kwashiorkor seems nowadays to be less common than it was when this story began. It seems to occur more often in a rural than an urban setting. Even in Calcutta, probably one of the world's poorest cities, kwashiorkor is now less often seen (A. K. Bhattacharyya, personal communication). It was described more frequently in regions where the staple cereal is low in protein or contains protein of poor quality: in Mexico, Central America and South Africa where the staple is maize; in Uganda, where it is plantain; in Jamaica, where a common weaning diet is refined cornmeal and sugar. This list could be extended, but what is really needed is a world-wide epidemiological survey. On the other hand, kwashiorkor was much less often described in regions where the staple is wheat, such as Northern India and the Middle East. McLaren (1966), one of the few who attempted a systematic estimate of relative prevalence, reported that in Jordan 85 per cent of cases of PEM were marasmus and only 15 per cent kwashiorkor or marasmic kwashiorkor. Annegers (1973) observed that in West Africa, as one proceeds from north to south, the prevalence of kwashiorkor was low in the Sahel, where the staple is millet, and much higher on the coast, where the staple is cassava.

This, in brief, is the case for the protein deficiency theory, a theory now described as outdated and 'effete' (Landman and Jackson, 1980). The first serious attack on it was mounted by Gopalan (1968), ironically at a meeting organized by McCance, who on the basis of his experiments on pigs and his observations in Uganda, was a firm believer in protein deficiency (McCance, 1968). Gopalan described a prospective study on some 2000 children, of whom about 1.5 per cent developed kwashiorkor and a somewhat higher proportion marasmus. No quantitative or qualitative differences were found in the diets of these two groups of children. Gopalan re-emphasized the point made earlier (Waterlow *et al.*, 1960), that the two conditions are inter-convertible. The essence of Gopalan's view is that the outcome is determined not by the diet but by the child's response. He went on to describe marasmus as an adapted state and kwashiorkor as a dysadaptation, but this terminology does little to clarify the issue. Rao (1974) suggested that the difference in the clinical picture could be explained by inborn differences in the pattern of endocrine changes. This explanation seems to be putting causality the wrong way round, in view of the well established experimental evidence on endocrine responses to different diets (Waterlow, 1974; Alleyne *et al.*, 1977).

Laditan and Reeds (1976) studied a series of cases of PEM in Nigeria, classified according to the Wellcome system. In both marasmus and kwashiorkor, the diets fed after weaning were identical and consisted solely of a maize-starch gruel. They commented: 'The similarity in the dietary histories suggests some uncertainty concerning a specific role for protein deficiency in the development of kwashiorkor'. They did, however, note differences in the pattern of infection: children with marasmus had a longer history of *chronic* diarrhoea.

Gopalan's basic point, however, is valid; children differ in their nutrient requirements (Chapter 16) and therefore may be expected to differ in their response to the same marginal intake. Energy may be limiting for one child, who will thus become marasmic; protein may be limiting for another who, on the classical theory, would develop kwashiorkor. In every community in which it has been described, kwashiorkor occurs in only a small proportion of children, who perhaps represent the upper tail of the distribution of protein requirements. If this is correct, Gopalan's observations could be accommodated by the protein deficiency theory.

The next hole in the argument was driven by McLaren (1975) in an important article with the title 'The great protein fiasco'. The thrust of the paper was an attack on the wasteful expenditure of time and money by the UN Agencies in the unnecessary promotion of high protein weaning foods (United Nations, 1968). The ammunition was provided by the publication in 1973 of a report on energy and protein requirements by a committee of FAO/WHO. On the basis of these estimates it was argued that no diets of pre-school children anywhere in the world could be deficient in protein (Waterlow and Payne, 1975). Published figures for the intakes of young children were and still are regrettably scanty, but they consistently showed intakes of protein above the 1973 requirements and intakes of energy below them. This seemed to spell the end of the protein deficiency theory.

However, such a judgement may be premature. In the more recent UN report (WHO, 1985) estimates of energy requirements were somewhat reduced and more recent work suggests that even those lower estimates may be too high (Chapter 16). Protein requirements of young children were maintained at about the same level as in 1973. In my opinion the pendulum swung too far in the 1970s, and it is entirely possible that some Third World children have food intakes that fail to meet their protein needs. If that conclusion is correct it has practical implications. We need to look again, without preconceived ideas, at the condition of children in regions where the weaning diet is particularly low in protein.

Before leaving the subject it should be noted that the protein deficiency theory of kwashiorkor has to cope with a paradox: it is contended later (Chapter 13) that stunting in linear growth may be caused by deficiency of good quality protein. How can this be reconciled with the fact that children with kwashiorkor are typically less stunted than those with marasmus or marasmic kwashiorkor? If the hypothesis about stunting is correct, one way of resolving the contradiction is to suppose that stunting results from a long-standing and continuing marginal deficiency, whereas the development of kwashiorkor is a more acute process.

In conclusion, I see no reason to abandon the essential concepts put forward many years ago of the pathogenesis of kwashiorkor and marasmus, which, at the risk of some repetition, may be summarized as follows.

1. Kwashiorkor develops when the diet has a low protein-energy (P/E) ratio (Chapter 16), so that protein and the vitamins and minerals associated with protein in foods are limiting.
2. Since children vary in their requirements for nutrients, if the P/E ratio is marginal, protein may be a limiting factor for some children but not for others.
3. As we have seen in Chapter 8, the initial endocrine responses to such a diet in which energy is not limiting are a high plasma insulin and a low plasma cortisol level. The effect of this hormonal pattern is to promote the uptake of amino acids in muscle and to divert them from the liver.
4. As a consequence, there is a reduced synthesis of albumin, leading to hypoalbuminaemia, and of apolipoproteins, leading to fatty liver. These effects are exaggerated by an acute infection, which further diverts amino acids to the synthesis of acute phase proteins.
5. When energy is limiting, either primarily because of an inadequate food intake, or secondarily because of repeated and long-continued infections, there is the opposite hormonal pattern—low insulin and high cortisol. Amino acids are released from muscle and are available for the synthesis of specific proteins in the liver, so that the characteristic features of kwashiorkor do not develop and the end result is marasmus. As Trowell put it succinctly, 'the marasmic lives on his own meat'.

The free radical theory

Golden and his colleagues have developed the theory of free radicals as a cause of kwashiorkor in a number of reviews (Golden, 1985; Golden and Ramdath, 1987; Golden *et al.*, 1990). It is summarized by Golden *et al.* (1990) as follows.

> We have put forward the argument that kwashiorkor results from an imbalance between the production of free radicals and their safe disposal. The proposed unifying hypothesis, which would account for all the factors described, is that the various noxae to which these children are ubiquitously exposed, produce an oxidative toxic stress which leads to excess free radical, peroxide and carbonyl generation. These toxic products cause damage because the mechanisms for their safe disposal are generally compromised. The impaired state of the body's anti-oxidant defence is directly caused by the inadequate diets that these children consume.

The theory is described as 'holistic' because it implicates a wide range of nutritional deficiencies on the one hand and of environmental noxae on the other. This diversity is a source of strength and of weakness. It is satisfying to bring together so many different factors operating through a final common pathway of free radical damage. Whereas the protein deficiency theory concerns itself principally with one feature, oedema, and to a lesser extent with fatty liver, the free radical theory aims to explain the whole range of characteristics of kwashiorkor. The diversity, however, makes it more difficult to define clearly the causal sequence.

As with the protein deficiency theory, we can postulate three links in the causal chain.

A. First link   Children with kwashiorkor, compared to those with marasmus, have been more exposed to noxae that generate oxidative stress (A1); or to factors that compromise defence against free radicals (A2). As regards A1, it has never been shown, as far as we know, that children who develop kwashiorkor have been more exposed to infections, although the pattern of infections may be different. Measles is often mentioned as precipitating kwashiorkor, particularly in Africa, whereas diarrhoeal disease is prominent in the background of marasmus. It is not clear that this difference has any relevance for free radical generation. One could speculate that if children with kwashiorkor had had a higher energy intake, there would have been more substrate for bacterial overgrowth in the bowel. Hendrickse and his colleagues have proposed that kwashiorkor results from aflatoxin poisoning, but their results do not show any very clear difference between kwashiorkor and marasmus in the amounts of aflatoxin or its metabolites present in urine, plasma or tissues (Hendrickse, 1984; Coulter *et al.*, 1988).

As far as A2 is concerned no evidence has been adduced that diets of children with kwashiorkor are more deficient in factors that protect against free radical damage, such as β-carotene, vitamin E, selenium or zinc. However, if in relation to Gopalan's findings cited above, we accept that children may differ in their requirements for protein and energy, we must also accept differences in their requirements for other essential nutrients.

B. Second link   There should be evidence of greater free radical damage in kwashiorkor than in marasmus. Of the measurements that have been made so far (Chapter 10), four fulfil this criterion: red cell glutathione, serum ferritin, urinary excretion of mercapturic acids and the proportion of red cell NADP that is in the oxidized form. Considering the rough and ready nature of the clinical classification, this is an impressive set of differences. It should not be taken as evidence against the free radical theory that in kwashiorkor and marasmus no difference was found in some of the other variables measured, such as enzymes concerned with the disposal of toxic products, e.g. glutathione peroxidase. Enzyme activity measured *in vitro* does not tell one very much about the flux through the pathway *in vivo*.

C. Third link   Free radicals should be demonstrable causes of the specific features of kwashiorkor. It is an important part of the theory that free radicals or their products cause damage to cell membranes. Ways have been proposed in the previous chapter by which such damage might produce oedema. Free radicals have also been held responsible for the fatty liver, by analogy with Reye's disease and with the effects of infections and poisons (Golden *et al.*, 1990), but this, we have argued in Chapter 5, is a misconception, which does not take account of the detailed pathology.

Golden has also suggested that ultraviolet radiation, which generates free radicals, may be responsible for the skin lesions of kwashiorkor. They do tend to occur in exposed parts, which is why some workers originally attributed them to pellagra. The skin lesions are one of the more variable features of kwashiorkor; this suggests that more than one factor may be involved, and the other factor is probably zinc deficiency (Golden *et al.*, 1980*b*).

In my view the causal links in the free radical theory of kwashiorkor are not yet very firmly established, but these are early days; so far kwashiorkor has been studied from this point of view in only one centre, Jamaica. The theory has also not yet been subjected to the test of animal experiments. Perhaps, however, it is not so important whether damage by free radicals can account for the classical features of kwashiorkor; what is more important is whether this sequence of events can explain the undue severity and fatal outcome in some cases of PEM, particularly those described as marasmic kwashiorkor. The free radical theory has done a service in drawing attention to factors and processes in the pathogenesis of severe PEM that have previously been neglected, and it has important implications for treatment. The implications of the protein deficiency theory are different; they lie more in the field of nutrition policy and public health.

References

Abbrecht, P. H., Vandar, A. J. (1970). Effects of chronic potassium deficiency on plasma renin activity. *Journal of Clinical Investigation* **49**: 1510–1516.

Alleyne, G. A. O. (1966). The excretion of water and salt by malnourished children. *West Indian Medical Journal* **15**: 150–154.

Alleyne, G. A. O., Hay, R. W. *et al.* (1977). *Protein-energy malnutrition*. Edward Arnold, London.

Annegers, J. F. (1973). Ecology of dietary patterns and nutritional status in West Africa. *Ecology of Food and Nutrition* **2**: 107–119.

Bearn, A. G., Litwin, S. G. (1978). Deficiencies of circulating enzymes and plasma proteins. In Stanbury, J. B., Wyngaarden, J. B., Frederickson, D. S. (eds) *The metabolic basis of inherited disease*. McGraw Hill, New York, pp. 1712–1725.

Beattie, J., Herbert, P. H., Bell, D. J. (1948). Famine oedema. *British Journal of Nutrition* **2**: 47–65.

Bose, J. P., De, U. N., Mukerjee, P. (1946). A preliminary study of the biochemical changes in starvation cases. *Indian Journal of Medical Research* **34**: 143–150.

Bras, G., Hill, K. R. (1956). Veno-occlusive disease of the liver: essential pathology. *Lancet* **2**: 161–163.

Brock, J. F., Hansen, J. D. L. *et al.* (1955). Kwashiorkor and protein malnutrition: a dietary therapeutic trial. *Lancet* **2**: 355–360.

Coulter, J. B. S., Suliman, G. I. *et al.* (1988). Protein-energy malnutrition in Northern Sudan: clinical studies. *European Journal of Clinical Nutrition* **42**: 787–796.

Coward, W. A. (1975). Serum colloidal osmotic pressure in the development of kwashiorkor and in recovery: its relationship to albumin and globulin concentrations and oedema. *British Journal of Nutrition* **34**: 459–467.

Dean, R. F. A., Whitehead, R. G. (1964). Plasma aminograms in kwashiorkor. *Lancet* **2**: 98–99.

Fiorotto, M. L., Nichols, B. L. (1982). Oedema of malnutrition. *Lancet* **2**: 871.

Fleck, A., Raines, G., Hawker, F. (1985). Increased vascular permeability: a major cause of hypoalbuminaemia in disease and injury. *Lancet* **1**: 781–784.

Food and Agriculture Organization (1973). *Energy and protein requirements.* Report of a Joint FAO/WHO *Ad Hoc* Expert Committee. FAO Nutrition Meetings Report Series No. 52. FAO, Rome.

Frood, J. D. L., Whitehead, R. G., Coward, W. A. (1971). Relationship between pattern of infection and development of hypoalbuminaemia and hypo-β-lipoproteinaemia in rural Ugandan children. *Lancet* **2:** 1047–1049.

Godard, C. M., Muñoz, M. *et al.* (1986). A study of the renin-aldosterone system in severe infantile malnutrition. *International Journal of Pediatric Nephrology* **7:** 39–44.

Golden, M. H. N. (1982). Protein deficiency, energy deficiency and the oedema of malnutrition. *Lancet* **1:** 1261–1265.

Golden, M. H. N. (1985). The consequences of protein deficiency in man and its relationship to the features of kwashiorkor. In Blaxter, K. L., Waterlow, J. C. (eds) *Nutritional adaptation in man.* John Libbey, London, pp. 169–188.

Golden, M. H. N., Ramdath, D. (1987). Free radicals in the pathogenesis of kwashiorkor. *Proceedings of the Nutrition Society* **46:** 53–68.

Golden, M. H. N., Golden, B. E., Jackson, A. A. (1980*a*). Albumin and nutritional oedema. *Lancet* **1:** 114–116.

Golden, M. H. N., Golden, B. E., Jackson, A. A. (1980*b*). Skin breakdown in kwashiorkor responds to zinc. *Lancet* **1:** 1256.

Golden, M. H. N., Ramdath, D. D., Golden, B. E. (1991). Free radicals and malnutrition. In Dreosti, I. E. (ed) *Trace elements, micronutrients and free radicals.* Humana Press, Clifton, New Jersey. In press

Gopalan, C. (1950). Antidiuretic factor in the urines of patients with nutritional oedema. *Lancet* **1:** 304–306.

Gopalan, C. (1968). Kwashiorkor and marasmus. Evolution and distinguishing features. In McCance, R. A., Widdowson, E. M. (eds) *Calorie deficiencies and protein deficiencies.* Churchill, London, pp. 49–58.

Gopalan, C., Venkatachalam, P. S. *et al.* (1952). Studies on nutritional oedema. *Indian Journal of Medical Science* **6:** 277–295.

Gounelle, H. (1962). Carence protéiques. *Gazette Médicale de la France* **69:** 3–47.

Gürson, C. T., Yüksel, T., Saner, G. (1976). The short-term prognosis of protein-calorie malnutrition in Marmara region of Turkey. *Journal of Tropical Pediatrics and Environmental Child Health* **22:** 59–62.

Guyton, A. C. (1981). Capillary dynamics and exchange of fluid between the blood and interstitial fluid. In Guyton, A. C. (ed) *Textbook of medical physiology*, 6th edn. W. B. Saunders, Philadelphia, pp. 358–382.

Hansen, J. D. L. (1956). Electrolyte and nitrogen metabolism in kwashiorkor. *South African Journal of Laboratory Clinical Medicine* **2:** 206–231.

Hay, R. W., Whitehead, R. G., Spicer, C. C. (1975). Serum albumin as a prognostic indicator in oedematous malnutrition. *Lancet* **2:** 427–429.

Hendrickse, R. G. (1984). The influence of aflatoxins on child health in the tropics with particular reference to kwashiorkor. *Transactions of the Royal Society of Tropical Medicine and Hygiene* **78:** 427–435.

Jackson, A. A. (1986*a*). Severe undernutrition in Jamaica. Kwashiorkor and marasmus: the disease of the weanling. *Acta Paediatrica Scandinavica* Suppl. **323:** 43–51.

Jackson, A. A. (1986*b*). Blood glutathione in severe malnutrition in childhood. *Transactions of the Royal Society of Tropical Medicine and Hygiene* **80:** 911–913.

Jackson, A. A. (1990). The aetiology of kwashiorkor. In Harrison, G. A., Waterlow, J. C. (eds) *Diet and disease in traditional and developing societies.* Cambridge University Press, pp. 76–113.

Joles, J. A., Jansen, E. H. J. M. *et al.* (1989). Plasma proteins in growing analbuminaemic rats fed on a diet of low protein content. *British Journal of Nutrition* **61:** 485–495.

Klahr, S., Alleyne, G. A. O. (1973). Effects of chronic protein-calorie malnutrition on the kidney. *Kidney International* **3**: 129–141.

Kritzinger, E. E., Kanengoni, E., Jones, J. J. (1972). Effective renin activity in plasma of children with kwashiorkor. *Lancet* **1**: 412.

Kurnick, N. B. (1948). War oedema in the civilian population of Saipan. *Annals of Internal Medicine* **28**: 782–791.

Laditan, A. A. O., Reeds, P. J. (1976). A study of the age of onset, diet and the importance of infection in the pattern of severe protein-energy malnutrition in Ibadan, Nigeria. *British Journal of Nutrition* **36**: 411–419.

Landman, J., Jackson, A. A. (1980). The role of protein deficiency in the aetiology of kwashiorkor. *West Indian Medical Journal* **29**: 229–238.

McCance, R. A. (1951). The history, significance and aetiology of hunger oedema. In *Studies of undernutrition, Wuppertal, 1946–49*. Medical Research Council Special Report Series No. 275. HM Stationery Office, London, pp. 21–82.

McCance, R. A. (1968). The effect of calorie deficiencies and protein deficiencies on final weight and stature. In McCance, R. A., Widdowson, E. M. (eds) *Calorie deficiencies and protein deficiencies*. Churchill, London, pp. 319–328.

McLaren, D. S. (1966). A fresh look at protein-calorie malnutrition. *Lancet* **2**: 485–488.

McLaren, D. S. (1975). The protein fiasco. *Lancet* **2**: 93–96.

Migeon, C. J., Beitins, I. Z. *et al.* (1973). Plasma aldosterone concentration and aldosterone secretion rates in Peruvian infants with marasmus and kwashiorkor. In Gardner, L. I., Arnacher, P. (eds) *Endocrine aspects of malnutrition*. Kroc Foundation, Santa Ynez, California, pp. 399–424.

Mönckeberg, F. (ed). *Desnutricion infantil: fisiopatología, clínica, tratamiento y prevención: nuestra experiencia y contribución*. Instituto de Nutricion y Tecnologia de los Alimentos, Santiago, Chile.

Montgomery, R. D. (1963). The relation of oedema to serum proteins and pseudocholinesterase levels in the malnourished infant. *Archives of Disease in Childhood* **38**: 343–348.

Mukherjee, K. L., Chaudhuri, R. N., Werner, G. (1954). Plasma volume and thiocyanate space in nutritional oedema. *Proceedings of the National Institute of Science, India* **20**: 151–156.

Patrick, J. (1979). Oedema in protein energy malnutrition: the role of the sodium pump. *Proceedings of the Nutrition Society* **38**: 61–68.

Ramalingaswami, V., Deo, M. G. *et al.* (1971). Studies of the Bihar famine of 1966–67. In *A symposium dealing with nutrition and relief operations in times of disaster*. Studies of the Swedish Nutrition Foundation IX. Almqvist and Wiksell, Stockholm.

Ramdath, D., Golden, M. H. N. (1989). Non-haematological aspects of iron nutrition. *Nutrition Research Reviews* **2**: 29–50.

Rao, K. S. J. (1974). Evolution of kwashiorkor and marasmus. *Lancet* **1**: 709–711.

Rhodes, K. (1957). Two types of liver disease in Jamaican children. *West Indian Medical Journal* **6**: 1–161.

Simpson, F. O. (1988). Sodium intake, body sodium and sodium excretion. *Lancet* **2**: 25–29.

Sinatra, F. R., Merritt, R. J. (1981). Iatrogenic kwashiorkor in infants. *American Journal of Diseases in Children* **135**: 21–23.

Sinclair, H. M. (1948). Nutritional oedema. *Proceedings of the Royal Society of Medicine* **41**: 541–544.

Srikantia, S. G., Gopalan, C. (1959). Role of ferritin in nutritional oedema. *American Journal of Applied Physiology* **14**: 829–833.

Srikantia, S. G., Mohanham, S. (1970). Antidiuretic hormone values in plasma and urine of malnourished children. *Journal of Clinical Endocrinology* **31**: 312–314.

Still, G. F. (1909). *Common disorders and diseases of childhood*, 1st edn. Oxford University Press, London, p. 141.

Thomson, J. (1908). *Clinical examinations of sick children*, 2nd edn. William Green, Edinburgh and London, p. 176.

Tripathi, R. M., Agrawal, K. K., Agarwal, K. N. (1983). Oedema fluid composition in childhood disorders. *Acta Paediatrica Scandinavica* **72:** 741–745.

Trowell, H. C., Muwazi, E. M. K. (1945). Severe and prolonged underfeeding in African children. (The kwashiorkor syndrome of malignant malnutrition.) *Archives of Disease in Childhood* **20:** 110–116.

Trowell, H. C., Davies, J. N. P., Dean, R. F. A. (1954). *Kwashiorkor.* Part IV. Protein malnutrition in adults. Academic Press, London. (Reprinted 1982).

United Nations (1968). *International action to avert the impending protein crisis.* Report to the Economic and Social Council of the Advisory Committee on the Application of Science and Technology to Development. United Nations, New York.

Vis, H. L. (1985). On the treatment of certain forms of protein-energy malnutrition in childhood with respect to fatal complications (an example from rural Central Africa). *Annales Nestlé* **43:** 19–30.

Walter, S. J., Shore, A. C. *et al.* (1988). Effect of potassium depletion on renal tubular function in the rat. *Clinical Science* **75:** 621–628.

Waterlow, J. C. (1974). Evolution of kwashiorkor and marasmus. *Lancet* **2:** 712.

Waterlow, J. C. (1984). Kwashiorkor revisited: the pathogenesis of oedema in kwashiorkor and its significance. *Transactions of the Royal Society of Tropical Medicine and Hygiene* **78:** 436–441.

Waterlow, J. C., Alleyne, G. A. O. (1971). Protein malnutrition: advances in knowledge in the last 10 years. *Advances in Protein Chemistry* **25:** 117–242.

Waterlow, J. C., Payne, P. R. (1975). The protein gap. *Nature (London)* **258:** 113–117.

Waterlow, J. C., Cravioto, J., Stephen, J. M. L. (1960). Protein malnutrition in man. *Advances in Protein Chemistry* **15:** 131–238.

Weech, A. A. (1939). The significance of the albumin fraction of the serum. *Bulletin of the New York Academy of Medicine* **15:** 63–91.

Weech, A. A., Ling, S. M. (1931). Nutritional edemas: observations on the relation of the serum proteins to the occurrence of edema and to the effect of certain inorganic salts. *Journal of Clinical Investigation* **10:** 869–887.

Weech, A. A., Snelling, C. E., Goeltsch, E. (1933). Relation between plasma protein content, plasma specific gravity and edema in dogs maintained on a protein-inadequate diet and in dogs rendered edematous by plasmaphoresis. *Journal of Clinical Investigation* **12:** 193–216.

Whitehead, R. G., Coward, W. A., Lunn, P. G. (1973). Serum albumin concentration and the onset of kwashiorkor. *Lancet* **1:** 63–66.

Whitehead, R. G., Coward, W. A. *et al.* (1977). A comparison of the pathogenesis of protein-energy malnutrition in Uganda and The Gambia. *Transactions of the Royal Society of Tropical Medicine and Hygiene* **71:** 189–195.

World Health Organization (1985). *Energy and protein requirements.* Report of a Joint FAO/WHO/UNU Expert Consultation. Technical Report Series No. 724. WHO, Geneva.

12

Treatment of severe PEM

Where should children be treated?

In 1971 Cook asked the question: 'Is hospital the place for the treatment of malnourished children?' Sadre and Donoso (1969) expressed the view that hospital treatment of PEM was a waste of time and money, because about one-third of the children died in hospital and a further one-third after discharge. Table 12.1 shows figures for case-fatality rates in hospital. Comparisons between different centres are clearly inappropriate, because of differences in the criteria for admission and the prevalence and type of infec-

Table 12.1 Death rates in hospital of children with PEM

Place	Date of publication	Death rate (% of cases)	Author
Mexico	1956	31	Gómez et al.
South Africa	1959	20	Kahn
India, Calcutta	1961	15	Chaudhuri et al.
Jamaica	1962	16	Garrow et al.
Mexico	1965	30	Ramos-Galván and Calderón
Lebanon	1969	28	McLaren and Shirajian
India, Tamil Nadu	1974	10.5	Pereira and Begum
Sudan	1975	16	Omer et al.
Nigeria	1976	28	Reeds and Laditan
	1983	32	Laditan and Tineimebwa
Bangladesh	1981	21	Brown et al.
Zaïre	1985	{ 37 in 1977 13 in 1982	Vis
Tanzania	1986	9	Van Roosmalen-Wiebenga
Lesotho	1986	25	Tolboom et al.
Guyana	1987	{ 51 in 1982 29 in 1986	Sinha
Sudan	1988	20	Coulter et al.
Niger	1989	14.5	Soutif

In all studies the data were collected over varying periods of time, which are usually not stated exactly. When comparative data are given for more than one period, they have been indicated separately (Zaïre, Guyana).

tions, as well as in the facilities. Measles, for example, will completely distort the picture, because when it supervenes in a severely malnourished child, the case-fatality rate may be as high as 60 per cent (Vis, 1985). The distribution of deaths in relation to time in hospital is shown in Table 12.2. Some children reach hospital in such a precarious state that perhaps the stress of being transported and examined is the last straw and they die almost immediately. This is not an argument against hospital treatment; it is an argument for earlier referral. We believe that the great majority of deaths after the first day are preventable.

Table 12.2   Distribution of deaths: days after admission to hospital

	% of all deaths	
	Mexico[a]	Jamaica[b]
Day 1	30	39
Days 2–7	48	48
Days > 7	22	13

[a] Gómez *et al.* (1956)
[b] Garrow *et al.* (1962)

The disadvantages of hospital treatment are obvious: expense, risk of cross-infection, emotional deprivation if the mother is not able to be with the child. Moreover, the results after discharge are often very unsatisfactory. Almost 20 years after Cook's paper, follow-up studies have shown a death rate of 10 per cent or more after discharge from hospital, with extremely high rates in those who absconded before they had completed the hospital treatment (Table 12.3).

The alternatives that have been proposed to hospital treatment are nutrition rehabilitation centres (NRC), which are discussed below, and treatment in the home. Khare *et al.* (1976) reported the results of domiciliary treatment of kwashiorkor with monthly visits from primary health care workers. No children died and modest gains in nutritional status were recorded over 15 months. A more recent study in Indonesia (Husaini *et al.*, 1982) of the results of treating children with PEM as out-patients at a nutrition clinic is less

Table 12.3   Deaths after discharge from hospital

Country	Period of follow-up after discharge (months)	% died after discharge or absconding	Average duration of stay in hospital (days)
Zaïre[a]	12	9.5	79
Tanzania[b]	6–36		
discharged		9	15
absconded		41	10
Niger[c]	3–16		
discharged		17	20
absconded		47	13

[a] Hennart *et al.* (1987)
[b] Van Roosmalen-Wiebenga (1986)
[c] Soutif (1989)

encouraging (Table 12.4). It is to be noted that these children were described as 'third degree malnutrition but not severely ill'.

Treatment in hospital or outside hospital should not be regarded as alternatives but complementary. I believe that some children with PEM are so gravely ill that they will almost inevitably die without paediatric and nursing care. Admittedly the outcome of hospital treatment has often been very unsatisfactory, but the response should not be to abandon hospital treatment, but wherever facilities are available, to improve it. The function of treatment in clinics or through the primary health care system is to prevent children getting into the state where they need hospital care.

Table 12.4   Out-patient treatment of severe PEM

	No. of cases	
Initially seen	108	
Drop outs	41	
		% of total
Total in whom outcome known	67	100
Died	18	27
Completed the study (6 months)	49	73
Condition at 6 months:		
unchanged	9	13
mild/moderate PEM	33	50
well-nourished	7	10

Adapted from Husaini *et al.* (1982)

Criteria for admission to hospital

Since hospital facilities are everywhere limited, criteria are needed for selecting those most at risk. Suggested guidelines are listed in Table 12.5. Like all guidelines, these have to be interpreted flexibly, according to local conditions. It may be difficult to decide about the admission of marasmic children when they do not present complications. The Wellcome cut-off point for marasmus, 60 per cent of expected weight for age (Chapter 1) is not entirely suitable for screening for admission to hospital. Weight for length is a better predictor of *acute* risk than weight for age (Chapter 14); since marasmic

Table 12.5   Criteria for selection of cases to be admitted to hospital

Substantial weight deficit, e.g. < 70% of standard weight for height or < 60% of standard weight for age, with:
   oedema (marasmic kwashiorkor)
   severe dehydration
   persistent diarrhoea and/or vomiting
   extreme pallor, hypothermia, clinical evidence of 'shock'
   signs of systemic, respiratory tract or other localized infection
   severe anaemia (Hb < 5 g/dl)
   jaundice
   purpura
   persistent loss of appetite
   age < 1 year

children are often severely stunted, weight for age will overestimate the severity of acute malnutrition.

Oedema without other complications also presents a problem. It has been suggested that all children with oedema should be classified as third degree, i.e. severe, PEM. However, the general experience (see below) is that oedema in itself is not an important risk factor. The most urgent risks that demand medical attention are the complications.

Treatment

Detailed accounts of the treatment of severe PEM in hospital are to be found in Picou *et al.* (1975), Waterlow *et al.* (1978), WHO (1981), Jackson and Golden (1987), Golden (1988) and Mönckeberg (1988). Treatment can be divided into three phases: (1) initial, mainly of complications; (2) intermediate, or initiation of cure; (3) rehabilitation. Phases (1) and (2) require close supervision in hospital; for phase (3) a nutrition rehabilitation unit should be quite adequate.

The underlying physiological changes, as compared with values found after recovery, are shown in Table 12.6, which summarizes results presented in previous chapters. The table shows how profound and widespread are the deviations from normal function and illustrates the difficulty of the task with which the clinician is confronted.

The principal causes of early death are listed in Table 12.7. These very ill children are intolerant of being handled, so clinical examination, blood sampling and other procedures should be kept to a minimum.

Table 12.6 Physiological changes in malnourished children and in children after recovery to normal weight for height

Physiological change	Malnourished (M)	Recovered (R)	$\frac{M-R}{R}$ (%)
Metabolic rate, kJ/kg$^{0.75}$/day	315	417	−24
Sodium pump activity, turnover of pool per hour	3.62	4.94	−27
Intracellular sodium, mmol/kg DS[a]	169	109	+55
Intracellular potassium, mmol/kg DS[a]	341	387	−12
Protein synthesis, g/kg/day	4.0	6.3	−37
Protein breakdown, g/kg/day	3.7	6.4	−42
Cardiac output, l/min/m^3	4.77	6.90	−31
Stroke volume, ml/beat/m^3	44.1	53.0	−22
Circulation time, seconds	13.7	10.5	+30
Glomerular filtration rate, ml/min/m^3	47.1	92.4	−41
Renal blood flow, ml/min/m^3	249	321	−22
H$^+$ excretion after NH$_4$Cl, μequiv/min	10.4	28.4	−63
Osmolal clearance rate, ml/min	0.20	0.66	−70
Sodium excreted, % of infused	22.3	48.7	−54
Sodium excreted, % of sodium filtered			
normal ECF	0.50	1.23	−59
expanded ECF	0.82	11.07	−93
Response to temperature change	poikilotherm	homoeotherm	

These values, reproduced by permission of Golden (1988), in some instances differ slightly from those presented in previous chapters.
a DS = dry solids

Table 12.7   Causes of death in severe PEM

Dehydration and electrolyte disturbances
Over-treatment with fluids
Cardiac failure
Undiagnosed and untreated infections
Severe anaemia
Liver failure (massive hepatomegaly and jaundice)
Hypoglycaemia and hypothermia

Phase 1: treatment of acute complications

Fluid and electrolyte disturbances

Dehydration as a result of diarrhoea and vomiting is a common complication of PEM. The clinical signs are summarized in Table 12.8. In cases of marasmic kwashiorkor evidence of dehydration may co-exist with oedema. Estimates of the severity of dehydration from clinical signs alone are not very reliable, but in most cases that is all that we have to go on. The severity can be determined retrospectively from the gain in weight over 24 hours; by this criterion clinicians tend to overestimate it (Mackenzie *et al.*, 1989).

Some guidelines for fluid therapy in the first 24 hours are shown in Table 12.9. The intravenous route should be avoided unless dehydration is severe

Table 12.8   Signs of severe dehydration in children with PEM

Child limp, apathetic or unconscious
Rapid weak pulse
Skin pale and cold, with decreased turgor
Sunken eyes and fontanelle
Dry mucosae
Absence of tears when crying
Urine volume decreased

Table 12.9   Intravenous fluid replacement for dehydration in children with PEM

Time period	Fluid administered	Rate of infusion
1–2 hours	Hartmann's solution or Ringer-lactate or glucose (50 g/l) in 0.5N saline (4.5 g NaCl/l) with NaHCO$_3$ (2.8 g/l)	20 ml/kg/hour
2–12 hours	glucose (50 g/l) in 0.2N saline (1.8 g NaCl/l)	10 ml/kg/hour
12–24 hours	glucose (50 g/l) in 0.2N saline	5 ml/kg/hour
After 24 hours	glucose (50 g/l) in 0.2N saline	75 ml/kg/day (maintenance requirement)
After urine has been passed	1.5 g KCl/l added to infusion solution	

and should be continued for the shortest possible time because of the danger
of overloading the heart. The earliest sign of overload is an increase in the
respiration rate, which should be monitored frequently in children on an
intravenous drip. In the early days in Jamaica, when fluids were frequently
given intravenously, many children at autopsy had pulmonary oedema.

Severely malnourished children, particularly if young, are often too weak
to take fluids from a cup or bottle, so the preferred method is by nasogastric
drip. The solution recommended by WHO (1976) (Table 12.10) for oral
rehydration is the same as that used in the field (Chapter 17). However, in
Jamaica we have preferred to give less sodium and more glucose, on the
grounds that these children have a sodium overload (Chapter 4), and they
desperately need glucose as a fuel for maintaining basic processes such as
heat production, protein synthesis and ion pumps. We have not found that this
amount of glucose leads to malabsorption and osmotic diarrhoea (Chapter 6).

Table 12.10 Composition of glucose-electrolyte solutions for oral therapy in mildly or
moderately dehydrated children with PEM

	WHO, 1976		TMRU, Jamaica	
	(g/l)	(mmol/l)	(g/l)	(mmol/l)
Sodium chloride	3.5	60	1.8	31
Sodium bicarbonate	2.5	30	–	–
Potassium chloride	1.5	20	1.5	23
Glucose	20	110	50	280

Most workers accept that children with severe PEM are deficient in both
potassium and magnesium (Chapter 4), although Vis (1985) has said that
these deficiencies have not been observed in Zaïre. Potassium supplements
(4 mmol/kg/day) should be provided as a routine from the earliest stages of
treatment. Some paediatricians have been concerned that it may be dangerous
to give potassium until a good urine flow has been established, but in our
experience there have been no ill effects. The clinical signs of magnesium
deficiency have been described (Chapter 4). Treatment is to give magnesium
sulphate, 25 per cent w/v intravenously in a dose of 0.5 ml/kg. Magnesium,
like potassium, should be added to the rehydration solution even in the
absence of clinical signs. Golden (1988) has suggested that magnesium chloride or sulphate may promote acidosis and therefore recommends that magnesium chloride should be balanced by an appropriate amount of potassium
acetate. Unless diarrhoea is severe, rehydration should be complete in 24
hours.

Persistent vomiting and diarrhoea are not in themselves indications for
parenteral treatment. Vomiting is best dealt with by a nasogastric drip. It is
now generally accepted that 'resting the gut' is not the best way of treating
diarrhoea. Roediger (1986) has suggested that in grossly malnourished children diarrhoea is in large measure due to mucosal malnutrition. Glucose
or dilute milk formulae given by mouth stimulate regeneration of the gut
epithelium. It would be logical to give glutamine, which is an important
substrate for nitrogen and energy metabolism in the gut, but to our knowledge
this has not been tried. Malabsorption is minimized if the feeds are given

continuously by nasogastric drip, or frequently and in small amounts by mouth.

More often than not no specific pathogens are isolated from the stools. The most probable cause of diarrhoea is bacterial colonization of the small intestine (Chapter 5). The treatment recommended is metronidazole, 300 mg/day for six days, and in Jamaica this is now given routinely to all children with severe PEM. The drug is also effective against *Giardia*.

Local and generalized infections

Infections such as bronchopneumonia, otitis media, pyelitis and septicaemia are frequently present but often not diagnosed because the child is unable to mount a pyrexia or a leucocytosis; clinical signs are difficult to elicit, X-rays may not be available and there is no time to wait for the results of microbiological tests on blood or urine. Most clinicians nowadays therefore give broad-spectrum antibiotics routinely from the time of admission, on the presumption that there is an infection.

Septicaemia is often caused by gram-negative organisms such as *Klebsiella sp.* and *Salmonella sp.* and urinary tract infections by *Proteus sp.* or *Klebsiella sp.* Unfortunately they are often resistant to antibiotics. Chest infections are sometimes caused by *Pneumococcus* or *Haemophilus* but mixed cultures are usually obtained. The possibility of organisms such as *Pneumocystis carnii* should be considered whenever there is a possibility of malnutrition secondary to AIDS. Skin infections are usually due to a mixed infection of *Streptococci* and *Staphylococci* and otitis media is usually caused by a mixed flora of *Haemophilus sp.* and *Streptococcus*. Unfortunately many children with severe malnutrition are likely to have been ill for some time before they come to a centre where their complications can be adequately diagnosed and managed.

For 'pre-emptive' therapy ampicillin has been found useful. Suskind (1975) recommended a triple regime of ampicillin, methicillin and gentamycin or kanamycin. Golden (1988) used penicillin plus gentamycin, or, if this is not available, chloramphenicol or tetracycline. Gentamycin is widely used because of its effectiveness in *Pseudomonas* infections. However, the details of antibiotic treatment will depend on local circumstances. It will at least give a breathing space for cultures and drug-resistance tests to be carried out if the facilities are available.

If the child does not respond and remains very ill, tuberculosis should be suspected and treated in the appropriate way. Malaria may be missed if there is no fever; the presenting feature is often diarrhoea. Therefore a blood film should always be examined in regions where malaria is endemic.

Drug metabolism is likely to be altered in PEM, as a result of delayed absorption, reduced protein binding, changes in the volume of distribution, decreased conjugation or oxidation in the liver, and decreased renal clearance. The literature has been reviewed by Krishnaswamy (1989). For example, in malnourished children the half-life of gentamycin was found to be increased by 25 per cent and its clearance decreased by 50 per cent. Free drug concentrations tend to be higher in malnutrition and detoxification mechanisms compromised. However, in the present state of knowledge it is not possible to make definitive recommendations for changes in standard dose regimes.

Hypothermia and hypoglycaemia

As described in Chapter 6, the body temperature in severe PEM is low and the capacity to maintain it when the environmental temperature falls is impaired. It may be for this reason that death often occurs in the small hours of the night. It is therefore very important that at night the child should be kept well-covered up. This is an advantage of allowing the mother to be with the child in hospital. Hypothermia is sometimes associated with a gram-negative septicaemia (Alleyne *et al.*, 1977).

Hypoglycaemia may occur (Chapter 8) and unless there are convulsions is difficult to differentiate from circulatory collapse. A blood sugar below 3 mmol/l (50 mg/dl) carries a high mortality. It may not be possible to monitor the blood sugar on the spot, and therefore it is better to prevent hypoglycaemia by providing a fairly high concentration of glucose (50 g/l) in the fluid that is given in the initial phase. If hypoglycaemia is suspected and the child is not on an intravenous or nasogastric drip, small quantities of the glucose solution should be given by mouth every hour.

Anaemia

Occasionally children present with very severe anaemia (Hb < 5 g/dl) caused by dysentery, malaria or folic acid deficiency. The malnourished child seems to be able to tolerate anaemia remarkably well, perhaps because the demand for oxygen is so low, and blood transfusion should only be undertaken as a last resort. To keep the volume low, packed red cells should be given; 30–50 ml will produce a significant increase in haemoglobin concentration. Golden (1988) records that in severely ill children who do not respond to treatment small transfusions of whole blood (10 ml/kg) may have a dramatic effect, possibly by supplying essential micronutrients, even though the amounts will be very small.

Other indications for urgent treatment

Vitamin A

In a child with low vitamin A stores PEM predisposes to the development of keratomalacia, which may progress with devastating speed. Therefore in areas where vitamin A deficiency is prevalent the vitamin should be given immediately to all children with severe PEM, preferably as water-dispersible, retinol palmitate, 30 mg intramuscularly daily for three days (D. S. McLaren, personal communication). Since marginal vitamin A deficiency may be commoner than has been supposed, and vitamin A supplements may reduce mortality and morbidity from infections (Chapter 17), perhaps this treatment should be given more generally, not only in areas where the deficiency is known to be common.

Folic acid deficiency

In Jamaica folic acid deficiency used often to be seen (McIver and Back, 1960). The bone marrow is typically atrophic and megaloblastosis only becomes apparent after there has been a response to treatment. Therefore the practice was adopted of giving folic acid 5 mg/day routinely, without waiting for a haematological diagnosis.

No other needs have yet been defined for urgent treatment in the initial stage. The treatments discussed above are directed mainly to complications rather than to the underlying state of malnutrition. If the free radical theory of kwashiorkor (Chapter 11) is correct, it would be logical in these cases to provide as a matter of urgency antioxidants and nutrients that play a role in free radical scavenging, such as vitamin E, glutathione, selenium, copper and zinc. However, the benefit of the anti-free radical therapy in the initial phase has not yet been evaluated (Golden, 1988). Vitamins of the B complex have not been of any use, and in the experience of Veghelyi (1950) were actually harmful.

Phase 2: Initiation of cure

Once electrolyte and water imbalances and infections have been brought under control, the child enters the phase that has been called the initiation of cure. Brock *et al.* (1955) considered that cure had started when oedema was lost, but this approach is too simplistic. In our view oedema, which may persist for one or two weeks, is of no great relevance. Metabolic activity is reduced, as judged by the low BMR and low rate of protein turnover (Chapter 6). It is altered or distorted in other ways also; examples are the reduction in capacity for urea formation, and the changes in metabolism of aromatic amino acids described by Dean and Whitehead (1963). Therefore it is necessary to proceed with caution to avoid overloading the system at both the physiological and the biochemical levels. Food should never be forced, and recovery of appetite is crucial. Table 12.11 shows the energy intakes of Mexican children with PEM who were fed on 'self-demand' (Gomez *et al.*, 1958).

If feeding is too vigorous death may occur in the first week, often with signs of heart failure (Wharton *et al.*, 1967). Several mechanisms have been proposed; the first is an excessive amount of salt in the food, causing expansion of the ECF volume. The second is that restoration of albumin synthesis causes an increase in the circulating albumin mass and expansion of the plasma volume at the expense of ECF. A third possibility is that with increased energy supply the sodium pump becomes more active and extrusion of sodium that has accumulated in cells (Chapter 10) again leads to expansion of extracellular and plasma volumes. Fourthly, it has been observed that at

Table 12.11 Average energy intakes of children fed by 'self-demand' at different stages of recovery from PEM

Days	Energy (kcal/kg/day)
0– 5	35
6–10	61
11–15	110
thereafter	190

From Gomez *et al.* (1958)

the start of high energy feeding there is an increase in body water (Chapter 4). Whatever the mechanism, prompt treatment with digoxin or frusemide is usually effective.

A suitable regime in this stage of cure is one that provides no more than the maintenance requirements of energy and protein: about 80 kcal and 0.7 g protein/kg/day (Chapter 15). Supplements of potassium and magnesium should be continued, to make good specific deficits and to allow for growth, and trace elements may also be added. Suskind (1975) added virtually the whole range of known trace elements. The amounts suggested by Golden (1988) are shown in Table 12.12.

Although most children with severe PEM have some degree of iron-deficiency anaemia, with haemoglobin levels of 7–9 g/dl, it is wise not to give iron at this stage because of the danger of promoting free radical generation and bacterial proliferation (Chapter 10). In Jamaica mortality was higher in children who received iron supplements within three days of admission than in those to whom it was given later on (Smith *et al.*, 1989*a*).

The stage of initiation of cure may last about a week. During this time a child who is oedematous will usually lose weight and one who is not clinically oedematous gain little or nothing. This need be no cause for concern, because measurements of body water have shown that there are gains in tissue, but they are masked by loss of excess water.

The indication for moving on to the next stage, that of rehabilitation, is

Table 12.12 Typical feeding regime of a milk-based mixture during initiation of cure (phase 2)

Composition	g/l	
Dried skimmed milk powder	17	
Sugar	90	
Oil	30	
Provides approximately 700 kcal and 6 g protein/l		

Amounts	Day 2 (approx)	Days 3–7 (approx)
Number of feeds/day	12	8 → 6
Volume of feed, ml/kg body weight	10	15 → 20
Total volume, ml/kg/day	120	120
These volumes may be increased a little if there is dehydration and decreased if there is oedema.		
120 ml/kg provides approximately 85 kcal and 0.7 g protein/kg		

Additions	per litre of feed	
Potassium chloride	1.2–2.4 g	These may be made
Magnesium chloride	300–600 mg	up as a solution which
*Zinc acetate	20 mg	is added routinely
*Copper acetate	2 mg	to the feed

	per day	
Ferrous sulphate	70 mg, not before 7th day	
Folic acid	5 mg	
*Selenium as sodium selenate	6–10 μg/kg/day if deficiency expected	

* After Golden (1988)

that the child recovers its appetite. Persistent anorexia is probably most often the result of psychological deprivation, but it should also give rise to the suspicion of zinc deficiency.

Logistics of treatment in the early phases

It might seem that successful treatment of these severe and complicated cases must require all the resources of an intensive care unit, but this is not so. The essentials are as follows.

i.   A doctor is needed to examine the child and decide on the line of treatment. The basic decisions are on the amount and route by which fluid is to be given and the type and dosage of antibiotics.

ii. If intravenous infusion is considered necessary an experienced nurse will probably do a better job of setting it up than a junior doctor and disturb the child less. If a vein is being cannulated the opportunity should be taken to obtain a blood sample for measurement of haemoglobin, electrolytes (particularly sodium), sugar and perhaps albumin.

iii. When fluids are given by the nasogastric route, if the child is pale and collapsed, it may be wise to take a sample of blood by heel-prick, for measurement of haemoglobin and sugar and, if appropriate, to screen for malaria. Thus only minimal laboratory investigations are needed.

iv. Once treatment has been started, careful and frequent observation is essential: of the rate of drip if fluids are being given intravenously or by nasal tube; of the respiration and pulse rate, at least hourly; of rectal temperature, perhaps three-hourly. The passage of urine and stools should, of course, be noted. They could be collected on a large pad of cottonwool and weighed, as a guide to the amount of fluid replacement needed.

v.   When the child is able to take fluids by mouth, they should be given frequently and in small amounts. Patience is essential; each feed may take half an hour, but it may be given by a nursing-aid or by the mother, if she is told what to do. It is important to record the volumes taken.

Thus the requirement for equipment, drugs and special investigations is not very great, but the care of these gravely sick children is labour-intensive, and the limiting factor is often pairs of hands. If feeds are to be two-hourly and each takes half an hour, one person can only look after four children. However, that person need not be a highly trained nurse. All that is necessary for feeding and keeping the child clean is what Cicely Williams refers to as TLC—tender loving care.

Prognosis in the early stages

Death may occur in the first few days even if the initial treatment has been successful in overcoming dehydration and infection. Gürson *et al.* (1976) analysed the clinical features considered important for prognosis in six separate studies. Their main findings are summarized in Table 12.13. Some authors, but not all, have found the age of the child to have an important effect, as one might expect. Data from Ramos-Galván and Calderón (1965) are shown

Table 12.13 Factors affecting prognosis in PEM according to various authors

Author and country	No. of subjects	Factors for prognosis	
		Important	Not important
Gomez *et al.* (1956) Mexico	753	Weight loss Electrolyte imbalance Diarrhoea Bronchopneumonia	Oedema Skin lesions
Kahn (1959) South Africa	100	Weight loss Skin lesions Low serum Na Low serum K Hepatomegaly Hypothermia	Oedema
Smith (1960) Jamaica	129	Age Low serum Na Low serum K Pulmonary oedema	Oedema
Ramos-Galván and Calderón (1965) Mexico	2401	Age Electrolyte imbalance Infection	Oedema
Garrow and Pike (1967) Jamaica	248	Raised serum bilirubin Low serum Na	Oedema Age Weight loss
Gürson *et al.* (1976) Turkey	200	Weight for age Height for age Low serum Na Age Weight for height Low Hb	Hepatomegaly Oedema Skin changes Hair changes Serum K, HCO_3 concentrations Serum total protein

From Gürson *et al.* (1976)

in Table 12.14. This is probably the largest series (2401 cases) that has ever been published. There is remarkable agreement in Gürson's summary that oedema is not a good indicator of outcome.

There is no consistency in the literature about whether death rates are higher in kwashiorkor, marasmic kwashiorkor or marasmus. Some authors, but not all, have recorded the highest fatality rates in marasmic kwashiorkor,

Table 12.14 Effect of age on mortality from PEM in hospital

Age (months)	Number	% of total number	% who died at each age	% with oedema at each age
1–12	291	12	39.5	19
13–24	1142	48	33.8	61
25–36	509	21	28	75
37–48	234	10	19.5	83
49+	225	9	17	72
Total	2401	100	overall mortality 30.2%	

Note lack of correlation of oedema with mortality
From Ramos-Galván and Calderón (1965)

e.g, Vis (1985) in Zaïre, Van Roosmalen-Wiebenga *et al.* (1986) in Tanzania and Coulter *et al.* (1988) in Sudan. That has also been our experience in Jamaica. Laditan and Tineimebwa (1983) in Nigeria found the highest fatality rate in marasmus, which is unusual, but their marasmic children were younger than those with kwashiorkor.

Paradoxically, although the presence of oedema may not be important for prognosis, several workers have found a close relation between mortality rate and plasma albumin concentration. The results of the Zaïre group are shown in Fig. 12.1. The figure also illustrates the remarkable improvement in Zaïre between 1977 and 1982. In Jamaica Garrow *et al.* (1962) recorded that 36 per cent of children with plasma albumin less than 1.5 g/dl died, against an overall mortality of 16 per cent. In Uganda there was a linear relation between mortality and albumin concentration (Hay *et al.*, 1975); in South India 30 per cent of children with albumin less than 1 g/dl died, compared to less than 4 per cent of children with albumin above 2 g/dl (Pereira and Begum, 1974).

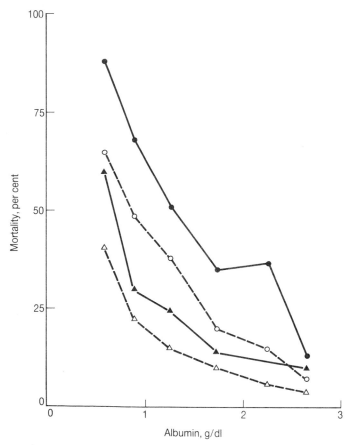

Fig. 12.1 Relation between mortality rate and serum albumin concentration in children in Zaïre with PEM. Comparison between kwashiorkor and marasmic kwashiorkor and between two studies, in 1977 and 1982. ●——● 1977, marasmic kwashiorkor; ▲——▲ 1977, kwashiorkor; ○---○ 1982, marasmic kwashiorkor; △---△ 1982, kwashiorkor. Reproduced by permission from Vis (1985).

Other biochemical indicators of a bad prognosis are a high bilirubin level (>6 mg/l), which presumably reflects the degree of fatty liver, and a low serum sodium (Garrow *et al.*, 1962; Garrow and Pike, 1967). In Garrow's series 72 per cent of children with serum sodium < 120 mmol/l died. McLaren and Shirajian (1969) found significant differences in the initial serum concentrations of vitamins A and E between those who recovered and those who died. In Liberia low levels of fibronectin correlated with poor survival, and children destined to recover had rapidly increasing fibronectin levels before there were other overt signs of recovery (Fredell *et al.*, 1987).

For most of these pathological changes that carry a bad prognosis there is unfortunately no specific treatment. No way has yet been found of increasing the rate of clearance of fat from the liver. For hyponatraemia it is important to avoid overloading with sodium and to give supplementary potassium; the body must then be left to itself to adjust the composition of the extracellular fluid, once any volume deficit due to dehydration has been overcome.

Phase 3: Rehabilitation

The aim in this phase is to restore normal weight for height. This should be achieved as quickly as possible in order to reduce the length of stay in hospital or nutrition rehabilitation unit (NRU). The indications that the child is ready to enter this phase are recovery of appetite and a change of expression. It is often said that the best sign is the first smile replacing the original apathy and misery. During this phase the child is recovering emotionally and psychologically as well as physically. It is therefore important that some members of the staff should have time to make human contact with the children, if the mothers are not with them. Toys should be provided and the children encouraged to play with them and to socialize with each other. These matters are considered in more detail in Chapter 19.

Once the appetite is restored children recovering from PEM eat voraciously and should be fed *ad libitum*. Rates of weight gain of 10–20 g/kg/day can be obtained (Fig. 12.2); these are 10–20 times the normal rate of gain between one and two years. Thus a child weighing 6 kg, if properly fed, could put on 3 kg in a month. Gains tend to be more rapid in the early part of the recovery phase and later to fall off (Ashworth, 1969). In these later stages there is a tendency to lay down more fat. It seems likely that repletion of protein takes precedence over that of fat (Standard *et al.*, 1959), although it is possible that some nutrient other than energy or protein has become limiting (see p. 180). We consider the child to be fully rehabilitated when the expected weight for height has been reached. At this stage most children show a voluntary reduction in food intake and their weight reaches a plateau (e.g. RG, Fig. 12.3), although in a minority of cases (e.g. PF, Fig. 12.3) this does not happen: they continue to gain and become obese. Ashworth (1969) remarked on the sensitivity of the mechanism of regulating body weight in these children through reduction of appetite. We have no idea what the signal is.

The theoretical energy and protein requirements for such rapid catch-up growth are discussed in Chapter 16. In practice there are two limiting factors: the first in the capacity of the stomach, which puts an upper limit on the size of the feeds. Stomach volume has been estimated as 3 per cent of body weight

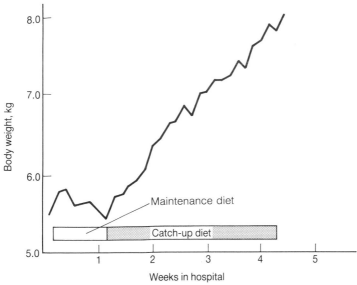

Fig. 12.2 Catch-up growth of a child on a high energy diet; expected weight for height 8.70 kg. Reproduced by permission from Waterlow *et al.* (1978).

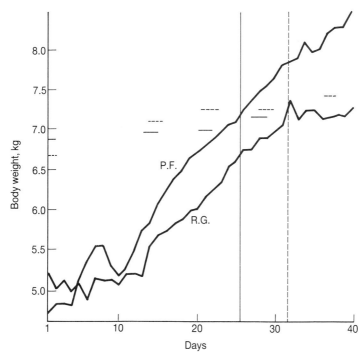

Fig. 12.3 Weight curves of two children during recovery from malnutrition. When expected weight for length has been reached RG's weight maintains a plateau, whereas that of PF continues to rise. ---- , expected weight for length of PF, aged 8 months; ⎯ , expected weight for length of RG, aged 14 months; ⎸ , time when PF reached expected weight for length; ⋮ , similarly for RG.

(National Research Council, 1985). Thus in a child weighing 6 kg with a stomach capacity of 180 ml, a feed at least every four hours would be needed to achieve an intake of 1 litre per day.

The second limiting factor is the energy density of the feeds. It was some time before it was recognized that energy intake is more likely to be limiting than that of protein (Waterlow, 1961; Ashworth *et al.*, 1968). If a milk-based formula is used it is easy to supply enough protein as skimmed milk powder, but to achieve the necessary energy density fat has to be added. In Jamaica this has usually been in the form of coconut oil, which is locally available and cheap, but other vegetable oils appeared to be equally effective and well-tolerated. In coconut oil the fatty acids are highly saturated; Golden (1988) has suggested that it may be wise to avoid vegetable oils rich in polyunsaturated fatty acids, because they may provide substrates for peroxidation reactions.

Table 12.15 shows the proximate composition of the milk-based diet that has been used successfully in Jamaica, with a typical feeding schedule. As the child gains weight the feeds become progressively larger and more widely spaced. In the later stages the formula diet should be gradually replaced by or supplemented with the kind of foods that the child will receive at home.

With a liquid formula it is simple to calculate the amounts needed to fulfil the requirements for catch-up growth and to measure intakes accurately. Several authors have reported on the results of feeding vegetable mixtures: for the most part weight gains and regeneration of serum albumin were slower than with milk diets (Venkatachalam *et al.*, 1956; Graham *et al.*, 1966; Pereira and Begum, 1974). However, good weight gains have been achieved on diets composed of ordinary foods. For example, the children with kwashiorkor

Table 12.15 Composition of feeds and example of a feeding schedule during the phase of nutritional rehabilitation (phase 3)

A. *Estimated requirement for catch-up growth at the rate of 20 g weight gain/kg/day[a]*
      Energy   175 kcal
      Protein   5.75 g/kg/day

B. *Composition of feed*
      Dried skimmed milk (35% protein)   110 g/l = 38.5 g protein/l
      Sugar   50 g/l
      Oil   60 g/l
      Total energy   1180 kcal/l
This feed will provide the requirements at A if fed at the rate of 150 ml/kg/day

C. *Feeding regime for a child initially weighing 6 kg*

Days from admission	Weight (kg)	Total intake (ml/day)	Number and volume (ml) of feeds/day
7	6.0	900	6 × 150
10	6.36	960	6 × 160
15	7.0	1050	6 × 175
20	7.7	1150	5 × 230
30	9.2	1400	5 × 280

The feed volume approaches the capacity of the child's stomach. The feeds can be made more concentrated if required, but the proportions of the components should be maintained the same.

[a] See Table 15.16, p. 252

described by Smith *et al.* (1989*b*) gained an average of 14 g/kg/day in a diet of local staples with meat, fish, vegetables and palm oil. For older children, such as those in Zaïre, whose average age was four years, a mixed diet is undoubtedly more suitable (Vis, 1985). The disadvantage of such diets is that it is much more difficult to know exactly how much the children are eating, and when they are reported as not recovering well in hospital the reason may simply be that they are not getting the very large amounts of food needed for rapid catch-up. The solution is to feed *ad libitum* and to use the weight gain as a check on the adequacy of the intake.

The recovery diet must not only correct any specific deficiencies that remain from the earlier stages of treatment, but also provide amounts of all the constituents of normal tissue—minerals, trace elements and other micronutrients—in amounts adequate to match the rapid rate of gain. If any one component is limiting, appetite decreases and growth falls off (Chapter 2). Therefore supplements of potassium and magnesium should be continued. Zinc was found to be limiting in children who, because of cow's milk intolerance, were fed a soya-based formula. Growth fell off and was promptly restored by the addition of zinc (see Fig. 9.1). Golden and Golden (1985) suggested that weight gain alone is not an adequate criterion of recovery because the tissue laid down on the high energy diet may contain an excessive amount of fat. They showed that zinc supplements promoted the deposition of lean tissue and increased the rate of protein turnover (Golden and Golden, 1990). Simmer *et al.* (1988) found that the addition of zinc (10 mg/kg/day) to a mixed diet almost doubled the rate of weight gain. At the same time there was an increase in the zinc content of leucocytes. There is therefore good reason for including zinc with potassium and magnesium as essential supplements to the recovery diet. Other trace elements, particularly copper and selenium, may fall into the same category, but the evidence that they are ever limiting is less clear.

Iron salts are necessary to provide for an increase in red cell mass and may safely be given at this stage ($FeSO_4$, 70 mg daily). There is no indication for intramuscular iron, although this was used in Thailand without adverse effects (Suskind, 1975).

It has already been mentioned that folic acid may be limiting for haemopoiesis once growth begins. The same applies to vitamin D. Rickets is common in a geographical belt that runs from North Africa through the Middle East and North India to China. In Ethiopia clinical rickets with high alkaline phosphatase and low serum calcium and phosphate has been described in children who were quite severely stunted (91 per cent height for age) but not particularly wasted (80 per cent weight for height) (Höjer *et al.*, 1977). In Calcutta children with more severe PEM showed neither the clinical nor the radiological signs of rickets, but once growth started the typical broadening and cupping of the epiphyses became apparent (Bhattacharyya and Dutta, 1976).

It has been observed in Jamaica that after several weeks on the high energy formula some children developed an eczematous rash, lost their appetite and stopped gaining weight. The rash cleared up on a mixed diet which supplied an adequate ratio of vitamin E to polyunsaturated fatty acids, suggesting that this vitamin might have become limiting (Waterlow *et al.*, 1978). All these are examples of a new limiting factor emerging during rapid growth.

Duration of stay

Catch-up growth in height tends to start later than in weight, but once it begins the rate of linear growth may be two to three times the normal rate for a child of the same age (Walker and Golden, 1988). Thus the target of 100 per cent weight for height is continuously receding and may take some two months to reach.

Two related questions arise: is it necessary for the child to reach 100 per cent weight for height before discharge? Is it necessary for the child to remain in hospital until this target has been reached? The answer to the second question is clearly No. Such a prolonged stay is not practical in a busy paediatric ward, nor is it even beneficial, because rehabilitation is an exercise in applied nutrition, not in medicine. A long stay in hospital is not a guarantee of successful long-term results. In Zaïre Hennart *et al.* (1987) found that one year after discharge 10 per cent of children admitted with PEM had died (see Table 12.3). There was no significant difference between those who survived and those who died in the average duration of their stay in hospital (72 *versus* 78 days).

The other question is more difficult: whether there is any benefit in keeping children in hospital or a nutrition rehabilitation centre (NRC) until they have reached normal weight for height. Cooper *et al.* (1980) in St Lucia attempted to study this problem. One group of children was kept in hospital for an average of three weeks, until their appetite had recovered and they were eating voraciously; a second group was discharged after a few days, once acute illnesses had been treated. The mean weight on admission was 6.0 kg at a mean age of 13 months; all were less than 75 per cent of reference weight for age and many of them below 60 per cent. At six and 12 months after discharge there was no difference in the weight gains of the two groups. Cooper concluded that the contribution to subsequent weight gain made by in-patient care with high energy feeding was negligible. More studies of this kind are badly needed.

In a more recent study in Jamaica (G. T. Heikens, personal communication) malnourished children admitted to hospital were divided into two groups. One group remained in hospital until weight for height was fully restored, with a mean stay of 40 days. The other group was discharged after a mean stay of 18 days, but were followed up at home by community health aides and for three months received from the public health service a supplement providing about 200 kcal and 20 g protein per day. The mortality rate after discharge was less than 1 per cent. Both stunting and wasting were fully corrected, though more slowly in the short stay group. Both groups were anthropometrically normal after three years.

If achieving a certain weight for height or weight for age is to be the factor determining the time of discharge, the target weight should be one that does not carry an unacceptable risk of morbidity or death under the conditions of life in the community. As far as present knowledge of risk goes (Chapter 18), it seems reasonable to accept 80 per cent of reference weight for height or 75 per cent of reference weight for age as cut-off points for discharge. The child whose weight curve is shown in Fig. 12.2 might be taken as an example. Initially he was 62 per cent of expected weight for height. After two weeks in hospital followed by only two weeks in an NRC he would have reached 86 per cent weight for height and be ready to go home, provided that the same rate of gain was achieved in the NRC as was in fact obtained in hospital. There is no reason why it should not be.

Nutrition rehabilitation centres

The ideal would be, once Phase 3 has begun, after perhaps two weeks in hospital, for children to be moved to a nutrition rehabilitation centre (NRC) attached to the hospital. Cases of severe PEM who do not fulfil the criteria for admission to hospital could also be treated there. A staff member with training in applied nutrition/dietetics is needed to supervise the feeding and progress of each child, and enough pairs of hands to carry out the feeding properly. If mothers are not able to stay with the children, it is important that there should be facilities for play and stimulation (Chapter 19). If mothers do stay, the opportunity can be taken to provide some instruction in child feeding and hygiene.

There was great enthusiasm for NRCs in the 1970s, stimulated by Bengoa, who was at that time head of the Nutrition Unit of WHO. Cook (1971), Beghin and Viteri (1973), Cutting (1983) and others have reviewed the operation of these centres and made recommendations about how they should be organized. Alleyne *et al.* (1977) point out that the whole approach of NRCs, in which the mothers and the community become involved, is very different from the aloof, authoritarian approach of hospitals, and much more likely to achieve prevention as well as cure. In the centres examined by Beghin and Viteri the cost per day ranged from one-quarter to one-fifteenth of the cost per day in hospital.

It is clearly very difficult to make any general evaluation, because of differences in the clinical state of children on admission, in the duration of their stay and in the operation of the centres. On the whole the results seem to be modest. Table 12.16 gives an example of what was achieved in an NRC in South India (Cutting *et al.*, 1973). In this centre the staff for ten children admitted with their mothers was a graduate nutritionist, two health-demonstrators, a part-time nurse and a part-time doctor. It is probable that the results were not better because the need was not appreciated for securing every day the kind of intakes recommended in Table 12.15.

On the other hand, a study by Mönckeberg and his colleagues in Chile (1988) had a most impressive outcome. A comparison was made between two

Table 12.16 Results of treatment of PEM in a Nutrition Rehabilitation Centre in India

Grade	Weight for age (%)	Percentage of children in each grade of malnutrition		
		Admission	Discharge	Follow-up
0	> 80	0	1	1
I	80–71	3	7	24
II	70–61	14	32	43
III	60 or less	83	60	32

Sample size 140. All but 13 of the children were initially oedematous
Follow-up time: 3–26 months
From Cutting *et al.* (1973)

groups of marasmic children, with an average initial age of five months and weight 3.5 kg. Both groups were maintained for five months, one in a paediatric hospital and the other in a special treatment centre. In the hospital group there were 29 deaths, in the other group none. The incidence of infections was 15 times greater in the hospital group. Gains in weight, height and psychomotor development were much better in the treatment centre. The main difference between the two treatments was that in the centre special attention was given to psychomotor stimulation and to producing the right kind of environment for the childrens' development.

The fact that experience of NRCs in the past has not always been entirely satisfactory does not diminish the need for them, as a half-way house for severe cases between the hospital and the primary health care system of the community. Not only do NRCs relieve the burden on hospitals and reduce the costs of treatment, but if well organized they can provide a better environment for recovery, as the Chilean experience shows.

In conclusion, the responsibility for treating children with severe PEM is in principle shared between the hospital, the NRC and the primary health care system. The child when 'cured' is returning to the environment which allowed it to become malnourished, and to prevent a recurrence, continuing supervision for some time is needed at the community level.

References

Alleyne, G. A. O., Hay, R. W. *et al.* (1977). *Protein-energy malnutrition*. Edward Arnold, London.

Ashworth, A. (1969). Growth-rates in children recovering from protein-energy malnutrition. *British Journal of Nutrition* **23**: 835–845.

Ashworth, A., Bell, R. *et al.* (1968). Calorie requirements of children recovering from protein-energy malnutrition. *Lancet* **2**: 600–603.

Beghin, I. D., Viteri, F. E. (1973). Nutritional rehabilitation centres: an evaluation of their performance. *Environmental Child Health*, Monograph No. 31, 403–416.

Bhattacharyya, A. K., Dutta, K. N. (1976). Atrophic rickets in children with protein-energy malnutrition. *Indian Journal of Radiology* **30**: 267–270.

Brock, J. F., Hansen, J. D. L. *et al.* (1955). Kwashiorkor and protein malnutrition: a dietary therapeutic trial. *Lancet* **2**: 355–360.

Brown, K. H., Gilman, R. H *et al.* (1981). Infections associated with severe PEM in hospitalized infants. *Nutrition Research* **1**: 33–46.

Chaudhuri, R. N., Bhattacharyya, A. K., Basu, A. K. (1961). Kwashiorkor and marasmus in Calcutta. *Journal of the Indian Medical Association* **36**: 557–565.

Cook, R. (1971). Is hospital the place for the treatment of malnourished children? *Environmental Child Health* **17**: 15–25.

Cooper, E., Headden, G., Lawrence, C. (1980). Caribbean children, thriving and failing in and out of hospital. *Journal of Tropical Pediatrics* **26**: 232–238.

Coulter, J. B. S., Suliman, G. I. *et al.* (1988). Protein-energy malnutrition in Northern Sudan: clinical studies. *European Journal of Clinical Nutrition* **42**: 787–796.

Cutting, W. A. M. (1983). Nutritional rehabilitation. In McLaren, D. S. (ed) *Nutrition in the community*. John Wiley, New York, pp. 321–326.

Cutting, W. A. M., Cutting, M. McL., Paul, N. (1973). Nutrition rehabilitation. *Archives of Child Health* **15**: 23–33.

Dean, R. F. A., Whitehead, R. G. (1963). The metabolism of aromatic amino acids in kwashiorkor. *Lancet* **1**: 188–191.

Fredell, J., Takyi, Y. *et al.* (1987). Fibronectin as possible adjunct in treatment of severe malnutrition. *Lancet* **2**: 962.

Garrow, J. S., Pike, M. C. (1967). The short-term prognosis of severe primary infantile malnutrition. *British Journal of Nutrition* **21**: 155–165.

Garrow, J. S., Picou, D., Waterlow, J. C. (1962). The treatment and prognosis of infantile malnutrition in Jamaican children. *West Indian Medical Journal* **11**: 217–227.

Golden, B. E., Golden, M. H. N. (1985). Effect of zinc supplementation on the composition of newly synthesized tissue in children recovering from malnutrition. *Proceedings of the Nutrition Society* **44**: 110A.

Golden, B. E., Golden, M. H. N. (1990). Zinc and muscle growth during recovery from malnutrition. *West Indian Medical Journal* **39**: Supplement, 41.

Golden, M. H. N. (1988). Marasmus and kwashiorkor. In Dickerson, J. W. T., Lee, M. A. (eds) *Nutrition in the clinical management of disease*, 2nd edn. Edward Arnold, London, pp. 88–109.

Gomez, F., Ramos-Galván, R. *et al.* (1956). Mortality in second and third degree malnutrition. *Journal of Tropical Pediatrics* **2**: 77–83.

Gomez, F., Ramos-Galván, R. *et al.* (1958). Prevention and treatment of chronic severe infantile malnutrition (kwashiorkor). *Annals of the New York Academy of Sciences* **69**: 969–981.

Graham, G. G., Baertl, J. M., Cordano, A. (1966). Studies in infantile malnutrition. The effect of dietary protein source on serum proteins. *American Journal of Clinical Nutrition* **18**: 16–19.

Gürson, C. T., Yüksel, T., Saner, G. (1976). The short-term prognosis of protein-calorie malnutrition in Marmara region of Turkey. *Journal of Tropical Pediatrics and Environmental Child Health* **22**: 59–62.

Hay, R. W., Whitehead, R. G., Spicer, C. C. (1975). Serum albumin as a prognostic indicator in oedematous malnutrition. *Lancet* **2**: 427–429.

Hennart, P., Beghin, D., Bossuyt, M. (1987). Long-term follow-up of severe protein-energy malnutrition in Eastern Zaïre. *Journal of Tropical Pediatrics* **33**: 10–12.

Höjer, B., Gebre-Medhin, M. *et al.* (1977). Combined vitamin D deficiency rickets and PEM in Ethiopian infants. *Journal of Tropical Pediatrics* **23**: 73–79.

Husaini, Y. K., Sulaeman, Z. *et al.* (1982). Outpatient rehabilitation of severe protein-energy malnutrition (PEM). *Food and Nutrition Bulletin* **8**: 55–59.

Jackson, A. A., Golden, M. H. N. (1987). Severe malnutrition. In Weatherall, D. J., Ledingham, J. G. G., Warrell, D. A. (eds) *Oxford textbook of medicine*. Oxford University Press, pp. 8.12–8.28.

Kahn, E. (1959). Prognostic criteria of severe protein malnutrition. *American Journal of Clinical Nutrition* **7**: 161–165.

Khare, R. D., Shah, P. M., Junnarkar, A. R. (1976). Management of kwashiorkor in its milieu: a follow-up for 15 months. *Indian Journal of Medical Research* **64**: 1119–1127.

Krishnaswamy, K. (1989). Drug metabolism and pharmacokinetics in malnourished children. *Clinical Pharmacokinetics* **17**: (Suppl. 1) 68–88.

Laditan, A. A. O., Tineimebwa, G. (1983). The protein-energy malnourished child in a Nigerian teaching hospital. *Journal of Tropical Pediatrics* **29**: 61–64.

McIver, J. E., Back, E. H. (1960). Megaloblastic anaemia of infancy in Jamaica. *Archives of Disease in Childhood* **35**: 134–145.

Mackenzie, A., Barnes, G., Shann, F. (1989). Clinical signs of dehydration in children. *Lancet* **2**: 605–607.

McLaren, D. S., Shirajian, E. (1969). Short-term prognosis in protein-calorie malnutrition. *American Journal of Clinical Nutrition* **22**: 863–870.

Mönckeberg, F. (ed) (1988). *Desnutricion infantil. Fisiopathología, clínica, tratamiento y prevención: neustra experiencia y contribución*. Institute of Nutrition and Food Technology, University of Chile, Santiago.

National Research Council Subcommittee on Nutrition and Diarrheal Diseases Control (1985). *Nutritional management of acute diarrhea in infants and children.* Food and Nutrition Board, National Research Council. National Academy Press, Washington, DC.

Omer, H. O., Omer, M. I. A., Khalifa, O. O. (1975). Pattern of protein energy malnutrition in Sudanese children and comparison with some other Middle East countries. *Journal of Tropical Pediatrics* 21: 329–333.

Pereira, S. M., Begum, A. (1974). The manifestations and management of severe protein-calorie malnutrition (kwashiorkor). *World Review of Nutrition and Dietetics* 19: 1–50.

Picou, D., Alleyne, G. A. O. *et al.* (1975). *Malnutrition and gastroenteritis in children: a manual for hospital management.* Caribbean Food and Nutrition Institute, Kingston, Jamaica.

Ramos-Galván, R., Calderón, J. M. (1965). Deaths among children with third degree malnutrition. *American Journal of Clinical Nutrition* 16: 351–355.

Reeds, P. J., Laditan, A. O. (1976). Serum albumin and transferrin in protein-energy malnutrition. Their use in the assessment of marginal undernutrition and the prognosis of severe undernutrition. *British Journal of Nutrition* 36: 255–263.

Roediger, W. E. W. (1986). Metabolic basis of starvation diarrhoea: implications for treatment. *Lancet* 1: 1082–1084.

Sadre, M., Donoso, G. (1969). Treatment of malnutrition. *Lancet* 2: 112.

Simmer, K., Khanum, S. *et al.* (1988). Nutritional rehabilitation in Bangladesh. *American Journal of Clinical Nutrition* 47: 1036–1040.

Sinha, D. P. (1987). Hospital admissions for malnutrition: trends in the English-speaking Caribbean. *Cajanus* 20: 179–190.

Smith, I. F., Taiwo, O., Golden, M. H. N. (1989*a*). Plant protein rehabilitation diets and iron supplementation of the protein-energy malnourished child. *European Journal of Clinical Nutrition* 43: 763–768.

Smith, I. F., Taiwo, O., Payne-Robinson, H. M. (1989*b*). Plasma somatomedin in Nigerian malnourished children fed a vegetable protein rehabilitation diet. *European Journal of Clinical Nutrition* 43: 705–713.

Smith, R. (1960). Total body water in malnourished infants. *Clinical Science* 19: 275–285.

Soutif, C. (1989). *Étude de la recuperation nutritionelle dans le centre de renutrition intensive de Tahona au Niger.* Médecins sans Frontières, Paris.

Standard, K. L., Wills, V. G., Waterlow, J. C. (1959). Indirect indicators of muscle mass in malnourished infants. *American Journal of Clinical Nutrition* 7: 271–279.

Suskind, R. (1975). The in-patient and out-patient treatment of the child with severe protein-calorie malnutrition. In Olson, R. E. (ed) *Protein-calorie malnutrition.* Academic Press, New York, pp. 404–410.

Tolboom, J. J. M., Ralitapole-Maruping, A. P. *et al.* (1986). Severe protein-energy malnutrition in Lesotho, death and survival in hospital, clinical findings. *Tropical Geographical Medicine* 38: 351–358.

Van Roosmalen-Wiebenga, M. W., Kusin, J. A. (1986). Nutrition rehabilitation in hospital—a waste of time and money? Evaluation of nutritional rehabilitation in a rural district hospital in South-west Tanzania. I. Short-term results. *Journal of Tropical Pediatrics* 32: 240–243.

Van Roosmalen-Wiebenga, M. W., Kusin, J. A., de With, C. (1987). Nutrition rehabilitation in hospital—a waste of time and money? Evaluation of nutritional rehabilitation in a rural district hospital in South-west Tanzania. II. Long-term results. *Journal of Tropical Pediatrics* 33: 24–28.

Veghelyi, P. V. (1950). Nutritional oedema. *Annals of Paediatrics* 175: 349–377.

Venkatachalam, P. S., Srikantia, S. G. *et al.* (1956). Treatment of nutritional oedema syndrome (kwashiorkor) with vegetable protein diets. *Indian Journal of Medical Research* 44: 539–545.

Vis, H. L. (1985). On the treatment of certain forms of protein-energy malnutrition in childhood with respect to fatal complications (an example from rural Central Africa). *Annales Nestlé* **43:** 19–30.

Walker, S. P., Golden, M. H. N. (1988). Growth in length of children recovering from severe malnutrition. *European Journal of Clinical Nutrition* **42:** 395–404.

Waterlow, J. C. (1961). The rate of recovery of malnourished infants in relation to the protein and calorie levels of the diet. *Journal of Tropical Pediatrics* **7:** 16–22.

Waterlow, J. C., Golden, M. H. N., Patrick, J. (1978). Protein-energy malnutrition: treatment. In Dickerson, J. W. T., Lee, H. A. (eds) *Nutrition in the clinical management of disease*. Edward Arnold, London, pp. 49–71.

Wharton, B. A., Howells, G. R., McCance, R. A. (1967). Cardiac failure in kwashiorkor. *Lancet* **2:** 384–387.

World Health Organization (1976). *Treatment and prevention of dehydration in diarrhoeal diseases*. WHO, Geneva.

World Health Organization (1981). *The treatment and management of severe protein malnutrition*. WHO, Geneva.

13
Nutrition and growth

Introduction

It has been said that '. . . growth, however fascinating a phenomenon it may be in itself, will be for many people no more than a proxy either for nutritional state or for a more general measure of overall health' (Healy, 1989). However, we cannot say that growth status is a *proxy* for nutritional status, because in the usual situation, when there are no specific clinical signs, there is no way of defining nutritional status. It is not like saying that growth retardation is a proxy for poverty, because poverty can be defined by independent criteria. Fifty years ago, at the height of the slump in Britain, an economist was trying to find ways of assessing the nutritional status of schoolchildren (Huws Jones, 1938). He got a number of clinicians to grade the children's status on purely clinical grounds and compared the findings with the children's heights and weights. He was forced to the conclusion that there was no clinical 'gold standard' against which height and weight could be calibrated; they had to stand on their own as measures of nutritional state. We are still grappling with this problem today.

There is always the danger of a circular argument: growth failure is caused by an inadequate intake of food and nutrients; therefore growth failure represents a state of malnutrition; therefore the food intake that caused that state was inadequate. The only way out of this circle is to start from the premise that growth failure, however we define it, is in its own right an undesirable state. Beaton (1989) in an important article on the conceptional basis of nutritional anthropometry, with the sub-title 'are we asking the right questions?', summarized his position as follows: '. . . we have been mistaken in labelling the problem "malnutrition" rather than what it is, "growth failure consequent to environmental constraints."'. In this passage Beaton implicitly accepts the premise that growth failure is undesirable, otherwise he would not refer to it as a 'problem'.

The next step in developing the concept of *nutritional anthropometry* is to show that growth failure is associated with some particular pattern of the diet. Again in Beaton's words: '. . . it is to be argued equally strongly that food and nutrition are an obligatory part of the situation. By itself food may not be enough to change the situation; without food other interventions are likely to fail.' This link, if it can be established, is the justification for moving from growth status to nutritional status.

Most people will probably have no difficulty with this argument in so far as it concerns deficits in body weight. The 'Road to Health' charts introduced by Morley (1973) for use in the Third World rely on weight or weight gain as measures of a child's health. The interpretation of retardation in linear growth is much more difficult. A child's attained length or height reflects the whole of his past history, and for this reason height is often used as a measure of biological age. Graham (1968) has defined a developmental quotient (DQ) as the ratio of biological age to chronological age. Height, therefore, has a wider significance than weight and in most of the auxological literature (from the Greek αὐξἕιν, to increase) the word 'growth' is used specifically to refer to increases in length or height (Tanner, 1976).

Growth, whether in weight or height, is not, of course, a simple process. A child does not just increase in size, like a balloon being inflated; it develops as it grows and this involves qualitative as well as quantitative changes. As a child grows it changes in shape (Cole, 1991). There are also changes in body composition: the fetus puts on a great deal of fat in the third trimester. As the infant develops into a child it exchanges fat for lean tissue. At puberty girls gain more fat, boys more muscle. Karlberg *et al.* (1987, 1988) have suggested that the growth curve can be separated into three components— infancy, childhood and puberty, each under a different control or drive. The childhood component normally begins to take over at about six months of age, when growth hormone comes into operation.

Auxologists have devoted much attention to developing smoothed curves to describe the growth in height of children from birth to the end of puberty and Healy (1989) has summarized the various mathematical approaches that have been used for this purpose. However, the growth process seems in reality not to be so smooth. A new very accurate method of measuring linear growth (knemometry) has shown that mid-childhood growth spurts occur, and that even in normal children height gains fluctuate over shorter or longer periods in a way that cannot be attributed to seasonal effects or illnesses (Harrison, 1984; Hermanussen *et al.*, 1988*a*, *b*). Marshall (1971) concluded that 'a child's growth rate over the 3 months of fastest growth is most frequently 2–3 times the slowest growth rate, so that a satisfactory assessment of a child's growth cannot be made over less than 1 year'. These fluctuations clearly have important implications for the use of growth velocity as a measure of health status.

Classification of growth deficits

The traditional method of assessing growth deficits in young children is on the basis of weight for age, as in the growth charts of individual children that are widely used in child health clinics. Gomez and his colleagues in Mexico were the first to divide deficits in weight for age into three categories of severity, as a basis for the prognosis of malnourished children in hospital (Gomez *et al.*, 1956). Three categories of malnutrition were recognized, based on the so-called 'Harvard' growth standards (see below):

Normal: more than 90 per cent of standard weight for age
Grade I: 90–75 per cent—mild malnutrition
Grade II: 75–60 per cent—moderate malnutrition
Grade III: less than 60 per cent—severe malnutrition

The drawback to this system is that it combines in one number two different kinds of deficit: in weight for height and in height for age. Figure 13.1 shows two children with the same weight for age who are clearly quite different: one is tall and thin, the other short and even fat. Growth retardation is a rather cumbersome term. Some years ago it was proposed, for brevity, to describe a child with a deficit in height for age as 'stunted' and one with a deficit in weight for height as 'wasted' (Waterlow, 1973). The corresponding processes leading to the deficits are 'stunting' and 'wasting'. These terms were preferred to 'short' and 'thin' because they imply deficits outside the normal range in healthy children. They are preferred to 'acute' and 'chronic' malnutrition because they represent what is observed, without begging questions about cause.

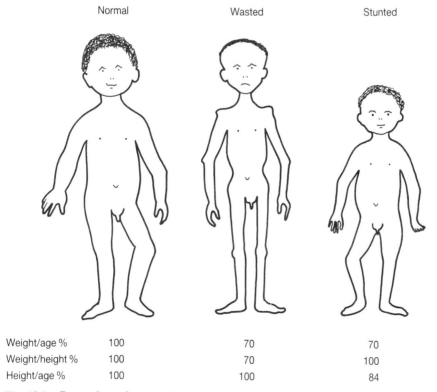

	Normal	Wasted	Stunted
Weight/age %	100	70	70
Weight/height %	100	70	100
Height/age %	100	100	84

Fig. 13.1 Comparison of a normal, a wasted and a stunted child, all aged one year.

If it is accepted that wasting and stunting represent different biological processes, as discussed below, then the simple Gomez classification of severity based on weight for age has to be replaced by a two-way classification in which wasting and stunting are recorded separately. Originally a system was proposed in which both variables had four degrees of severity, from normal

to grade III. Such a tabulation had 16 cells, which was clearly far too complicated for practical use. It was therefore replaced by the simple 2 x 2
classification shown as an 'action diagram' in Fig. 13.2 (Waterlow, 1974).
Prevalences of wasting and stunting can easily be compared in such a system.

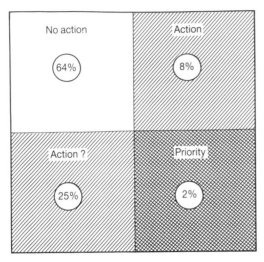

Fig. 13.2 Two-by-two classification of wasting and stunting, arranged as an 'action diagram'.
The cut-off point for wasting is 80 per cent of reference weight for height and for stunting
90 per cent of reference height for age. The prevalences in each cell are from unpublished
data of Dr H. J. L. Burgess for boys aged 24–35 months in Malawi. Reproduced by
permission from Waterlow and Rutishauser (1974).

Table 13.1 shows that, taking age three years as representative of the
pre-school period as a whole, stunting is many times commoner than wasting.
There is no dispute that a wasted child is a malnourished child. However, the
position about stunting is not so clear. If being stunted is not regarded as a
state of malnutrition, then it is evident from Table 13.1 that the prevalence
of malnutrition world-wide would be reduced several-fold. The nature, causes
and consequences of linear growth retardation therefore have important
implications for policy, and much of the rest of this chapter is devoted to
discussion of these matters.

When the wasting/stunting system was first proposed by WHO (Waterlow
et al., 1977) it was emphasized that data must be disaggregated by age,
because, as illustrated in the next chapter (Fig. 14.5), the relative prevalences
of wasting and stunting vary greatly with age. The peak prevalence of wasting
is in the second year; thereafter children who do not die mostly recover more
or less normal weight for height. The pattern for stunting is different: the
prevalence rises sharply and then levels off. These age-related differences
have an obvious bearing on public health policy.

Before going on to consider in more detail the significance of stunting in
particular, something has to be said about the references or standards, according to which deficits in weight and height are defined as 'wasting' and
'stunting'.

Table 13.1 Prevalence of stunting in samples of children aged 3 years in representative countries by WHO region

Region	Date	Prevalence, %	
		Stunting	Wasting
Africa			
Ethiopia	1982	42	10
Zambia	1970–72	42	4
Niger	1980	28	10
South America & Caribbean			
Bolivia	1981	60	0
Peru	1985	52	1
Jamaica	1976	9	4
Haiti	1978	52	6
South-east Asia			
Bangladesh	1982–83	79	16
Indonesia	1977	79	6.5
Thailand	1983	27	3
Eastern Mediterranean			
Egypt	1978	37	0.1
Pakistan	1984	14	N.A.
Palestinian refugees	1984	17	1.3
West Pacific			
Philippines	1982	43	4
Papua-New Guinea	1970	57	2.5

Source: WHO (1987)

Growth standards and references

In the preceding discussion words like 'normal', 'satisfactory', 'retarded', 'deficit', etc., have been used which imply some standard of comparison. In theory it is important to distinguish between a reference and a standard, but in practice it is almost impossible to do this. A reference should be neutral, carrying no value judgements, acting simply as a yardstick for making comparisons, whereas in many languages, including English, the word 'standard' does imply a value judgement, a target or a level that ought to be met.

A set of reference measurements of weight and height is very useful for normalizing data, e.g. for grouping together results from children of different ages. The average weight of a group of children means nothing, because it depends on the age-distribution. On the other hand, indices showing the extent to which each child differs from the reference median child of the same age or height can be averaged and treated statistically. However, even this use can be dispensed with by modern methods of covariance analysis, in which age is treated as a covariant. A reference based on a sufficient number of measurements allows calculation of the dispersion in a population in terms of standard deviations and centiles, and a point in the distribution, e.g. − 2 SD, is often used as a cut-off, to distinguish between satisfactory and unsatisfactory growth (see Chapter 14). However, this use implies that the reference is being regarded as a standard, based on 'normal' healthy children.

In the early days of nutritional anthropometry most workers used the so-called 'Harvard' standards, based on measurements made in Iowa (USA)

in the 1930s and published by Stuart and Meredith in 1946. Their tables were reproduced in Nelson's *Textbook of Pediatrics* (Stuart and Stevenson, 1959) and again in Jelliffe's well-known monograph on the assessment of nutritional state (Jelliffe, 1966). When it became apparent that to assess wasting it was necessary to have standards of weight for height, it was a serious drawback of the Harvard data that they did not contain this information. In 1977 the available data-bases were reviewed (Waterlow *et al.*, 1977) to see how this gap could best be filled, and the data from the US National Center for Health Statistics (NCHS) were accepted by WHO for use as an international reference. The choice was made principally on technical grounds because the NCHS had large numbers in each age-group and the data had been very thoroughly worked out statistically. The detailed tables have been published by WHO (1983).

It is a disadvantage of the NCHS reference that the data were collected many years ago. Some of those for infants date back as long as 60 years. More recent studies on healthy children (e.g. Whitehead and Paul, 1984) show a pattern that differs somewhat from the NCHS, with average weights beginning to fall below the NCHS median at four to six months. It is suggested that this results from changes in methods of infant feeding in industrialized countries, with breast feeding becoming more common. To the extent that the international reference is supposed to represent the growth of healthy children in a healthy environment it would be logical to pool the large amounts of more recent data now available from Britain, The Netherlands, Sweden and Switzerland as well as the USA. However, we are in a dilemma: any reference will in due course become out of date, but to change the international reference would produce chaos. For the time being we must make do with what we have.

Many people feel that in this sense it is inappropriate to use the NCHS growth pattern as a standard for the Third World. There is no certainty that the growth of North American infants and young children is optimal—they may well be too fat; and bigger is not necessarily better. However, Habicht *et al.* (1974) in an important paper summarized evidence that pre-school children from well-to-do families of different ethnic groups had the same growth potential as American children, and later studies in several countries supported this conclusion (Graitcer and Gentry, 1981; Kow *et al.*, 1991). Martorell (1985), in a very thoroughly documented analysis, extended these observations to children of school-age (Fig. 13.3). There certainly are genetic differences in growth potential and stature, since in well-off societies the height of children is related to that of their parents, but Martorell's figure shows that the environmental effects are far larger.

Figure 13.3 also shows, as Martorell emphasized, that well-to-do Asiatic children had a mean height that falls on about the 25th centile of the American reference. Data collected by Davies (1988) on Asiatic children 'brought up in what were generally considered to be favourable socioeconomic conditions' showed that their mean length at one to two years was more than 1 SD below the NCHS mean. If the difference is genetic rather than environmental, it would be logical to adopt an 'Asiatic' reference. That would have the effect of reducing several-fold the enormously high prevalences of stunting in the Asian region shown in Fig. 13.3 (see Chapter 14). However, it would be rash to assume that the difference really is genetic. A group of Asian infants in a

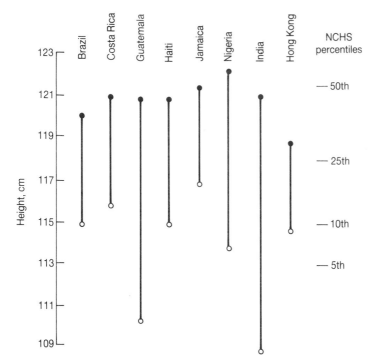

Fig. 13.3 Mean heights of seven-year old boys of high (●) and low (○) socioeconomic status in representative countries. Reproduced by permission from Martorell (1985).

depressed industrial town in the UK showed no significant difference in length growth from matched Caucasian controls: in fact, at 12 and 24 months their length was 0.25 SD greater (Warrington and Storey, 1988).

The debate between international and national growth standards has been long and hotly contested. Gopalan (1989) has summarized very cogently the drawbacks of the national approach. If a standard is to represent a target, it has to be derived from well-to-do groups, and as Gopalan points out, it is no easier to define affluence than to define poverty. If the object of local standards is to take account of ethnic differences, then in India and in many Latin American countries it would be necessary to have several sets of standards. Another use of a local standard is to give a picture of the average in a country, in order to identify groups or individuals who are above or below the average. Goldstein and Tanner (1980) and Van Loon *et al.* (1986) have argued strongly for this approach, saying that 'the selection of malnourished children by anthropometric variables can only be done successfully by "local references", which represent "acceptable growth in a given environment" '. There is force in this argument, but also great practical difficulties; there would apparently have to be a separate reference for each tribal group and Van Loon *et al.* admit that the references would have to be upgraded periodically.

When it comes to the practical application of anthropometric data, it begins to look as if the debate may be a non-controversy. As discussed in the next chapter, for the purpose of screening individual children it will often be necessary to be flexible about cut-off points based on the international reference. For the purpose of comparisons between populations, as Goldstein and Tanner (1980) point out, a reference is not really necessary. Nevertheless, an international reference will probably be useful for a long time to come to provide an easily understood picture of world-wide prevalences of growth deficit, in the way that is being done by WHO (1987) and UNICEF (Carlson and Wardlaw, 1990).

Growth velocity

In recent years there has been increasing interest in growth velocity as perhaps providing a more sensitive indicator of retardation than deficits in attained weight or height.

Tanner and his colleagues were the first to establish velocity standards well defined in the statistical sense, with centiles and standard deviations (Tanner *et al.*, 1966). Other velocity standards are now available, e.g. Prader *et al.* (1989). Velocity data from the Fels study, which provided the basis of the NCHS reference up to the age of three years, have recently been published (Baumgartner *et al.*, 1986; Roche *et al.*, 1989). In these velocity standards the data points for infants and young children are at intervals of three months or longer.

If a falling off in velocity is to provide early warning of growth failure, it must be detected over much shorter periods than three months. The expected velocity over any given month can indeed be obtained by interpolation, but the standard deviations (SD) of three-month gains cannot be applied to gains over one month. The shorter the interval, the larger the SD. Fomon and co-workers (1971) have recorded measurements made at intervals of two or four weeks up to six months. The coefficients of variation (CV) of gains in length over four weeks are of the order of 20–30 per cent. No calculations have been made to separate the variability between children from that within children, but the variability of linear growth in any individual child is certainly quite large. In Fomon's series a child might easily, within four weeks, move from the 50th to the 25th or to the 75th centile of attained weight. As might be expected, the variability tends to be even greater in Third World children who are subjected to a wider range of environmental insults (Zumrawi *et al.*, 1987; Harrison and Schmitt, 1989). The latter authors have indeed proposed that the variability of height gain could be used as an index of environmental stress.

This high variability makes it difficult to predict impending malnutrition from velocity data. In studies on the adequacy of exclusive breast feeding (Zumrawi *et al.*, 1987; Hijazi *et al.*, 1989) 'faltering' was defined as a gain in weight below −2 SD of the standard gain. However, because the SD is so large, such a definition is very insensitive. Nevertheless, Healy *et al.* (1988) have proposed a systematic way of using short-term gains in length for early warning or screening.

An important use of velocity measurements is to help in identifying causal factors. One example is the responsiveness of gains in weight and length to seasonal influences. Another is the effect of infections on growth, which is difficult to quantify except in terms of gains (see Chapter 17).

Natural history of stunting

Growth in length is proportionally slower than growth in weight; a baby trebles its birth weight in the first year, while its length increases by only 50 per cent. Deficits in length thus tend to develop more slowly and are restored more slowly, if at all, whereas deficits in weight can be rapidly reversed. In a limited sense, therefore, it may be justifiable to regard wasting as an acute process, stunting a chronic one, i.e. continuing for a long time. However, in my view it is not correct to call stunting 'chronic malnutrition'. This implies that it is simply a continuation of the process of acute malnutrition represented by wasting. It also begs the highly debatable question, discussed below, of whether being stunted can in any meaningful way be regarded as a state of malnutrition. Statistically the two states of being wasted and stunted are not significantly associated (Keller and Fillmore, 1983). I believe that they represent different biological processes which often, but by no means always, occur together. Their being different processes does not rule out the possibility of a biological relationship. There is some indication that during catch-up growth gain in weight takes precedence over gain in height. Walker and Golden (1988) showed that in children recovering from severe malnutrition height growth did not take off until weight had been restored to 85 per cent of expected weight for height. In Nepal Costello (1989) observed a very interesting inverse relationship between initial weight deficit and subsequent height velocity (Fig. 13.4). Nabarro *et al.* (1988), also working in Nepal, found that seasonal changes in height gain followed those in weight gain with a lag of about three months, confirming earlier findings of Brown and co-workers in Bangladesh (1982).

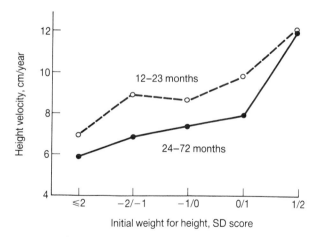

Fig. 13.4 Effect of initial nutritional status (weight for height) on subsequent mean height velocity in the period after harvest in Nepal for age-groups 12–23 and 24–72 months. Reproduced by permission from Costello (1989).

Prevalences of stunting in different parts of the world have been tabulated by Keller (1988). Longitudinal or semi-longitudinal data from a number of countries suggest that the processes of stunting and wasting both start very early, within the first three months of life (Waterlow *et al.*, 1980; Waterlow,

1988). This conclusion has been criticized on the grounds that the reference is inappropriate and that the growth of exclusively breast-fed healthy babies in well-to-do countries begins to fall below the reference at around four months (Ahn and MacLean, 1980; Whitehead and Paul, 1981; Hitchcock *et al.*, 1981; Salmenperä *et al.*, 1985). However, the deficits in both weight and height in Third World children are larger and last longer. The important point is that both deficits start in the early months of life.

Figure 13.5 shows average length/height increments between birth and five years recorded in 17 developing countries. Figure 13.6 shows height velocity

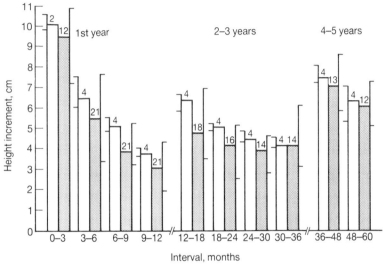

Fig. 13.5   Average increments in length/height over three months (first year), six months (second and third years) and one year (fourth and fifth years) in children from developing (shaded bars) and developed (open bars) countries. Numbers above the columns represent the number of studies and the error bars the range of variation between studies, not between individuals. Reproduced by permission from Waterlow (1988).

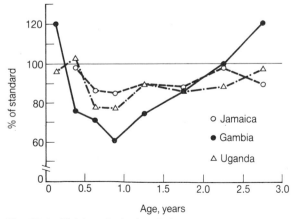

Fig. 13.6   Height velocity in relation to age in three longitudinal studies, expressed as a percentage of the normal velocity. Reproduced by permission from Waterlow and Rutishauser (1974).

related to age in three longitudinal studies, in The Gambia, Uganda and Jamaica. The pattern is the same in these three very different environments, although the extent of the growth deficit differs.

Growth in height is not only affected in the long term by environmental factors; it is also sensitive to short-term changes. A good example is provided by the seasonal fluctuations in height growth in Nepal, mentioned above and illustrated in Fig. 13.7. Thus stunting can be reversed and catch-up can occur if conditions become favourable. Very rapid increases in the rate of linear growth are found not only in children recovering from malnutrition (Hansen *et al.*, 1971; Walker and Golden, 1988), but also as a result of treatment for conditions such as coeliac disease (Prader, 1978), Crohn's disease (Kirschner *et al.*, 1981) and colitis caused by *Trichuris* infestation (Cooper *et al.*, 1990).

Several authors have found that at school-age children who had been severely malnourished in infancy were no shorter than their peers who had not been malnourished (Garrow and Pike, 1967; Keet *et al.*, 1971; Cameron *et al.*, 1986). Garrow and Pike invoked a kind of reverse genetic effect, that the ex-patients had a genetically greater growth potential, and hence greater food requirements, and for that reason became malnourished. A most striking example of recovery from stunting has been described from Peru. A small group of severely growth-retarded children were discharged from hospital to well-off foster parents. At nine years they had reached the US 25th centile for height, whereas those who had returned to their poor homes were still below the third centile (Graham and Adrianzen, 1971, 1972). It is interesting that in Ethiopia survivors from kwashiorkor had the same stature at school age as children who had not been malnourished in infancy, whereas survivors from marasmus were significantly shorter (Branko, 1979). All these experiences, taken together with the normal fluctuations in growth referred to at the beginning of this chapter, show that growth in length is a much more plastic process than has sometimes been thought.

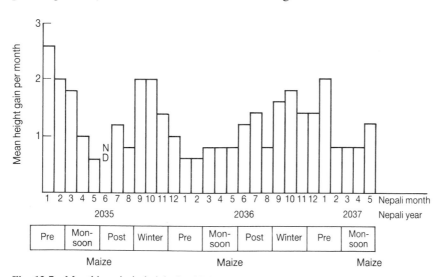

Fig. 13.7 Monthly gain in height in children aged 12–23 months in Chuliban village, Nepal, in relation to season and the maize harvest. Reproduced by permission from Nabarro *et al.* (1988).

It is not entirely clear how far stunting in childhood influences adult height. Undernutrition and poor social conditions cause delay in skeletal maturation and in the onset of puberty (Satyanarayana *et al.*, 1989), so that the time available for continuing growth will be extended. However, this may not be enough for full catch-up, because skeletal maturation or bone-age is less retarded than height-age (Martorell *et al.*, 1979).

In girls the onset of menarche is delayed by malnutrition (Galler *et al.*, 1987). Frisch and Revelle (1971) suggested that a critical weight might have to be achieved before menarche starts. However, they found that the gain in height was the same, whether girls entered menarche early or late. Thus the pattern seems to be similar to that in boys: development is delayed, but growth is continued for longer.

Keet *et al.* (1971) summarized the results of 11 studies in which previously malnourished children had been followed for varying periods, but not beyond the age of puberty. In five of the studies the weights and heights of ex-patients at follow-up were the same or slightly greater than those of controls; in the other six they were lower. Presumably the discrepancies result from the conditions during childhood. The catch-up of malnourished children who were returned to good homes has already been mentioned.

Table 13.2 shows the results of five studies in which the growth of children was followed from five years to adult or nearly adult age. These differ from those described by Keet *et al.* (1971), in that although many of the children were initially stunted, they were not, as far as is known, severely malnourished. It is remarkable how uniform the pattern is in such very different ecological settings. In all cases the increment in height was very much the same as that of American children, and it was similar regardless of the degree of stunting at five years. Initially stunted children grew along a curve parallel to those who were less stunted, but they did not catch up.

Martorell *et al.* (1990) suggest that these children were irreversibly pro-

Table 13.2 Height gains from five years to maturity

Study and group	Height at 5 years (% of reference)	Interval (years)	Mean total gain, cm	
			Boys	Girls
Hyderabad[a]				
poor	81	5–20	68	–
better-off	95	5–20	68	–
Guatemala[b]				
1st tercile	86	5–20	64	53
3rd tercile	94	5–20	64	53
Gambia[c]	92	5–20	65	57
South Africa[d]				
ex-kwashiorkor	88.5	5–17	65	55
siblings	88	5–17	64	53
Berkeley, USA[b]	100	5–adult	68	56.5
NCHS[e]	100	5–18	67	55

References: [a] Satyanarayana *et al.* (1986)
 [b] Martorell *et al.* (1990)
 [c] Billewicz and McGregor (1982)
 [d] Bowie *et al.* (1980)
 [e] WHO (1983)

grammed by environmental stresses to become adults of short stature. McCance's (1976) experimental work suggested that if growth is retarded at a critical period, full catch-up can never occur, however well an animal is fed. Dobbing (1990) contends that the critical period for determining somatic growth coincides with the growth-spurt of the brain, which in humans extends from the last trimester of pregnancy to about the end of the second year (Dobbing and Sands, 1973). However, he points out that the long-term effect depends not only on the timing but on the duration and severity of the insult. In general, babies who are small for gestational age and have perhaps been undernourished *in utero* do tend to catch up (Cruise, 1973; Davies, 1980), so that although small for dates babies are common in the Third World, this does not seem an adequate explanation of postnatal stunting. In a prospective study in Thailand, children who later became stunted were of nearly normal length at birth (P. Somnasang *et al.*, personal communication).

The hypothesis of programming does not account for the rapid catch-up growth in height observed in the clinical situations already mentioned, since many of these children were well over five years old. Graham and Adrianzen (1972) showed continuing catch-up in height for seven years or more in the severely marasmic stunted children who were adopted into privileged homes. The effects of supplementary feeding trials described later in this chapter also argue against the hypothesis.

If we move from individuals to communities, secular changes in height, with a reduction in the difference between upper and lower social classes, have been documented in Britain (Boyne *et al.*, 1957; Cone, 1961; Cameron, 1979) and other countries also, as in the well-known example of Japan (Matsumoto, 1982). Historical research suggests that in Europe and the USA over the last two centuries adult height may have been quite a sensitive indicator of prevailing social and economic conditions (Floud, 1989; Steckel, 1989; Sandberg, 1989). Going back 3000 years, the anthropologist Angel (1946) regarded better nutrition as the cause of a 6 cm increase in height of Mediterranean men that occurred between the Mycenaean and late classical eras.

In more recent times Tanner (1982) quotes Vaillarmé, who wrote in 1828:

> Human height becomes greater, and growth takes place more rapidly, other things being equal, in proportion as the country is richer, comfort more general, houses, clothes and nourishment better, and labour, fatigue and privations during infancy and youth less: in other words, circumstances which accompany poverty delay the age at which complete stature is reached and stunt adult height.

Tanner, indeed, regards height as a proxy for health in population groups.

How then are we to explain the differences in adult height in different ethnic groups recorded by Eveleth and Tanner (1976) in their synopsis of world-wide variations in human growth? In the extreme case the difference between the pygmies of the Congo and the Dinka of Sudan amounts to 36 cm. There are large, though not so pronounced differences between other ethnic groups. It seems unlikely that these can all be explained on the basis of adverse influences in the first few years of life. Perhaps there are genetic determinants which come into play at puberty, provided that conditions are favourable. Such a hypothesis would reconcile large differences in adult height with a relatively uniform growth potential in young children. Steckel (1987) records that American slaves, as children, were about at our modern 1st centile, but after puberty had caught up to more than the 25th centile. It has been reported that in pygmies acceleration of growth at adolescence was blunted or absent and that in adolescent pygmy boys IGF1 levels were only one-third of those of controls, whereas before puberty they were the same (Fig. 13.8). Perhaps, therefore, puberty is the critical period for determining adult stature.

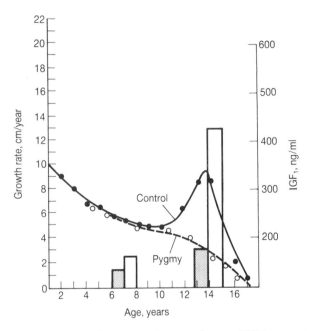

Fig. 13.8   Mean linear growth rate and serum IGF 1 concentrations in pygmy boys and controls; ●——●, growth rate, controls; ○---○ , growth rate, pygmies; ▢ , serum IGF 1, controls; ▨ , serum IGF 1, pygmies. Reproduced by permission from Merimee *et al.* (1987).

Causes of retardation of linear growth

Many conditions are associated with a reduction in linear growth: deficiency of almost any nutrient, particularly those that, like protein, are components of body tissue, described by Golden (1988) as type II nutrients (Chapter 2); endocrine disturbances, particularly growth hormone deficiency and hypothyroidism; many chronic diseases of childhood, such as cystic fibrosis, congenital heart disease, chronic nephritis, etc.; repeated or continuing infections; inadequate psychosocial stimulation; finally, poverty and deprivation, which are usually cited as the causes of stunting in discussions on nutrition policy.

At the level of the cell there are again a number of possible causal factors: not only a deficiency of nutrients but a lack of growth-promoting substances such as somatomedins (Root, 1990; see also Chapter 10); a decrease in the number of receptors; and the action of substances that suppress growth.

If inadequate nutrition is proposed as a primary cause of stunting, what is the nature of the inadequacy? It has been suggested that stunting could result from specific deficiency of good quality protein or of factors associated with protein in foods (Waterlow, 1978). Golden (1988) has marshalled the evidence in detail.

This idea has a long history. In the slump in the 1930s Boyd Orr was asked by the Ministry of Agriculture for advice on how to dispose of surplus milk which people were too poor to buy. He recommended that it should be fed to school children and organized trials to test whether the supplements had any effect. Leighton and Clark (1929) reported small but significant increases in height in the supplemented children, together with remarkable improvement in their general appearance. It is interesting to record some of the other observations made in this classical study:

> Dr C. A. Douglas examined all the children clinically . . . in practically every case it was noted that the children receiving milk showed, even where there was obviously poor maternal care, that sleekness peculiar to a well-fed animal. Their hair had a glossy and bright appearance. General alertness was common to all the children fed on milk . . . It was gathered from teachers and janitors that the children receiving milk were much more alert and very much more boisterous and difficult to control than the others. This was only too evident when they were waiting in small groups to be weighed.

Aykroyd and Krishnan (1937) followed up this work with similar trials in India. They showed that school children on a poor rice diet supplemented with skimmed milk showed better growth in height than unsupplemented controls. Aykroyd also mentions a transformation in the appearance of the children, particularly of the skin. Coming to more recent times, Lampl *et al.* (1978) in New Guinea found that a milk supplement given to school children produced an increase in height, whereas an energy supplement did not. Gopalan *et al.* (1973) gave a supplement providing 310 kcal and only 3 g protein daily for 14 months to children aged one to five years. The supplement produced very significantly greater gains in height, compared with controls, which were largest in the youngest age-groups. Fomon *et al.* (1977) fed infants on a skimmed milk mixture low in energy but high in protein. They gained in length almost as well as controls on a normal formula, although their weight gains were much less.

A different type of study that is very interesting in this context is that of Rutishauser and Whitehead (1969) on the children of two tribes in Uganda. Fig. 13.9 shows their weights and heights. The Karamoja, who are herdsmen, live on milk and meat and their children are tall and thin. The Buganda are farmers with plantains as their staple, and their children are short and of normal weight for height. In Peru Graham *et al.* (1981) noted in boys a strong association between protein intake and attained height.

All these results, taken together, are quite impressive. They do not, however, allow us to determine whether the stimulation of growth can be attributed to an increased intake of protein, or of other factors such as calcium

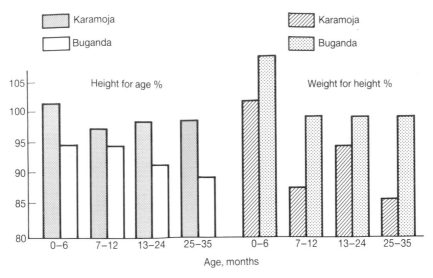

Fig. 13.9 Weights for height and heights for age, as percentages, of children from two Ugandan tribes, Karamoja and Buganda. Drawn from data of Rutishauser and Whitehead (1969).

or zinc (Chapter 4). Another suggestion is a deficiency of phosphate as a cause of growth retardation (Fraser, 1988).

At the biochemical level it seems entirely possible that the requirements for skeletal growth should be different from those for cellular growth. Thus sulphur intake might be limiting for the formation of the sulphated polysaccharides that are a major component of cartilage. This hypothesis of the nutritional cause of stunting fits in with the proposition that stunting and wasting are distinct and separate processes, since it is reasonable to regard wasting as a result of energy deficiency.

Karlberg *et al.* (1988), on the basis of a study in Pakistan, suggested that stunting beginning in the first year of life resulted from delay in the change-over from the infancy to the childhood component in their model of the determinants of growth (see p. 188). This is an interesting idea because it implies that stunting represents a qualitative departure from the normal pattern, rather than just a quantitative deficiency.

Functional consequences and associations of stunting

It may be contended that for practical purposes the nutritional cause of stunting is irrelevant; what matter are the handicaps and benefits of small body size.

There are some obvious benefits: small people need less food, less clothing, less space. The most direct disadvantage is a reduction in the absolute capacity for physical work, as defined by VO_2max (Spurr, 1984). Spurr's studies in Colombia on boys who were small for their age showed that their working capacity per kg body weight was normal (Spurr, 1988). This means that they had no impairment of cardio-respiratory fitness. However, according to Spurr, no task can be performed continuously at a rate greater than about 40 per cent of VO₂max. Therefore, with a given work load, people who are small, even though fit, will be at a disadvantage. For rural cultivators this could be a severe handicap.

Satyanarayana *et al.* (1979, 1980) in India showed that in a culture in which it is usual for boys to be employed in agricultural work, those who were small in stature had less chance than their better grown peers of getting employment and earning money. So the problem perpetuates itself. For women small size means an increased difficulty in childbirth. In Mayan women a striking relationship was found between maternal height and infant mortality (Martorell, 1989).

Other handicaps that are described in stunted children are not presumably direct effects of small body size, but associated effects of the environment that produced stunting. There is evidence of defects in phagocytic function and cell-mediated immunity (Reddy *et al.*, 1976; Bhaskaram *et al.*, 1980). In these studies the children were classified according to weight for age, but they probably were stunted. Tomkins (1988) concluded that there was no evidence for a higher incidence of infection in stunted children, but in the case of diarrhoeal disease the severity and duration of episodes were somewhat greater (Chapter 17).

By far the most important association of stunting, which has been well documented in school-age children, is with impairment of mental development (DQ) (Cravioto and DeLicardie, 1973, 1976; Richardson, 1976; Cravioto and Arrieta, 1986). This association is not found in well-to-do groups, where differences in the height of individual children are presumably genetic. In Richardson's study in Jamaica height accounted for 25 per cent of the variance in DQ. The relationship of stunting to DQ in younger children is discussed in Chapter 19. Little is known about the extent to which the deficit in mental development is reversible, although Grantham-McGregor's work in Jamaica (Chapter 19) suggests that it may be (Grantham-McGregor, 1982; Grantham-McGregor *et al.*, 1989). Cravioto and Cravioto (1990) have shown that by the age of ten years children who had survived an earlier episode of malnutrition did reach the same level of competence as those who had not been malnourished. Nevertheless, the lag in their development may have serious effects, e.g. on their placing in school, and so have a permanent influence on their future role and status in society.

The question of adaptation

It has been proposed that, since a small child needs less food, stunting is a useful adaptation, promoting survival when food is in short supply (Seckler, 1982). This is the concept of 'costless biological adaptation' (FAO, 1988) which has aroused a great deal of heated discussion (Gopalan, 1983; Martorell, 1989; Beaton, 1989; Waterlow, 1989).

Seckler postulates that above a certain limit stunted children are 'small but healthy'. This hypothesis has very serious implications for policy. If stunted children are adapted rather than malnourished, the global prevalence of malnutrition is reduced by some 80 per cent (Table 13.1). It is understandable, therefore, that Seckler's concept should have found favour with policy makers, but the consensus of opinion among nutritionists is that it does not stand up to critical examination. Beaton (1989) and Martorell (1989) in particular have provided thoughtful discussions of the question. In the words of Gopalan: 'Here was a plea for letting the magnitude of the problem determine the yardstick for its measurement, rather than using a yardstick to determine the magnitude of a problem.'

Payne (1986, 1987) in two important reviews, in effect supports Seckler. He does not question that stunted children may have impairments of function, but if I read his argument correctly, he believes that this occurs in a minority who have failed to adapt or who have been pushed by environmental stress beyond the limit of their capacity for adaptation. The validity of the argument depends on the nature of the relationship between depression of physical growth and the various functional impairments. If there is no increase of risk or handicap until a threshold—breakdown of adaptation—is reached, then the argument is valid. If, on the other hand, the relationship is continuous, so that every degree of growth deficit carries with it some degree of functional impairment, then it fails. It would probably be quite wrong to generalize about these relationships. In the case of mortality there does seem to be a threshold (Chapter 18); for physical work capacity the relationship is probably continuous. For functions such as resistance to disease or mental handicap, the information does not exist on which to reach a conclusion.

Thus the difficulty in discussing the Seckler-Payne point of view objectively is that the concept of adaptation is so hard to define (Waterlow, 1985, 1990). We might rephrase the general hypothesis as follows: stunting is a compromise with environmental stress, perhaps the best that can be achieved under the circumstances. In the same vein Ghesquière and D'Hulst (1988) wrote: 'Taking a more evolutionary viewpoint, we may ask ourselves if this condition of "nutrition at risk" is not the living condition for which nature has prepared the human race: setting a high genetic potential, knowing by experience that the environment will thwart some of this potential.'

When it comes to questions of policy and action, both sides in the debate run up against difficulty: if children are regarded as adapted until they have reached a level where adaptation breaks down, where is that level? On the other side, it is necessary to decide on a dividing line at the upper end of the scale, between normal/acceptable and abnormal/unacceptable. Without being too academic about these matters, some rough and ready decisions have to be made as a guideline for action. As discussed in the next chapter, in real life the decision will probably depend on what is feasible in a given situation. For example, in Glasgow children whose fathers were unemployed were found to be slightly less well grown than children whose fathers were working (Cole *et al.*, 1983). In the UK this finding might reasonably be regarded as a trigger for action, whereas in a Third World country such a deficit could be regarded as trivial.

It would also be naïve to regard stunting as a purely nutritional problem, to be prevented or reversed by nutritional measures alone, important though they are. A high prevalence of stunted children indicates the need for long-term programmes to counteract the effects of poverty and disadvantage and to improve future productivity and the quality of life (Martorell *et al.*, 1988;

Gopalan, 1988). We return to these matters at the end of the book (Chapter 20), but here it is worth summarizing the points that relate directly to the biology of stunting. First, if it is true that the process of stunting often starts in the first few months of life, special emphasis has to be given to protecting the health and nutrition of young children in the critical period up to two years of age. Secondly, if the hypothesis about the nutritional cause of stunting is true, improvement in the quality of life should include improvement in the nutritional quality as well as the quantity of food available for young children.

At a more general level, the United Nations Convention on the Rights of Children includes many rights which, because they cannot be enforced, might more realistically be regarded as goals. Among them is the right of a child to a diet which enables him to fulfil his genetic growth potential.

References

Ahn, C. H., MacLean, W. C. (1980). Growth of the exclusively breast-fed infant. *American Journal of Clinical Nutrition* **33:** 183–192.

Angel, L. J. (1946). Ancient Greek skeletal change. *American Journal of Physiological Anthropology* **NS4:** 69–97.

Aykroyd, W. R., Krishnan, B. G. (1937). The effect of skimmed milk, soya bean and other foods in supplementing typical Indian diets. *Indian Journal of Medical Research* **24:** 1093–1115.

Baumgartner, R. N., Roche, A. F., Himes, J. F. (1986). Incremented growth tables supplementary to previously published charts. *American Journal of Clinical Nutrition* **43:** 711–722.

Beaton, G. H. (1989). Small but healthy? Are we asking the right question? *European Journal of Clinical Nutrition* **43:** 563–575.

Bhaskaram, P., Satyanarayana, K. *et al.* (1980). Effect of growth retardation in early life on immunocompetence in later life. *Indian Journal of Medical Research* **72:** 519–526.

Billewicz, W. Z., McGregor, I. A. (1982). A birth-to-maturity longitudinal study of heights and weights in two West African (Gambian) villages (1951–1975). *Annals of Human Biology* **9:** 309–320.

Bowie, M. D., Moodie, A. D. *et al.* (1980). A prospective 15-year follow-up study of kwashiorkor patients. *South African Medical Journal* **58:** 671–676.

Boyne, A. W., Aitken, F. C., Leitch, I. (1957). Secular change in height and weight of British children, including an analysis of measurements of English children in primary schools, 1911–1953. *Nutrition Abstracts and Reviews* **27:** 1–17.

Branko, Z. (1979). Height, weight and head circumference in survivors of marasmus and kwashiorkor. *American Journal of Clinical Nutrition* **32:** 1719–1727.

Brown, K. H., Black, R. E., Becker, S. (1982). Seasonal changes in nutritional status and the prevalence of malnutrition in a longitudinal study of young children in rural Bangladesh. *American Journal of Clinical Nutrition* **36:** 303–313.

Cameron, N. (1979). The growth of London schoolchildren 1904–1966: an analysis of secular trend and intra-county variation. *Annals of Human Biology* **6:** 505–525.

Cameron, N., Jones, P. R. M. *et al.* (1986). Timing and magnitude of adolescent growth in height and weight of Cape Coloured children after kwashiorkor. *Journal of Pediatrics* **109:** 548–555.

Carlson, B. A., Wardlaw, T. (1990). A global, regional and country assessment of child malnutrition. UNICEF draft.

Cole, T. J. (1991). Weight-stature indices to measure underweight, overweight and obesity. In Himes, J. H. (ed) *Anthropometric assessment of nutritional status*. Wiley-Liss, New York, pp. 83–111.

Cole, T. J., Donnet, M. L., Stanfield, J. P. (1983). Unemployment, birthweight and growth in the first year. *Archives of Disease in Childhood* **58**: 717–721.

Cone, T. E. (1961). Secular acceleration of height and biologic maturation in children during the past century. *Journal of Pediatrics* **59**: 736–740.

Cooper, E. S., Bundy, D. A. P. *et al.* (1990). Growth suppression in the *Trichuris* dysentery syndrome. *European Journal of Clinical Nutrition* **44**: 285–291.

Costello, A. M. de, L. (1989). Growth velocity and stunting in rural Nepal. *Archives of Disease in Childhood* **64**: 1478–1482.

Cravioto, J., Arrieta, F. (1986). Nutrition, mental development and learning. In Falkner, F., Tanner, J. M. (eds) *Human growth, Vol. 3*. Baillière Tindall, London, pp. 501–536.

Cravioto, J., Cravioto, P. (1990). Some long-term psychobiologic consequences of malnutrition. *Annales Nestlé* **48**: 93–102.

Cravioto, J., DeLicardie, E. R. (1973). Nutrition and behaviour and learning. *World Review of Nutrition and Dietetics* **16**: 80–96.

Cravioto, J., DeLicardie, E. R. (1976). Malnutrition in early childhood and some of its later effects at individual and community levels. *Food and Nutrition* **2**: 2–32.

Cruise, M. O. (1973). A longitudinal study of the growth of low birth weight infants. *Pediatrics* **51**: 620–628.

Davies, D. P. (1980). Size at birth and growth in the first year of life of babies who are overweight and underweight at birth. *Proceedings of the Nutrition Society* **39**: 25–33.

Davies, D. P. (1988). The importance of genetic influences on growth in early childhood with particular reference to children of Asiatic origin. In Waterlow, J. C. (ed) *Linear growth in less developed countries*. Nestlé Nutrition, Vevey/Raven Press, New York, pp. 75–86.

Dobbing, J. (1990). Early nutrition and later achievement. *Proceedings of the Nutrition Society* **49**: 103–118.

Dobbing, J., Sands, J. (1973). The quantitative growth and development of the human brain. *Archives of Disease in Childhood* **48**: 757–767.

Eveleth, P. B., Tanner, J. M. (1976). *Worldwide variation in human growth*. Cambridge University Press.

Floud, R. (1989). Changes in the mean stature of the British male population, 1750–1912. In Tanner, J. M. (ed) *Auxology 88: perspectives in the science of growth and development*. Smith-Gordon, London, pp. 167–174.

Fomon, S. J., Filer, L. J. *et al.* (1977). Skim milk in infant feeding. *Acta Paediatrica Scandinavica* **66**: 17–30.

Fomon, S. J., Thomas, L. N. *et al.* (1971). Food consumption and growth of normal infants fed milk-based formulas. *Acta Paediatrica Scandinavica* Suppl. **223**: 1–36.

Food and Agriculture Organization (1987). The fifth world food survey. FAO, Rome.

Fraser, D. R. (1988). Nutritional growth retardation: experimental studies with special reference to calcium. In Waterlow, J. C. (ed) *Linear growth retardation in less developed countries*. Nestlé Nutrition, Vevey/Raven Press, New York, pp. 127–135.

Frisch, R. E., Revelle, R. (1971). Height and weight at menarche and a hypothesis of menarche. *Archives of Disease in Childhood* **46**: 695–701.

Galler, J. R., Ramsey, F. C. *et al.* (1987). Long term effects of early kwashiorkor compared with marasmus. I. Physical growth and sexual maturation. *Journal of Pediatrics, Gastroenterology and Nutrition* **6**: 841–846.

Garrow, J. S., Pike, M. C. (1967). The long-term prognosis of severe infantile malnutrition. *Lancet* **1**: 1–4.

Ghesquière, J., D'Hulst, C. (1988). Growth, stature and fitness of children in tropical areas. In Collins, K. J., Roberts, D. F. (eds) *Capacity for work in the tropics*. Cambridge University Press, pp. 165–179.

Golden, M. H. N. (1988). The role of individual nutrient deficiencies in growth retardation of children, as exemplified by zinc and protein. In Waterlow, J. C.

(ed) *Linear growth retardation in less developed countries.* Nestlé Nutrition, Vevey/ Raven Press, New York, pp. 143–164.

Goldstein, H., Tanner, J. M. (1980). Ecological considerations in the creation and use of child growth standards. *Lancet* **1:** 582–585.

Gomez, F., Ramos-Galván, R. *et al.* (1956). Mortality in second and third degree malnutrition. *Journal of Tropical Pediatrics* **2:** 77–83.

Gopalan, C. (1983). 'Small is healthy?' For the poor, not for the rich. *Nutrition Foundation of India Bulletin* October 1983.

Gopalan, C. (1988). Stunting: significance and implications for public health policy. In Waterlow, J. C. (ed) *Linear growth retardation in less developed countries.* Nestlé Nutrition, Vevey/Raven Press, New York, pp. 265–279.

Gopalan, C. (1989). Growth standards for Indian children. *Nutrition Foundation of India Bulletin* **10:** No. 3, July 1989.

Gopalan, C., Swaminathan, M. C. *et al.* (1973). Effect of calorie supplementation on growth of undernourished children. *American Journal of Clinical Nutrition* **26:** 563– 566.

Graham, G. G. (1968). The later growth of malnourished infants: effects of age, severity and subsequent diet. In McCance, R. A, Widdowson, E. M. (eds) *Calorie deficiencies and protein deficiencies.* Churchill, London, pp. 301–315.

Graham, G. G., Adrianzen, T. B. (1971). Growth, inheritance and environment. *Pediatric Research* **5:** 691–697.

Graham, G. G., Adrianzen, T. B. (1972). Late 'catch-up' growth after severe infantile malnutrition. *Johns Hopkins Medical Journal* **131:** 204–211.

Graham, G. G., Creed, H.M. *et al.* (1981). Determinants of growth among poor children: nutrient intake-achieved growth relationships. *American Journal of Clinical Nutrition* **34:** 539–554.

Graitcer, P. L., Gentry, E. M. (1981). Measuring children: one reference for all. *Lancet* **2:** 297–299.

Grantham-McGregor, S. (1982). The relationship between developmental level and different types of malnutrition in children. *Human Nutrition:Clinical Nutrition* **36C:** 319–320.

Grantham-McGregor, S., Powell, C., Walker, S. (1989). Nutritional supplements, stunting and child development. *Lancet* **2:** 809–810.

Habicht J-P., Martorell, R. *et al.* (1974). Height and weight standards for pre-school children. How relevant are ethnic differences in growth potential? *Lancet* **1:** 611– 615.

Hansen, J. D. L., Freesemann, C. *et al.* (1971). What does nutritional growth retardation imply? *Pediatrics* **47:** 299–313.

Harrison, G. G. (1984). Application of incremental growth standards. *Food and Nutrition Bulletin* **6(2):** 18–21.

Harrison, G. A., Schmitt, L. H. (1989). Variability in stature growth. *Annals of Human Biology* **16:**45–51.

Healy, M. J. R. (1989). Growth curves and growth standards. In Tanner, J. M. (ed) *Auxology 88: Perspectives in the science of growth and development.* Smith-Gordon, London, pp. 13–22.

Healy, M. J. R., Yang, M. *et al.* (1988). The use of short-term increments in length to monitor growth in infancy. In Waterlow, J. C. (ed) *Linear growth retardation in less developed countries.* Nestlé Nutrition, Vevey/Raven Press, New York, pp. 41– 55.

Hermanussen, M., Geiger-Benoit, K. *et al.* (1988*a*). Knemometry in childhood: accuracy and standardization of a new technique of child leg measurement. *Annals of Human Biology* **15:** 1–16.

Hermanussen, M., Geiger-Benoit, K. *et al.* (1988*b*). Periodical changes of short-term growth velocity ('mini growth spurts') in human growth. *Annals of Human Biology* **15:** 103–110.

208   *Protein-energy malnutrition*

Hijazi, S. S., Abulaban, A. *et al.* (1989). The duration for which exclusive breast feeding is adequate. *Acta Paediatrica Scandinavica* **78**: 23–28.

Hitchcock, N. E., Gracey, M., Owles, E. N. (1981). Growth of healthy breast-fed infants in the first six months. *Lancet* **2**: 64–65.

Huws Jones, R. (1938). Physical indices and clinical assessments of the nutrition of school-children. *Journal of the Royal Statistical Society* **101**: 1–34.

Jelliffe, D. B. (1966). *The assessment of the nutritional status of the community*. WHO Monograph Series No. 53. WHO, Geneva.

Karlberg, J., Albertsson-Wikland, K. (1988). Infancy growth pattern related to growth hormone deficiency. *Acta Paediatrica Scandinavica* **77**: 385–391.

Karlberg, J., Engstrom, I. *et al.* (1987). Analysis of linear growth using a mathematical model. *Acta Paediatrica Scandinavica* **76**: 478–488.

Karlberg, J., Jalil, F., Lindblad, B. S. (1988). Longitudinal analysis of infant growth in an urban area of Lahore, Pakistan. *Acta Paediatrica Scandinavica* **77**: 392–401.

Keet, M. P., Moodie, A. D. *et al.* (1971). Kwashiorkor: a prospective ten-year follow-up study. *South African Medical Journal* **45**: 1427–1449.

Keller, W. (1988). The epidemiology of stunting. In Waterlow, J. C. (ed) *Linear growth retardation in less developed countries*. Nestlé Nutrition, Vevey/Raven Press, New York, pp. 17–29.

Keller, W., Fillmore, C. M. (1983). Prevalence of protein-energy malnutrition. *World Health Statistical Quarterly* **36**: 129–167.

Kirschner, B. S., Klich, J. R. *et al.* (1981). Reversal of growth retardation in Crohn's disease with therapy emphasizing oral nutritional rehabilitation. *Gastroenterology* **80**: 10–15.

Kow, F., Geissler, C., Balasubrimaniam, E. (1991). Are international anthropometric standards appropriate for developing countries? *Journal of Tropical Pediatrics* **37**: 37–44.

Lampl, M., Johnston, F. E., Malcolm, L. A. (1978). The effects of protein supplementation on the growth and skeletal maturation of New Guinean school children. *Annals of Human Biology* **5**: 219–227.

Leighton, G., Clark, M. L. (1929). Milk consumption and the growth of school-children. *Lancet* **1**: 40–43.

McCance, R. A. (1976). Critical periods of growth. *Proceedings of the Nutrition Society* **35**: 309–313.

Marshall, W. A. (1971). Evaluation of growth rate in height over periods of less than a year. *Archives of Disease in Childhood* **46**: 414–420.

Martorell, R. (1985). Child growth retardation: a discussion of its causes and of its relationship to health. In Blaxter, K. L., Waterlow, J. C. (eds) *Nutritional adaptation in man*. John Libbey, London, pp. 13–30.

Martorell, R. (1989). Body size, adaptation and function. *Human Organization* **48**: 15–20.

Martorell, R., Mendoza, F., Castillo, R. (1988). Poverty and stature in children. In Waterlow, J. C. (ed) *Linear growth retardation in less developed countries*. Nestlé Nutrition, Vevey/Raven Press, New York, pp. 57–74.

Martorell, R., Rivera, J., Kaplowitz, H. (1990). Consequences of stunting in early childhood for adult body size in rural Guatemala. *Annales Nestlé* **48**: 85–92.

Martorell, R., Yarbrough, C. *et al.* (1979). Malnutrition, body size and skeletal maturation interrelationships and implications for catch-up growth. *Human Biology* **51**: 371–389.

Matsumoto, K. (1982). Secular acceleration of growth in height of Japanese and its social background. *Annals of Human Biology* **9**: 399–410.

Merimee, T. J., Zapf, J. *et al.* (1987). Insulin-like growth factors in pygmies: the role of puberty in determining final stature. *New England Journal of Medicine* **316**: 906–911.

Morley, D. (1973). *Pediatric priorities in the developing world*. Butterworth, London.

Nabarro, D., Howard, P. *et al.* (1988). The importance of infections and environmental factors as possible determinants of growth retardation in children. In Waterlow, J. C. (ed) *Linear growth in less developed countries*. Nestlé Nutrition, Vevey/Raven Press, New York, pp. 165–184.

Payne, P. R. (1986). Appropriate indicators for project design and evaluation. In Greaves. J. P., Shaw, D. J. (eds) *Food aid and the well-being of children in the developing world*. United Nations Children's' Fund/World Food Programme, New York, pp. 105–141.

Payne, P. R. (1987). Malnutrition and human capital: problems of theory and practice. In Clay, E., Shaw, J. (eds) *Poverty, development and food*. Macmillan, Basingstoke, pp. 22–41.

Prader, A. (1978). Catch-up growth. *Postgraduate Medical Journal* **54:** Suppl.1, 133–146.

Prader, A., Largo, R. H. *et al.* (1989). Physical growth of Swiss children from birth to 20 years of age. *Helvetica Paediatrica Acta* **43:** Suppl. 52, 1–125.

Reddy, V., Jagadeesan, V. *et al.* (1976). Functional significance of growth retardation in malnutrition. *American Journal of Clinical Nutrition* **29:** 3–7.

Richardson, S. A. (1976). The relation of severe malnutrition in infancy to the intelligence of school-children with differing life-histories. *Pediatric Research* **10:** 57–61.

Roche, A. F., Guo, S., Moore, W. M. (1989). Weight and recumbent length from 1 to 12 months of age: reference data for 1 month increments. *American Journal of Clinical Nutrition* **49:** 599–607.

Root, A. W. (1990). Effects of undernutrition on skeletal development, maturation and growth. In Simmons, D. J. (ed) *Nutrition and bone development*. Oxford University Press, pp. 115–130.

Rutishauser, I. H. E., Whitehead, R. G. (1969). Nutritional status assessed by biological tests. *British Journal of Nutrition* **23:** 1–13.

Salmenperä, L., Perheentupe, J., Siimes, M. A. (1985). Exclusively breastfed healthy infants grow slower than reference infants. *Pediatric Research* **19:** 307–312.

Sandberg, L. G. (1989). Swedish height fluctuations during the 18th and 19th centuries in relation to the experiences of other European countries and the United States. In Tanner, J. M. (ed) *Auxology 88: Perspectives in the science of growth and development*. Smith-Gordon, London, pp. 187-198.

Satyanarayana, K., Naidu, A. N., Narasinga Rao, B. S. (1979). Nutritional deprivation in childhood and the body size, activity and physical work capacity of young boys. *American Journal of Clinical Nutrition* **32:** 1769–1775.

Satyanarayana, K., Nadamuni Naidu, A., Narasinga Rao, B. S. (1980). Agricultural employment, wage earnings and nutritional status of teenage rural Hyderabad boys. *Indian Journal of Nutrition and Dietetics* **17:** 281–286.

Satyanarayana, K., Prasanna Krishna, T., Narasinga Rao, B. S. (1986). Effect of early childhood malnutrition and child labour on growth and adult nutritional status of rural Indian boys around Hyderabad. *Human Nutrition:Clinical Nutrition* **40C:** 131–139.

Satyanarayana, K., Radhaiah, G. *et al.* (1989). The adolescent growth spurt of height among rural Indian boys in relation to childhood nutritional background: an 18 year longitudinal study. *Annals of Human Biology* **16:** 289–300.

Seckler, D. (1982). Small but healthy: a basic hypothesis in the theory, measurement and policy of malnutrition. In Sukhatme, P. V. (ed) *Newer concepts in nutrition and their implications for policy*. Maharashtra Association for the Cultivation of Science Research Institute, Pune, India, pp. 127–137.

Spurr, G. B. (1984). Physical activity, nutritional status and physical work capacity in relation to agricultural productivity. In Pollitt, E., Amante, P. (eds) *Energy intake and activity*. Alan Liss, New York, pp. 207–261.

Spurr, G. B. (1988). Body size, physical work capacity and productivity in hard work:

is bigger better? In Waterlow, J. C. (ed) *Linear growth retardation in less developed countries*. Nestlé Nutrition, Vevey/Raven Press, New York, pp. 215–244.

Steckel, R. H. (1987). Growth depression and recovery: the remarkable age of American slaves. *Annals of Human Biology* **14**: 111–132.

Steckel, R. H. (1989). Heights and health in the United States, 1710–1950. In Tanner, J. M. (ed) *Auxology 88: Perspectives in the science of growth and development*. Smith-Gordon, London, pp. 175–186.

Stuart, H. C., Meredith, H. V. (1946). Use of body measurements in the school health program. *American Journal of Public Health* **36**: 1365–1386.

Stuart, H. C., Stevenson, S. S. (1959). Physical growth and development. In Nelson, W. E. (ed) *Textbook of pediatrics, 7th edn*. W. B. Saunders, Philadelphia, p. 12.

Tanner, J. M. (1976). Growth as a monitor of nutritional status. *Proceedings of the Nutrition Society* **35**: 315–322.

Tanner, J. M. (1982). The potential of auxological data for monitoring economic and social well-being. *Social Science History* **6**: 571–581.

Tanner, J. M., Whitehouse, R. H., Takaishi, M. (1966). Standards from birth to maturity for height, weight, height velocity and weight velocity. British children, 1963, part II. *Archives of Disease in Childhood* **41**: 613–635.

Tomkins, A. M. (1988). The risk of morbidity in a stunted child. In Waterlow, J. C. (ed) *Linear growth retardation in less developed countries*. Nestlé Nutrition, Vevey/Raven Press, New York, pp. 185-195.

Van Loon, H., Vuylsteke, J. P. *et al.* (1986). Local versus universal growth standards: the effect of using NCHS as universal reference. *Annals of Human Biology* **13**: 347–357.

Walker, S. P., Golden, M. H. N. (1988). Growth in length of children recovering from severe malnutrition. *European Journal of Clinical Nutrition* **42**: 395–404.

Warrington, S., Storey, D. M. (1988). Comparative studies on Asian and Caucasian children. 1: growth. *European Journal of Clinical Nutrition* **42**: 61–67.

Waterlow, J. C. (1973). Note on the assessment and classification of protein-energy malnutrition in children. *Lancet* **2**: 87–89.

Waterlow, J. C. (1974). Some aspects of childhood malnutrition as a public health problem. *British Medical Journal* **4**: 88–90.

Waterlow, J. C. (1978). Observations on assessment of protein-energy malnutrition, with special reference to stunting. *Courrier* **5**: 455–463.

Waterlow, J. C. (1985). What do we mean by adaptation? In Blaxter, K. L., Waterlow, J. C. (eds) *Nutritional adaptation in man*, John Libbey, London, pp. 1–12.

Waterlow, J. C. (1988). Observations on the natural history of stunting. In Waterlow, J. C. (ed) *Linear growth retardation in less developed countries*. Nestlé Nutrition, Vevey/Raven Press, New York, pp. 1–16.

Waterlow, J. C. (1989). Observations on FAO's methodology for estimating the incidence of undernutrition. *Food and Nutrition Bulletin (UNU)* **11**: 8–13.

Waterlow, J. C. (1990). Nutritional adaptation in man: general introduction and concepts. *American Journal of Clinical Nutrition* **51**: 259–263.

Waterlow, J. C., Rutishauser, I. H. E. (1974). Malnutrition in man. In Cravioto, J., Hambraeus, L., Vahlquist, B. (eds) *Early malnutrition and mental development*. Swedish Nutrition Foundation Symposia, no. XII, Almqvist and Wiksell, Stockholm, pp. 13–26.

Waterlow, J. C., Ashworth, A., Griffiths, M. (1980). Faltering in infant growth in less developed countries. *Lancet* **2**: 1176–1178.

Waterlow, J. C., Buzina, R. *et al.* (1977). The presentation and use of height and weight data for comparing the nutritional status of groups of children under the age of 10 years. *Bulletin of the World Health Organization* **55**: 489–498.

Whitehead, R. G., Paul, A. A. (1981). Infant growth and human milk requirements. *Lancet* **2**: 161–163.

Whitehead, R. G., Paul, A. A. (1984). Growth charts and the assessment of infant feeding practices in the western world and in developing countries. *Early Human Development* **9**: 187–207.

World Health Organization (1983). *Measuring change in nutritional status. Guidelines for assessing the nutritional impact of supplementary feeding programmes for vulnerable groups.* WHO, Geneva.

World Health Organization (1987). *Global nutritional status: anthropometric indicators.* Document Nutr/Antref/3/87. WHO, Geneva.

Zumrawi, F. Y., Dimond, H., Waterlow, J. C. (1987). Faltering in infant growth in Khartoum Province, Sudan. *Human Nutrition:Clinical Nutrition* **41C**: 383–395.

14

Assessment of nutritional state in the community

Introduction

Methods of assessing the nutritional state of children in the field have generally been described under three headings: clinical, biochemical, and anthropometric. Jelliffe's monograph (1966), which has recently been very fully
updated (Jelliffe and Jelliffe, 1990), gives an excellent illustrated account of
the mild changes that may be seen in skin, hair and mucosae. Few of them
can be attributed with any confidence to a specific deficiency, except for the
eye signs of avitaminosis A and changes in lips and mucosae that are probably
caused by riboflavin deficiency. Changes in skin and hair are difficult to assess
and to interpret (Chapter 5). Oedema should always be looked for, because
although within the category of severe PEM the presence or degree of oedema
does not seem to have much prognostic importance, at the level of the community it is a sign of severity and carries an increased risk of death (Briend
et al., 1987).

Biochemical measurements or 'tests' were discussed in Chapter 7. Those
that need blood samples are not practical for surveys or large-scale screening,
though more use might be made of spot samples of urine to supplement
studies on dietary intake (Bingham, 1987).

We are left, then, with anthropometric assessment. The World Health
Organization (1986) published a detailed report on this subject, from which
much that follows is derived. An important earlier review is that of Keller *et
al.* (1976). Johnston and Lampl (1984) provide references to the history of
anthropometry and its various usages. Haas and Habicht (1990) and Cole
(1991) have given excellent reviews of the conceptual problems in the applications of anthropometry.

Measurements, indices and indicators

Indices, such as weight for height, are constructs from measurements, usually
relating an observed measurement to its counterpart in the reference popu-

lation. Some indices, however, are single ratios, such as chest circumference/ head circumference or the body mass index (weight/height^2) that is widely used for the assessment of adults.

The usual phrase 'weight for height' represents the weight of the observed child compared with that of the median reference child of the same height. This is often written W/H, but that is unsatisfactory because it may be confused with a ratio. It would be clearer to use a notation in which W for H is written with a double slash, W//H.

Whereas an index is simply a number, an *indicator* represents the use of an index, often in conjunction with a cut-off point, for making a judgement or assessment. Thus weight for height, with a cut-off at 80 per cent of the reference, is an indicator of wasting; or arm circumference, without correction for age or height, has been used as an indicator of risk of death (Briend *et al.*, 1987). An index has biological meaning; an indicator only has meaning in relation to some application or value judgement. It is useful to make this distinction.

The basic measurements are age (A), weight (W) and height, length or stature (H). Arm circumference (AC) is also of value, particularly when large numbers of children have to be measured quickly. Head circumference (HC) is often measured, but little use seems generally to be made of it. HC cannot be used as a proxy for H, because its pattern of change with time is quite different, HC increasing much more quickly and reaching almost its adult value by four years. The methods of making anthropometric measurements accurately have been described by Jelliffe (1966); WHO (1983) has set out schedules for testing reproducibility and making inter-observer comparisons, and detailed practical manuals have been published by the United Nations (1986, 1990).

The three indices most commonly used in anthropometric assessment are W//H, a measure of wasting, H//A, a measure of stunting, and W//A, which is referred to as a measure of 'undernutrition'.

The mid-upper arm circumference (AC) is widely used as a measure of thinness. The conventional cut-off points for AC are shown in Table 14.1. The advantages are its simplicity, particularly for screening children in emergency situations, and the fact that for normal children between one and five years it is virtually age-independent, increasing during that period by only about 1 cm (Burgess and Burgess, 1969). Jelliffe and Jelliffe (1969) collected together the results of studies with AC in a large number of different countries. If triceps skinfold thickness is measured at the same time it is possible to calculate fat area and muscle area in the cross-section of the arm, and so in theory to get some idea of which component is most affected. This approach, however, is more useful for research than for community surveys of nutri-

Table 14.1   Conventional cut-off points for mid-upper arm circumference

Arm circumference (cm)	Nutritional state
> 14.0	Normal
14.0–12.5	Mild/moderate undernutrition
< 12.5	Severe undernutrition

These cut-off points are supposed to be age-independent from one to five years.

tional status. A correlation has indeed been found between arm muscle area and creatinine excretion (Standard *et al.*, 1959; Trowbridge *et al.*, 1982). The latter authors stressed that there may be ethnic differences in body composition which have to be taken into account in interpreting measurements of AC. For example, Bolivian children living at high altitude had a higher proportion of muscle than the norms established by Frisancho (1981).

Correlations between indices

In a number of studies correlations have been calculated between different indices. In most populations W//A is fairly well correlated with H//A, for which it is often used as a proxy, to save the labour of measuring height. When this is done, wasting will be overlooked. Keller (1983) showed that there is no correlation whatever of W//H and H//A; however, between them these two indices explained more than 95 per cent of the variance in W//A. The two measures of thinness, W//H and AC, have usually shown a correlation of 0.6 – 0.7 (e.g. Margo, 1977), which is statistically significant, but still leaves plenty of room for disagreement. Anderson (1979) found marked ethnic differences in the strength of the correlation.

Problems and sources of error

Errors in measurement

Measurement errors, even when they show no consistent bias, increase the range of variability and hence the standard deviation of the sample. As will be shown later (p. 218), an increase in SD, without any change in the mean, results in an apparently greater prevalence of malnutrition, as judged by the proportion below a given cut-off point. Therefore careful training of field staff and inter-observer standardization are important.

Age

Gorstein (1989) has pointed out a source of error that may arise with indices related to age, when age is known. Very often the age of the reference child, with which an observed child is being compared, is taken as the nearest *attained* month. Thus any child aged between 10 and 10.9 months would be compared with a reference child of 10 months. This will lead to a systematic underestimate of deficits in the observed population. The error is not negligible, particularly for children under one year. It would be better to make comparisons with a reference at the nearest month. Thus a child aged 10.4 months should be compared with one of 10 months, and a child of 10.6 months should be compared with one of 11 months. Any errors will then cancel out. Ideally, the comparison should be made with the weight and height of a reference child of exactly the same age, obtained by interpolation in the tables, but this is a tedious procedure unless done by computer and probably an unnecessary refinement.

Height or length

Care must be taken over comparisons of length or height. The NCHS reference is made up of two data-sets, one of children from birth to three years in whom supine length was measured; the other of children from two to 18 years, in whom standing height was measured. In the overlapping period of two to three years, length is up to 2 cm greater than height. This problem has been discussed by Dibley *et al.* (1987). It is obviously important that in this age-range length should be compared with length and height with height.

Measurement of length in children under two years may be troublesome, but it is necessary that it should be done for the assessment of wasting and stunting at a very critical period.

Weight for height

When it was first proposed to use W//H as a measure of wasting (Seoane and Latham, 1971; Waterlow, 1973), it was argued that this index, except at extremes of height, is age-independent (Waterlow, 1973). Thus a younger child who is tall for his age and an older child who is short for his age, should have the same expected weight. This is an approximation; in reality in a normal child the relationship between W and H changes in the first two years of life and is not completely age-independent (McLaren and Read, 1972). Cole (1979, 1985) has proposed a method of calculating W//H, taking account of age. In his formulation,

$$\% \text{ W//H} = 100 \times \left(\frac{\text{observed W}}{\text{reference W//A}} \right) \div \left(\frac{\text{observed H}}{\text{reference H//A}} \right)^2$$

By comparison with Cole's method the conventional method will underestimate the prevalence of wasting in the first year of life and overestimate it in the second year. It is remarkable that although Cole's first paper was published in 1979, the impact of his approach on estimates of the prevalence of wasting has not been investigated.

From the practical point of view, in children who can stand, W//H can be estimated very simply with the Nabarro wall-chart (Fig. 14.1).

Relating observed measurements to the reference

There are three ways of relating observed measurements to the reference. The most widely used in the past has been to express the observed value as a percentage of the reference. The disadvantage of this method is that it has no precise statistical meaning. For example, 80 per cent W//A represents 1.5 SD below the mean at six months and 2 SD below at one year. For this reason the use of standard deviation units (Z-scores) was proposed (Waterlow *et al.*, 1977) and is gradually becoming more widely accepted. Z-scores, like percentages, can be averaged and analysed statistically. The third method of expression is to relate observed data to the centiles of the reference distribution. The proportion of children below the 3rd reference centile corresponds fairly closely to the proportion below −2 SD.

A commonly used cut-off point for the three main indices, W//A, W//H and H//A, is a Z-score of −2, i.e. 2 SD below the reference mean. When results are expressed as per cent of reference median or mean (the two are identical), the usual cut-off for W//A and W//H is 80 per cent, and for H//A 90 per cent. It is clearly more convenient to have a consistent system, as represented by the Z-score.

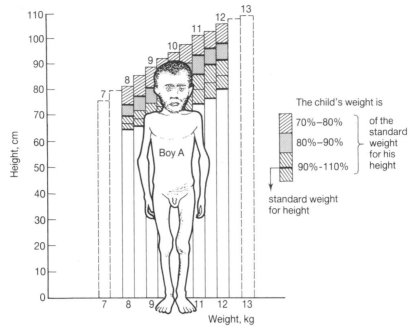

Fig. 14.1 The Nabarro wall-chart for estimating weight for height in the field. The chart consists of a series of vertical columns representing weight (kg) in half-kg intervals. The figure shows only a section of the chart from 7 to 13 kg. Each column has three coloured bands at the top. In descending order:

▨▨▨ = 70–80% of reference weight for height (in the real chart this would be shown as red)

▭▭▭ = 80–90% of reference weight for height (shown as yellow)

▨▨▨ = 90–110% of reference weight for height with a dividing line for 100% (shown as green).

The child is placed with his feet against the column corresponding to his weight and the top of his head indicates the range of weight for height in which he falls.

Analysis and presentation of data

Cut-off points

The World Health Organization tabulates in yearly age groups up to five years the prevalences of wasting, stunting and underweight (deficit in W//A) throughout the world (WHO, 1986). Prevalence is defined as the proportion of children below −2 SD of the reference median. Here the combination of index and cut-off point has become an indicator. This standardized method of presenting the data serves well for general information and comparisons and for advocacy.

There is, however, nothing immutable about the cut-off at −2 SD. When anthropometric measurements are being used for screening individual children, the cut-off should represent the dividing line between those who need intervention and those who do not.

If we have an independent measure of outcome, such as death, it is possible to choose the cut-off so as to provide the 'best' prediction of that outcome. Inevitably, however, there will be misdiagnosis: some malnourished children will be diagnosed as well-nourished and vice versa. As the cut-off point is lowered, the *sensitivity* decreases, which means that more truly malnourished children are missed; at the same time the *specificity* increases, which means that fewer well-nourished children are misdiagnosed as malnourished. The interrelationships of these variables are shown in Table 14.2. Table 14.3 illustrates the inverse relation between sensitivity and specificity. Habicht and his colleagues have discussed in detail the application of these concepts to the choice of cut-off point under different circumstances (Habicht, 1980; Habicht *et al.*, 1982; Haas and Habicht, 1990). Crudely, it is obvious that when resources are scarce, the cut-off point has to be low, even though some children who need treatment may be missed; when resources are generous, the cut-off can be high, because it does not matter if some children receive treatment when they do not need it.

A good analogy is the treatment of hypertension. We know something about the risks attached to each level of diastolic pressure. The level at which a decision is made to treat with hypotensive drugs depends partly on the cost of treatment. In the UK it was calculated that a national programme to treat

Table 14.2   Relationships between true prevalence and diagnosed prevalence

		Truly malnourished	
		Yes	No
	Yes	TP	FP
Diagnosed as malnourished:			
	No	FN	TN

TP = true positive diagnosis
FP = false positive diagnosis
FN = false negative diagnosis   S = sum of all 4 cells
TN = true negative diagnosis   (TP + FP + FN + TN)
Sensitivity   = TP/(TP + FN)
Specificity   = TN/(FP + TN)
Positive predictive value = TP/(TP + FP)
True prevalence   = (TP + FN)/S
Diagnosed prevalence = (TP + FP)/S

Modified from Habicht *et al.* (1982)

Table 14.3   Sensitivity, specificity and relative risk of death associated with various values for mid-upper arm circumference in children aged six to 36 months in Bangladesh

Arm circumference (mm)	Sensitivity (%)	Specificity (%)	Relative risk of death[a]
≤ 100	42	99	48
100–110	56	94	20
110–120	77	77	11
120–130	90	40	6

[a] The method for calculating relative risk is given in the original paper. Data from Briend *et al.* (1987)

everyone with a diastolic pressure above 90 mm Hg would be impossibly expensive. In clinical practice also the decision about whether or not to treat is influenced by the age of the patient and other factors, so that no single cut-off point is universally appropriate.

In using anthropometry to diagnose the need for intervention, the reality has so far not matched the theory. The only defined outcome for which the sensitivity and specificity of different indicators has been investigated is death and there has been very extensive discussion of their relative merits for short-term and long-term prediction (see, for example, correspondence in the *American Journal of Clinical Nutrition* (1981, 1982) and Bairagi *et al.*, 1985). Moreover, it appears that the predictive power of different indicators, i.e. the best trade-off between sensitivity and specificity, varies from one environment to another (Kasongo Project Team, 1983; Bairagi *et al.*, 1985; Haas and Habicht, 1990) (see also Chapter 18).

In any case, death is not the only outcome in which we are interested. For example, it would be very valuable if we had a cut-off point of H//A which predicted the likelihood of impairment of mental development.

Mean and standard deviation as descriptors

For describing populations the mean and SD are statistically more powerful than the prevalence below a cut-off point because they take account of all the data, not only the tail-end of the distribution. One can either use the mean and SD of the population or the mean Z-score with its SD. These measures provide a more sensitive estimate of changes or differences between populations, so that to establish a given difference a smaller sample is needed. For example, to establish a difference, significant at $P < 0.05$, between the growth of children in g/day in a particular population at two different seasons, a sample size of 620 was needed if the comparison was based on the percentages of children who gained no weight, but a sample of only 260 was needed if the comparison was between the mean weight gains in the two seasons (Briend *et al.*, 1989). From the biological as well as the statistical point of view the mean with SD is often more useful than cut-off points, since a small change in the population as a whole may be more revealing than a change in the prevalence of the frankly malnourished.

A further advantage of this approach is that it allows *direct* comparisons of different populations, or of the status of the same population at different times (Goldstein and Tanner, 1980); a reference is used not for comparative purposes but only to normalize for age or height.

The standard deviation is as important a part of the descriptor as the mean. The point was made earlier that the variability in heights and weights at a given age is greater in Third World children than in those from better-off countries, and this variability may be regarded as a measure of environmental stress (Harrison and Schmitt, 1989; Harrison *et al.*, 1990). Even if two populations have the same mean, it is obvious that the one with the larger SD will have a larger proportion below the cut-off point, wherever that point may be (Fig. 14.2). The disadvantage of the mean with SD as a descriptor is that it does not provide a number whose significance is self-evident, like the proportion below a cut-off point. Mora (1989) has proposed a method that helps to get over this difficulty. The prevalence of abnormality, as he puts it, is

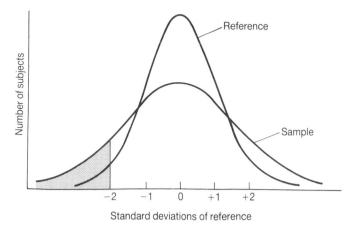

Fig. 14.2 The effect of increasing the standard deviation on the estimated prevalence of malnutrition. In the reference population the proportion below -2 SD is 2.3 per cent; in the observed population, with SD 1.6 x that of the reference, the proportion below the same cut-off point is 16 per cent.

represented by the black area in Fig. 14.3, where the observed distribution is outside the reference distribution. The prevalence depends only on the position of the mean and the size of the SD in the observed population compared to the reference and makes no use of cut-off points. Mora gives tables of prevalences for different values of mean and SD. These prevalences are substantially higher than those obtained by using a cut-off point of -2 SD. The reason is that Mora's estimate of prevalence includes 'false negatives'; these are children in the shaded area outside the reference curve, who in the standard method would not be counted among the

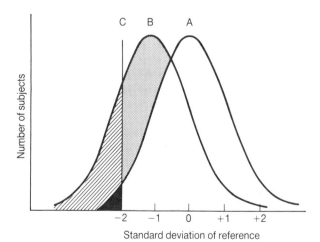

Fig. 14.3 Calculation of the prevalence of abnormality in an observed distribution (B) compared with the reference distribution (A). It is assumed that both distributions are Gaussian. C is the conventional cut-off point (-2 SD below the reference mean). ■■■, false positives; ▨▨, true positives; ▢▢, false negatives. For details see Mora (1989). Reproduced by permission from Mora (1989).

malnourished because they are above the cut-off point. Perhaps the easiest way to visualize these false negatives is to consider a child who is initially healthy, with a Z-score for weight of + 0.5. He becomes ill and loses weight equivalent to 2 standard deviations, so that his Z-score is now −1.5. By Mora's method he would be classified as malnourished, but by the conventional method he would not, because his weight has not fallen below −2 SD. This example is given by way of illustration. It will be interesting to see how far Mora's approach proves to be useful.

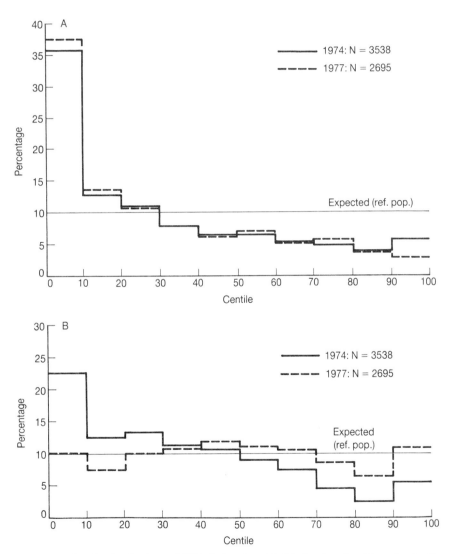

Fig. 14.4 Centile distributions of H//A (A) and W//H (B) showing the effect of a feeding scheme on W//H but not on H//A. The horizontal line at 10 per cent represents the reference population. Reproduced by permission from WHO (1983).

Centiles

Anthropometric data are sometimes related to centiles of the reference population. Centile charts have long been used for following the progress of individual children in a health centre. They present a picture which is very informative to an experienced person, though it is not readily quantified. Since the 3rd centile is close to −2 SD, any child who falls below it would, by the conventional system, be classified as malnourished. What is much less clear is the significance of a fall from e.g. the 50th to the 5th centile.

Population data can also be related to centiles. Charts such as those in Fig. 14.4 allow the state of a population and the effectiveness or otherwise of an intervention to be appreciated at a glance.

Applications of anthropometric data

The applications foreseen by the UN Agencies are listed in an abbreviated way in Table 14.4. The conclusions may be summarized as follows.

Indices

i.   W//H is the index of choice in all situations that involve short-term actions: screening, particularly in emergencies; the assessment of short-term interventions; early warning of impending food shortages. AC is also useful in these situations, particularly in emergencies.

ii.   H//A is the index of choice for assessments over the long term, e.g. for evaluating the effects of social and economic changes.

iii.   It would perhaps be going too far to say that W//A should never be used. It could be substituted for H//A for the purpose of long-term assessment, if it is already known that wasting is not prevalent and that there is no indication for short-term intervention. In principle, however, nothing should be done to discourage those who are planning anthropometric surveys from including height or length in their measurements. The only

Table 14.4   Summary of applications of indices and indicators

Index	Application	Indicator	Age-range
AC	Emergencies (screening)	CU[a] flexible	All children who can stand
W//H	Emergencies (screening)	CU flexible	All children who can stand
	One-time assessment of wasting	Mean (SD) or CU conventional	1–3 years
	Assessment of impact short-term programme	Mean (SD)	1–3 years
	Rapid targeting and timely warning	CU conventional	1–3 years
	Growth monitoring	None	1–3 years
W//A	Growth monitoring	None	0–1 year
H//A	Long-term planning	Mean (SD)	2–4 years
	Surveillance of trends (long term)	Mean (SD)	2–4 years
	Programme management	Mean (SD)	2–4 years
	Growth monitoring	None	1–3 years

[a] CU, cut-off; conventional CU, −2 SD.

exception is emergency screening, when it may be decided to use AC as
the indicator. For children who can stand, measurement of W//H with
the Nabarro wall chart (Nabarro and McNab, 1980) is simple and quick
(Fig. 14.1).

Analysis

iv.   Cut-off points and the associated estimates of the prevalence of malnutrition, particularly wasting, are best used for screening individuals and for
targeting programmes to individual children and families. The cut-off has
to be flexible according to resources. The method, although relatively
insensitive, may also be used for assessing the effects of short-term interventions, but only if the initial prevalence of malnutrition is high (Habicht *et al.*, 1982).

v.   In all situations that relate to populations or groups, particularly when
comparisons are being made, the descriptor of choice is the mean with
SD.

Anthropometric estimates of the prevalence of PEM

At the time of writing (1990) the main sources of information by country, by
region and globally are a summary produced by WHO (1986), a report produced by the UN Subcommittee on Nutrition (1987) and a report from
UNICEF (Carlson and Wardlaw, 1989). All these reports emphasize the
limitations of the data, in particular that they are not always nationally representative. A further report from the Subcommittee on Nutrition (1989)
illustrated marked seasonal changes in prevalence in some countries, even
though the index used was W//A. Clearly this effect has to be controlled for
when comparisons are being made.

Figure 14.5 brings together information collected worldwide by UNICEF
from WHO and other sources (Carlson and Wardlaw, 1989). Of course, too
much should not be made of this highly aggregated data. Within each region
there are large differences between countries. For some countries there is no
information and for others it is not nationally representative. Nevertheless,
some interesting points emerge.

Wasting

It is remarkable that the distribution of wasting with age shows the same
pattern in all regions in spite of their very different ecologies. Because of this
constancy of pattern it seems sensible that studies aimed at assessing the
prevalence of wasting should be concentrated on children aged six to 24 or
30 months. It is surely uneconomical to look for wasting in children four to
five years old, except in semi-famine conditions.

Stunting

Stunting presents more difficult problems, as discussed in the previous chapter. Whether one regards stunting as a form of malnutrition or as a marker
for poverty and deprivation, it is difficult to accept that the prevalence of
malnutrition or of poverty is really twice as great in South Asia as in Sub-

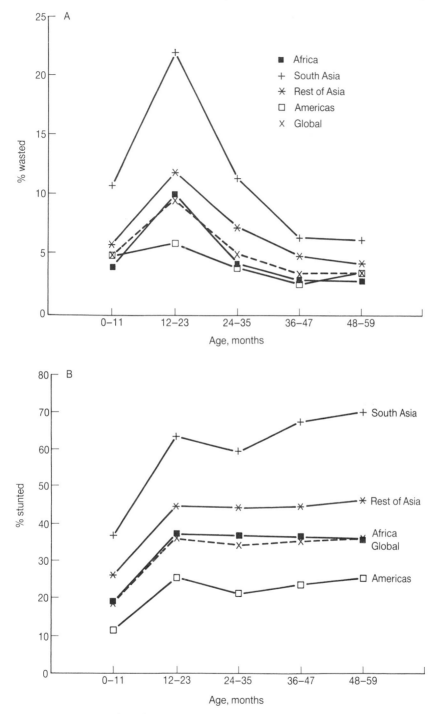

Fig. 14.5   Patterns of wasting and stunting by age. A, % wasted = % below −2 SD weight for height; B, % stunted = % below −2 SD height for age. Reproduced by permission from Carlson and Wardlaw (1990).

Saharan Africa. There is no comparable difference in infant mortality rates, which are somewhat higher in Africa than in South Asia.

Figure 14.6 shows that for a population with a 50 per cent prevalence of stunting by conventional standards, adoption of an 'Asian' reference with a mean 1 SD below that of the NCHS could reduce the apparent prevalence of stunting from 50 per cent to 16 per cent, a factor of three. Unless we are certain that a genetic difference is real—and we have no such certainty—such an adjustment could be regarded as an example of what Gopalan has called 'letting the magnitude of the problem determine the yardstick for its measurement, rather than using a yardstick to determine the magnitude of the problem'.

The only solution to this problem is to look at it from the point of view of action. An assertion that 70 per cent of children are malnourished is not helpful to policy makers, who are likely to respond that the method of assessment is inappropriate. If an intervention is planned directed to the most deprived families, as judged by the stunting of their children, then the cut-off point will have to be adjusted to the scale and resources of the programme. If stunting is being used to assess the impact of a more widespread and longer-term programme, then the appropriate indicator, as stressed above, is a change in the population mean. It is difficult to go further than this until we know more about the biology of stunting.

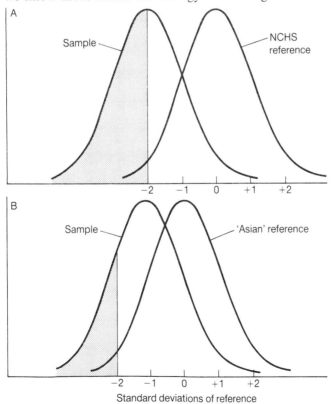

Fig. 14.6 Effect on the estimated prevalence of stunting (the percentage below −2 SD of height for age) of shifting NCHS reference by 1 SD.

Use of anthropometric indicators: their relationship to social and economic status

If stunting in particular is regarded as a proxy for poverty, there should be a demonstrable relationship between its prevalence and environmental and economic indicators of the quality of life. As an example, Table 14.5 shows correlations of wasting and stunting with infant mortality and various characteristics of the family environment. Both wasting and stunting were strongly correlated with the infant mortality rate; most of the other correlations were not significant, except for those between stunting and the availability of wells and a cement floor. Keller (1983) concluded from such data that infection played an important role in the causation of stunting. Many studies of this kind have been reported; usually the correlations observed have been quite weak.

Table 14.5 Coefficients of correlations of the prevalence of wasting or stunting with various socioeconomic variables in 15 health administrative districts of Sri Lanka

	Prevalence (% of sample)	
Variable	Stunting	Wasting
Infant mortality rate	0.85*	0.75*
Percentage of houses with:		
wells	−0.83*	−0.30
cement floor	−0.67*	−0.29
brick walls	0.05	0.26
latrines	0.30	0.04
electricity	−0.43	−0.30

* Significant at $P < 0.05$
From Keller (1983)

On a larger scale Haage *et al.* (1985) related the prevalence of underweight (W//A < -2 SD) in children aged six to 60 months to a variety of indicators listed in Table 14.6. On the whole the correlations were very low, which is not surprising considering the nature of the information. In the age-range studied underweight would mainly represent stunting. As might be expected from the previous section, the relationship between prevalence of underweight and most of the indicators was not the same in the South Asian countries as in other parts of the world. However, when allowance was made for this in a multiple regression analysis, it was found that child death rate

Table 14.6 Indicators that have been compared with prevalence of underweight (W//A < -2 SD) in children aged six to 60 months

Gross national product per head
Average energy consumption
Access to safe water supply
Adult female illiteracy
Child death rate
Infant mortality rate
Per cent of population with inadequate food intake

From Haage *et al.* (1985)

and average energy consumption between them 'explained' 80 per cent of the variance in the prevalence of underweight.

The second report of the UN Subcommittee on Nutrition (1989), based on a smaller number of countries, attempted to relate trends in the prevalence of undernutrition in the 1980s to trends in other indicators such as the debt ratio, the gross national product per head, the food production index and the consumer price index. This exercise is potentially very important, because the 1980s were a period of deteriorating economic conditions in many Third World countries, particularly in Africa (see Chapter 20). It is difficult to see any consistent relationship between the trends. In the nine African countries that were covered, there was little change in the prevalence of underweight in spite of a fall of nearly 10 per cent in the dietary energy supply per head and a large increase in outstanding debt. In most of the Asian and Latin American countries there were actually decreases in the prevalences of underweight, particularly in the cities, where they are usually lower than in rural districts. The authors rightly insist on the caution needed with such complex systems in tracing causal connections. Real relationships with economic and other indicators may be obscured when the only anthropometric information is W//A between six and 60 months, with no disaggregation of ages or distinction between wasting and stunting.

References

American Journal of Clinical Nutrition (1981). Nutritional anthropometry and mortality risk. Correspondence **34:** 2591–2598.

American Journal of Clinical Nutrition (1982). On best cut-off point for nutritional monitoring. Correspondence **35:** 769–778.

Anderson, M. A. (1979). Comparison of anthropometric measures of nutritional status in preschool children in five developing countries. *American Journal of Clinical Nutrition* **32:** 2339–2345.

Bairagi, R., Chowdhury, M. K. *et al.* (1985). Alternative anthropometric indicators of mortality. *American Journal of Clinical Nutrition* **42:** 296–306.

Bingham, S. A. (1987). The dietary assessment of individuals; methods, accuracy, new techniques and recommendations. *Nutrition Abstracts and Reviews Series A* **57:** 706–742.

Briend, A., Wojtynick, B., Rowland, M. G. M. (1987). Arm circumference and other factors in children at high risk of death in rural Bangladesh *Lancet* **2:** 725–728.

Briend, A., Hasan, K. Z. *et al.* (1989). Measuring change in nutritional status: a comparison of different anthropometric indices and the sample sizes required. *European Journal of Clinical Nutrition* **43:** 769–778.

Burgess, H. J. L., Burgess, A. P. (1969). A modified standard for mid-upper arm circumference in young children. *Journal of Tropical Pediatrics* **15:** 189–192.

Carlson, B. A., Wardlaw, T. (1990). *A global, regional and country assessment of child malnutrition.* Staff Working Paper No. 7, UNICEF, New York.

Cole, T. J. (1979). A method for assessing age-standardized weight-for-height in children seen cross-sectionally. *Annals of Human Biology* **6:** 249–268.

Cole, T. J. (1985). A critique of the NCHS weight for height standard. *Human Biology* **57:** 183–196.

Cole, T. J. (1991). Weight-stature indices to measure underweight, overweight and obesity. In Himes, J. H. (ed) *Anthropometric assessment of nutritional status.* Wiley-Liss, New York. pp. 83–111.

Cole, T. J., Paul, A. A. *et al.* (1989). The use of a multiple growth standard to highlight the effects of diet and infection on growth. In Tanner, J. M. (ed) *Auxology 88: perspectives in the science of growth and development.* Smith-Gordon, London, pp. 91–100.

Dibley, M. J., Goldsby, J. B. *et al.* (1987). Development of normalized curves for the international growth reference: historical and technical considerations. *American Journal of Clinical Nutrition* **46**: 736–748.

Frisancho, A. R. (1981). New norms of upper limb fat and muscle areas for assessment of nutritional status. *American Journal of Clinical Nutrition* **34**: 2540–2545.

Goldstein, H., Tanner, J. M. (1980). Ecological considerations in the creation and the use of child growth standards. *Lancet* **1**: 582–585.

Gorstein, J. (1989). Assessment of nutritional status: effects of different methods to determine age on the classification of malnutrition. *Bulletin of the World Health Organization* **67**: 143–150.

Graitcer, P. L., Gentry, E. M. (1981). Measuring children: one reference for all. *Lancet* **2**: 297–299.

Haaga, J., Kennick, C. *et al.* (1985). An estimate of the prevalence of malnutrition in developing countries. *World Health Statistics Quarterly* **38**: 331–347.

Haas, J. D., Habicht J-P. (1990). Growth and growth-charts in the assessment of pre-school nutritional status. In Harrison, G. A., Waterlow, J. C. (eds) *Diet and disease in traditional and developing societies.* Cambridge University Press, Cambridge, UK, pp. 160–183.

Habicht J-P. (1980). Some characteristics of indicators of nutritional status for use in screening and surveillance. *American Journal of Clinical Nutrition* **33**: 531–535.

Habicht J-P., Meyers, L. D., Brownie, C. (1982). Overview: indicators for identifying and counting the improperly nourished. *American Journal of Clinical Nutrition* **35**: (Suppl.) 1241–1254.

Harrison, G. A., Schmitt, L. H. (1989). Variability in stature growth. *Annals of Human Biology* **16**: 45–51.

Harrison, G. A., Brush, G. *et al.* (1990). Short-term variations in stature growth in Ethiopian and English children. *Annals of Human Biology* **17**: 407–416.

Jelliffe, D. B. (1966). *The assessment of the nutritional status of the community.* WHO Monograph Series No. 53, Geneva.

Jelliffe, D. B., Jelliffe, E. P. (1990). *Community nutritional assessment.* Oxford University Press.

Jelliffe, E. P., Jelliffe, D. B. (eds) (1969). The arm circumference as a public health index of protein-calorie malnutrition of early childhood. *Journal of Tropical Pediatrics* **15**: 177–260.

Johnston, E. F., Lampl, M. (1984). Anthropometric assessment. In Brožek, J., Schürch, B. (eds) *Malnutrition and behaviour: critical assessment of key issues.* Nestlé Foundation, Lausanne, pp. 51-70.

Kasongo Project Team (1983). Anthropometric assessment of young children's nutritional status as an indicator of subsequent risk of dying. *Journal of Tropical Pediatrics* **29**: 69–75.

Keller, W. (1983). Choice of indicators of nutritional status. In Schürch, B. (ed) *Evaluation of nutrition education in Third World communities.* Nestlé Foundation Publication Series No. 3. Hans Hüber, Bern, pp. 101–113.

Keller, W., Donoso, G., De Maeyer, E. M. (1976). Anthropometry in nutritional surveillance: a review based on results of the WHO collaborative study on nutritional anthropometry. *Nutrition Abstracts and Reviews* **46**: 591–606.

McLaren, D. S., Read, W. W. C. (1972). Classification of nutritional status in early childhood. *Lancet* **2**: 146–148.

Margo, G. (1977). Assessing malnutrition with mid-arm circumference. *American Journal of Clinical Nutrition* **30**: 835–837.

Mora, J. (1989). A new method for estimating a standardized prevalence of child malnutrition from anthropometric indicators. *Bulletin of the World Health Organization* 67: 133–142.

Nabarro, D., McNab, S. (1980). A simple new technique for identifying thin children. *Journal of Tropical Medicine and Hygiene* 83: 21–33.

Seoane, N., Latham, M. C. (1971). Nutritional anthropometry in the identification of malnutrition in childhood. *Journal of Tropical Pediatrics and Environmental Child Health* 17: 98–104.

Standard, K. L., Wills, V. G., Waterlow, J. C. (1959). Indirect indicators of muscle mass in malnourished children. *American Journal of Clinical Nutrition* 7: 271–279.

Trowbridge, F. L., Hiner, C. D., Robertson, A. D. (1982). Arm muscle indicators and creatinine excretion in children. *American Journal of Clinical Nutrition* 36: 691–696.

United Nations (1986). *How to weigh and measure children: assessing the nutritional status of young children in household surveys*. UN Department of Technical Co-operation for Development and Statistical Office, New York.

United Nations (1987). Subcommittee on Nutrition of the UN Administrative Committee on Co-ordination. *First report on the world nutrition situation*. ACC/SCN, WHO, Geneva.

United Nations (1989). Subcommittee on Nutrition of the UN Administrative Committee on Co-ordination. *Update on the nutrition situation*. ACC/SCN, WHO, Geneva.

United Nations (1990). *Assessing the nutritional status of young children*. Document DP/UN/INT-88-XO1/8E, Department of Technical Co-operation for Development and Statistical Office, United Nations, New York.

Van Lerberghe, W. (1990). *Kasongo: child mortality and growth in a small African town*. Smith-Gordon/Nishimura, London.

Waterlow, J. C. (1973). Note on the assessment and classification of protein-energy malnutrition in children. *Lancet* 2: 87–89.

Waterlow, J. C. (1976). Classification and definition of protein-energy malnutrition. In Beaton, G. H., Bengoa, J. M. (eds) *Nutrition in preventive medicine*. WHO, Geneva, pp. 530–555.

Waterlow, J. C., Buzina, R. *et al.* (1977). The presentation and use of height and weight data for comparing the nutritional status of groups of children under the age of 10 years. *Bulletin of the World Health Organization* 55: 489–498.

World Health Organization (1983). *Measuring change in nutritional status. Guidelines for assessing the nutritional impact of supplementary feeding programmes for vulnerable groups*. WHO, Geneva.

World Health Organization (1986). Report of a Working Group. Use and interpretation of anthropometric indicators of nutritional status. *Bulletin of the World Health Organization* 64: 929–941.

15

Energy and protein requirements of infants and young children

Energy requirements

Knowledge of the requirements of children for energy and protein is useful for the diagnosis of deficiency, in groups if not individuals; it is necessary for specifying infant formulae and post-weaning diets, and it sets targets for intervention programmes.

To the question 'requirement for what?' the answer must be: for health, activity and satisfactory growth—concepts that are vague but none the less real. There are two particularly critical periods in the early life of the young child. The first is at about four months, when in most cultures supplements to breast milk begin to be given if they have not been started before that (Chapter 16). At this stage also rates of gain in both weight and height of many Third World children are already falling off compared with the accepted international reference (Waterlow *et al.*, 1980).

The second critical period is between one and two years, when breast feeding will often have stopped completely, perhaps because of displacement by a new baby. Even if breast feeding is still continued at this age, it cannot be adequate as the sole source of food. The child is not yet able to take its full share of the family meal and its food may consist largely of starchy porridges or gruels which have a low energy density (see Chapter 16). It is just at this age that the young child needs to become more physically active. That it is a dangerous age is clear, since in most reports the highest incidence of severe PEM, at least as it presents at hospitals, is between one and two years of age. For looking at energy and protein requirements we have therefore concentrated on the ages of four months and one year as examples. It is the usual practice, which will be followed here, to establish first the requirements of supposedly normal healthy children and then, as a second stage, to examine later (in Chapter 17) the effects of infections and other stress.

Two ways have been used for estimating requirements for both energy and protein. One is based on intakes—measurements of what healthy well-growing children actually eat. The other is based on outputs, and requires physiological estimates of energy expenditure, of nitrogen losses and of the tissue laid down in growth. The two approaches provide a check on each other.

Measurements of energy intakes

It should be noted at the outset that the literature often does not state clearly exactly how energy intakes were calculated from the raw data. The *gross* energy content of foodstuffs is technically their enthalpy (Blaxter, 1989), which is most conveniently measured by complete oxidation in a bomb calorimeter. The enthalpies of carbohydrate, fat and protein are usually taken as 4, 9.3 and 5.7 kcal/g. The *metabolizable* energy is the energy available to the body after allowance has been made for the absorptive losses and, in the case of protein, incomplete oxidation. The factors generally used—the so-called Atwater factors—for calculating the metabolizable energy of carbohydrate, fat and protein are 4, 9 and 4 kcal/g. These values may not always be appropriate. In children who are malnourished or ill there is likely to be some malabsorption of fat, and if the diet is high in fibre, the absorption of both carbohydrate and protein may be reduced. In the case of breast milk a combined factor is commonly used, according to which metabolizable energy = gross energy x 0.92 (Southgate and Barrett, 1966).

Whitehead *et al.* (1981) analysed the literature on the energy intakes of healthy children, for the most part bottle-fed, in industrialized countries. Their findings were used by the FAO/WHO/UNU Expert Consultation in their most recent report on Energy and Protein Requirements (WHO, 1985), referred to for shortness as the Rome report. The results are shown in Table 15.1 and compared with the figures from an earlier report (WHO, 1973). The table shows an interesting phenomenon: a decline in average intake between three and nine months, with a rise again towards the end of the first year. The falling-off presumably reflects the decreasing requirement for growth and the later rise an increased level of physical activity. These average intakes are lower than those recorded by Fomon (1974) which were used in an earlier FAO/WHO report (WHO, 1973).

It would be more appropriate to use as a guideline the intakes of exclusively breast-fed children, at least as long as they are growing satisfactorily. It is a

Table 15.1   Average energy intakes of infants in industrialized countries

Age (months)	Intake, kcal/kg	
	WHO (1985)[a]	WHO (1973)[b]
0–3	116	120
3–6	99	115
6–9	95	110
9–12	101	112

[a] Based on data of Whitehead *et al.* (1981)
[b] Based on data of Fomon (1967)

remarkable inconsistency of the Rome report that this was done for protein but not for energy. The volume and composition of breast milk are considered in the following Chapter. For the present purpose it is enough to take average values that might be found in healthy well-fed mothers and babies.

Requirements at four months

Table 15.2 lists estimates of energy intake from breast milk by healthy normally growing children at four months. The median is about 90 kcal/kg/day. These intakes are lower than those of the bottle-fed children shown in Table 15.1, and there is some argument about whether or not they are optimal. Butte *et al.* (1990) reported that although formula-fed babies were ingesting more energy than a breast-fed group (96 *versus* 74 kcal/kg/day), they had identical weighs at four months. No differences were found in BMR or in skinfold thickness. On the other hand Fomon (1986) found that formula-fed infants gained more lean body mass than those who were exclusively breast-fed and has therefore questioned whether breast milk is really the ideal food for babies. It may represent a compromise between the interests of the baby and the mother. The point has already been made (Chapter 13) that even in the best circumstances, e.g. those of the children in Cambridge, UK, studied by Whitehead and Paul (1984), the growth of exclusively breast-fed infants tends to fall below the reference after about four months. Whitehead and Paul therefore suggested that the international reference is not an appropriate standard or target under modern conditions (for the distinction between reference and standard, see Chapter 13). However, the deviations are small compared with those found in the Third World (Waterlow *et al.*, 1980) and the Cambridge children had returned to the 50th centile of reference weight and height by the age of three years (Paul *et al.*, 1988).

Whitehead and Paul (1981) took the argument one step further. They asked: what are the energy intakes and hence the volumes of breast milk that would be needed to allow children to grow along the 50th—or any other centile—of the international reference? To answer this they derived from their data on energy intake and growth of Cambridge children a series of

Table 15.2   Estimates of metabolizable energy intake of breast-fed infants aged four months in affluent countries

Reference	Intake (kcal/kg/day)	Metabolizable energy of milk (kcal/dl)	
Wallgren (1945)	87	Assumed	70
Whitehead and Paul (1981)			
males	91	From food	
females	93	tables	69
Dewey and Lönnerdal (1983)	93	Proximate analysis, Atwater factors	79
Butte *et al.* (1984)	69	Proximate analysis, Atwater factors	62

In all cases the coefficient of variation of intakes is 20 per cent or more.
In the series of Dewey and Lönnerdal, the energy content of breast milk is substantially higher than the usual value of 67–70 kcal/100 g. In that of Butte *et al.* it was lower. This does not explain their very low figure for energy intake.

multiple regression equations relating energy intake to weight and weight gain; both have to be included, since actual weight determines the maintenance requirement and gain the growth requirement. The results are shown in Table 15.3.

Table 15.3 Predicted requirements for breast milk and energy for infant boys to grow along the 50th NCHS centile

Age (months)	Required breast milk intake (ml/day)	Required energy intake (kcal/kg/day)
2	780	104
3	840	97
4	880	91
5	950	89
6	980	87
8	1130	89

Predictions derived from regression of observed intakes on attained weight and weight gain
Predicted requirements for girls were 5–10 per cent less than for boys
From Whitehead and Paul, 1981

Factorial estimates of energy expenditure

Measurements of intake, with all their sources of error, can only provide guidelines. The requirement for energy, as of any nutrient, is the amount needed to balance expenditure or losses and to provide for growth. The physiological components of the energy requirement are listed in Table 15.4 in terms of metabolizable energy. The largest component is the basal metabolic rate (BMR), the values of which are very well established (Schofield *et al.*, 1985). The thermic effect of food can be taken with sufficient accuracy as 10 per cent of the intake. There are no direct measurements of energy expended on physical activity by such young children. When activity is minimal, as it is likely to be at this age, the sum of the components other than growth represents the expenditure for maintenance which in this calculation comes out as 1.34 x BMR. In adults the maintenance requirement has been estimated as 1.4 x BMR (WHO, 1985), and a similar value has been found

Table 15.4 Physiological (factorial) estimate of energy requirement at four months

Factor	Metabolizable energy (kcal/kg/day)
Basal metabolic rate	53[a]
Thermic effect of food	8[b]
Minimal activity	10[c]
Total for maintenance	71 = 1.34 × BMR
Growth	12[d]
Total requirement	83

[a] From Schofield *et al.* (1985)
[b] As 10 per cent of intake. Formerly called 'specific dynamic action (SDA)'.
[c] Little more than a guess
[d] See text

in a wide range of animals (Payne and Waterlow, 1971). If it is legitimate to apply this factor to infants, it would give a maintenance requirement of about 75 kcal/kg/day.

A more direct way of estimating the maintenance requirement is from the regression of weight gain on energy intake, the maintenance requirement being the intake at zero gain. This method is most reliable when gains are rapid, as in premature babies or young children recovering from malnutrition (Table 15.5). The results show a wide scatter, but the average is close to that given by the factorial calculation.

Table 15.5 Estimates of maintenance requirement for energy by regression of weight gain on intake

Reference	Infants	Maintenance requirement (kcal/kg/day)
Spady *et al.* (1976)	Infants aged about 1 year, recovering from malnutrition	85
Brooke *et al.* (1979)	Prematures	64
Duggan and Milner (1986)	Infants recovering from measles	64
Fjeld *et al.* (1988)	Infants aged ~ 15 months, recovering from malnutrition	77
	Mean	72.5 = 1.37 × BMR[a]

[a] Assuming that BMR = 53 kcal/kg/day

Energy cost of growth

The energy cost of growth has two components: the energy stored (E_s), calculated as its enthalpy (p. 230), and the energy used in the chemical reactions involved in storage (E_c). The amount of energy stored will depend on the composition of the tissue laid down. If it were adipose tissue containing 80 per cent fat, E_s would be about 7.5 kcal/g; if it were lean, containing 20 per cent protein, it would be 1.1 kcal/g. From the estimates of Fomon *et al.* (1982) on the body composition of the reference infant, it can be calculated that at four months of age the energy deposited would on average amount to 3.2 kcal/g gained. This corresponds to tissue containing 12 per cent protein and about 35 per cent fat. However, over short periods the composition and the energy content of the tissue laid down may be quite variable (Jackson *et al.*, 1977).

The other component of the energy cost of growth is the cost of synthesizing triglycerides from fatty acids and protein from amino acids (E_c). The former is negligible; the cost of protein synthesis and its associated processes (amino acid uptake, RNA turnover, etc.) can be estimated from what we know of the biochemistry of the reactions, and might amount to about 1 kcal/g protein deposited (Waterlow and Millward, 1989). This is small compared with the energy stored (E_s). These theoretical calculations give a total for ($E_s + E_c$) of about 4 kcal/g tissue gained.

A more direct estimate of the total energy cost of growth can be obtained from the regression of weight gain on energy intake, as shown in Fig. 15.1.

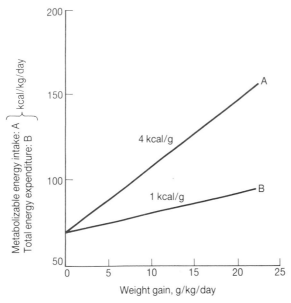

Fig. 15.1   Regression of energy intake on weight gain (line A). The intercept on the *y*-axis represents the maintenance requirement (intake for zero gain) and the slope of the line represents the total energy cost of growth [$(E_s + E_c)$ — see text]. In the same way the total energy expenditure by the doubly labelled water method can be plotted against weight gain (line B). The slope of the line then represents the energy cost of tissue deposition (E_c).

This approach is most satisfactory when there is a wide range of weight gains, as in children recovering from malnutrition (Spady *et al.*, 1976) or in premature babies (Brooke *et al.*, 1979). Studies of this kind have given values for ($E_s + E_c$) ranging from 4.4 to 6 kcal/g gained. A rounded-off figure often used is 5 kcal/g, but this may represent deposition of a somewhat excessive proportion of fat. Ashworth (1969) pointed out that the cost per g was much higher in recovered children who were gaining only 2 g weight/kg/day than in the early phase of recovery when they were gaining five times as much. She suggested that this may be because in the later stages the children were laying down more fat and even becoming obese.

In the same way, the component E_c of the energy cost of growth can be estimated from the regression of weight gain on total energy expenditure (Fig. 15.1). This has led to a value for E_c of 1.1 kcal/g tissue gained (Fjeld *et al.*, 1988).

If we adopt a figure of 4 kcal/g as a reasonable estimate of the total cost of depositing balanced tissue, and if the infant at four months is gaining 3 g/kg/day, then 12 kcal/kg has to be added to the maintenance expenditure (Table 15.4) to give a total requirement of 83 kcal/kg/day at this age.

Direct measurements of energy expenditure

The introduction of the doubly labelled water method makes it possible to check these somewhat theoretical calculations by direct measurements of total energy expenditure, which include the energy costs of tissue deposition, but not the energy deposited. The method, originally introduced by Lifson (1966), depends on the fact that the oxygen of water rapidly equilibrates with that of carbon dioxide under the influence of the enzyme carbonic anhydrase. If water is given in which both hydrogen and oxygen atoms are labelled with a stable isotope, the rate of disappearance of labelled oxygen from the body fluids, corrected for the disappearance rate of labelled hydrogen, is a measure of the rate of CO_2 production (Fig. 15.2). To convert CO_2 production to energy expenditure the respiratory quotient has to be measured or a value for it assumed. To get satisfactory slopes for the disappearance rates measurements have to be made over 7–14 days, and the final result is an integrated estimate of energy expenditure over that time. There are many good accounts in the literature of the theory and practice of the DLW method, e.g. the papers of Schoeller *et al.* (1986) and Coward (1988).

There remain some technical problems to be overcome in this method

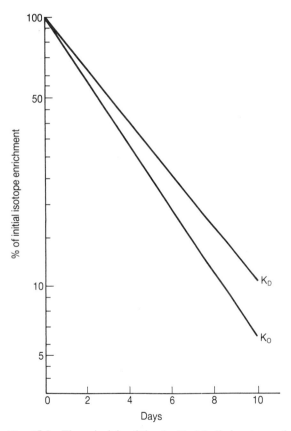

Fig. 15.2   The principle of the doubly labelled water method. A dose of $D_2{}^{18}O$ is given at zero time, and the isotopic abundance of D and ^{18}O is measured in water of saliva or urine for 10–15 days. The slope K_D represents the rate of loss of water. The slope K_O is the sum of the rates of loss of oxygen in water and in CO_2 that has equilibrated with water. The difference between these slopes represents the rate of CO_2 production. If V is the initial body water, the rate of CO_2 production is given in principle by $V(K_O - K_D)$. For corrections that have to be made, and for different methods of making the detailed calculations, see Coward (1988) and Wong *et al.* (1990). From data of Wong *et al.* (1990), infants four months old.

(James *et al.*, 1988). During rapid growth sequestration of labelled hydrogen into newly deposited fat may cause CO_2 production to be underestimated (Haggarty *et al.*, 1991) and there are differences of opinion about the most appropriate equation to be used (Wong *et al.*, 1990). Nevertheless, the results obtained so far in children, tabulated by Prentice *et al.* (1988), are encouraging. Those that apply in the age-range birth to six months are shown in Table 15.6. The mean is 73.5 kcal/kg/day. This value includes the energy cost of depositing new tissue ($E_c = \sim 1$ kcal/g) but not the energy deposited (E_s). If the total energy cost of growth ($E_s + E_c$) is taken as 4 kcal/g (see p. 233), then E_s would be 3 kcal/g. This is the appropriate figure to use when the requirement is being calculated from energy expenditure. If the average growth rate at four months is 3 g/kg/day, the total requirement then becomes 73.5 + (3 x 3) = approximately 83 kcal/kg/day.

Table 15.6 Total energy expenditure (TEE) of infants aged 0–6 months, measured by the doubly labelled water method

Reference	Method of feeding	Age (months)	TEE[a] (kcal/kg/day)
Lucas *et al.* (1987)	Breast and bottle-fed	1.5	70
Vasquez-Velasquez (1988)	Mixed fed	0–3	77
Vasquez-Velasquez (1988)	Mixed fed	3–6	77
Roberts and Young (1988)		3	73
Lucas, unpublished (cited in Prentice *et al.*, 1988)		3	73
Wong *et al.* (1990)	Formula-fed	4	70
		Mean	73.5

[a] Includes energy cost of growth (E_c) but not energy stored (E_s)

The agreement between three independent methods of estimating the energy requirement is satisfactory and indeed surprising. However, in the studies with doubly labelled water, within each group there is a rather wide variation in energy expenditure, which is probably not related to age, since there seems to be little change in total energy expenditure (TEE) up to the age of three years. The results of Wong *et al.* (1990) in babies aged four months showed a mean TEE of 70 kcal/kg/day and a range of 54–86. In that study they compared TEE measured isotopically (A) with energy expenditure estimated as the difference between intake and stored energy (B). The mean results by the two methods were identical, but the differences (A −B) ranged from +24 to −28 kcal/kg. A possible explanation is that the stored energy was calculated from weight gain, with a fixed composition (Fomon *et al.*, 1982), so that no allowance was made for individual variation in the composition of the tissue laid down.

Although difficulties remain, the results of the different approaches (Table 15.7) suggest that it would be reasonable to accept 85–90 kcal/kg/day as an estimate of the average energy requirement at four months of healthy children in a healthy environment. This is not a negligible decrease from the estimate of 101 kcal/kg/day proposed by FAO/WHO/UNU (WHO, 1985).

It seemed necessary to examine this subject in detail, because the implications of this decrease are clearly very important, as discussed in the next chapter.

Table 15.7   Summary of estimates by different methods of energy requirements at four months

Method			Requirement (kcal/kg/day)
Intakes of exclusively breast-fed infants			
	(Table 15.2)		90
Factorial estimate	(Table 15.4)		83
Total expenditure by doubly-labelled			
water method	(Table 15.6)	73.5	
add energy stored	(p. 236)	9	83

Energy requirements at one year onwards

By the end of the first year the rate of growth has become quite small: less than 1 g/kg, falling to 0.35 g/kg at three years, corresponding to energy costs of 4 and 1.4 kcal/kg. Since the BMR remains rather constant at 45–55 kcal/kg (Schofield *et al.*, 1985), the energy cost of growth accounts for only some 5 per cent of the total energy requirement at one year, falling to less than 2 per cent at three years. Weight gain is therefore not as sensitive a criterion of adequacy as it was at four months. This does not mean that the small requirement for growth is unimportant. In a child weighing 10 kg at one year, a deficit of only 1 kcal/kg/day over 12 months will lead to a cumulative deficit in attained weight of nearly 1 kg at two years. It is the obesity problem in reverse, that small deficits, like small excesses, mount up.

On the other hand, at one year physical activity becomes more important, but it is very difficult to measure. Moreover, there are no healthy standards for judging what constitutes an adequate or 'healthy' level of activity in a young child. In this situation the factorial method of computing the energy requirement is no longer very useful.

Another criterion that has been used in a few studies is nitrogen balance, since if the energy intake is inadequate, N balance on a fixed protein intake will be reduced or even become negative. In the main, however, it is necessary to rely on measurements of intake and expenditure in healthy children.

Intake

The estimates of FAO/WHO/UNU (WHO, 1985), based on figures from industrialized countries, are summarized in Table 15.8. Intakes reported by

Table 15.8   Average energy intakes of pre-school children in industrialized countries with some estimates by the doubly labelled water method of total energy expenditure (TEE). Sexes combined.

Age (years)	Energy, kcal/kg/day	
	Intake[a]	TEE[b]
1–2	106	
2–3	103 ⎱	
3–4	97 ⎰	80.5
4–5	93	83.5

[a] Intakes from WHO (1985)
[b] TEE from Davies *et al.* (1991)

Whitehead *et al.* (1981) in the UK are somewhat lower, about 95 kcal/kg/day at one year. Comparable data from Third World countries are hard to obtain, because many children in the second year of life are still being partially breast-fed. The difficulties of obtaining accurate estimates of intakes in free-living children are so great that the results have to be accepted with caution, but some figures from Third World countries are shown in Table 15.9.

Table 15.9   Energy intakes of pre-school children after weaning in various developing countries

Age (years)	Country	Intake (kcal/kg/day)
1–2	Ghana	86
	Guatemala	77
	Jamaica	83
	Polynesia	70
	Thailand	52
	Uganda	68
2–3	Ghana	74
	Guatemala	112
	Polynesia	60
	Thailand	71
	Uganda	76

From Waterlow and Rutishauser (1974)

Expenditure

Estimates of expenditure by the doubly labelled water method are probably more reliable than intakes. The results of a number of studies are summarized in Table 15.10. They are very similar, whether the children come from the UK, The Gambia or Guatemala and there is little change in expenditure/kg between one and five years. The table also shows the requirement for energy stored and hence the total requirement.

Table 15.10   Estimates by the doubly labelled water method of the total energy expenditure (TEE) of infants aged more than six months and of pre-school children in Cambridge, UK, The Gambia and Guatemala, together with estimates of energy stored

Age (months)	TEE (kcal/kg/day)	Energy stored (kcal/kg/day)	Total requirement (kcal/kg/day)
6–9	80	5.5	85.5
9–12	78	3.5 ⎫	
9–12	75	3.5 ⎬	80
12–24	80	1.7 ⎫	
12–24	83	1.7 ⎬	83
24–36	87	1.2 ⎫	
24–36	81	1.2 ⎬	85
36–60	82	1.0	83
Mean	81		

Note: The coefficient of variation in these series is of the order of 20 per cent.
From Vasquez-Velasquez (1988); Prentice *et al.* (1988); Davies *et al.* (1991)

Nitrogen balance

Measurements of N balance have to be made in a metabolic ward with inevitable restrictions on physical activity, so the results may underestimate the requirements of real life, but they provide some useful guidelines.

Table 15.11 shows results obtained by Jackson *et al.* (1983) in Jamaica. The expected N retention in children of one to two years is 20–30 mg N/kg/day. At the higher protein intake, which was above the protein requirement (see below), N retention was satisfactory even at an energy intake of 80 kcal/kg/day. At the lower protein intake, which is only enough for maintenance, decreasing the energy intake had a marked effect on N balance. In similar studies in Thailand and Guatemala, with a protein intake equivalent to the 'safe level', based on local weaning foods, N retentions were satisfactory at energy intakes of 80 kcal/kg (FAO, 1980). These results suggest that the capacity for growth, as reflected by N retention, is retained at this moderately low level of energy intake, provided that the protein intake is adequate. It has also been suggested that a period on a low level of energy intake may produce adaptive responses, so that weight can be gained at intake levels which were previously inadequate (Kennedy *et al.*, 1990).

Table 15.11   Effect of different levels of energy intake on nitrogen retention in children aged 7–22 months, fed on a milk-based diet

Protein intake (g/kg/day)	Energy intake (kcal/kg/day)	N rentention (mg N/kg/day)
1.7	102	+81
1.7	91	+55
1.7	82	+46
0.7	98	+11
0.7	87	+5
0.7	79	−32

From Jackson *et al.* (1983)

Physical activity

The doubly labelled water method gives an estimate of energy spent on physical activity as [total expenditure −(BMR + thermic effect of food)] but the difference between two larger numbers is not very reliable. Direct measurement of activity in young children is very difficult. In a pioneer study in 1972 Rutishauser and Whitehead recorded the activity of 20 Ugandan pre-school children over successive ten-minute periods for ten hours, and compared it with that of five European children. Activities were converted into estimates of energy expenditure by applying the standard values obtained in adults for the cost of standing, walking, etc. In the Ugandan children total daily expenditure came to 78 kcal/kg/day, in the Europeans to 98. These activity factors may not be appropriate for children (Torun *et al.*, 1983); however, the difference between the two groups is clear. The African children in this study, in spite of an energy intake that appears rather low, were growing at a normal rate. This is further evidence that activity may be sacrificed to maintain growth.

Meeks-Gardener *et al.* (1990) in Jamaica recorded activities minute by minute and showed that stunted children spent significantly less time on vigorous and moderate activities than those who were not stunted. A recent study by the activity-diary method has shown that Gambian children aged six to 18 months were significantly less active than their counterparts of the same age in Glasgow (Lawrence *et al.*, 1991). The authors attributed the difference to cultural factors rather than to the lower nutritional status of the Gambian children (average 85 per cent weight for age, compared with 100 per cent for the Glasgow children).

Only two studies have tackled directly the question whether in Third World children physical activity may be limited by energy intake. In Mexico Chavez and Martinez (1984) found that young children receiving a food supplement were more active than those who were not. They measured activity by the ingenious method of recording the number of times that the child's foot touched the ground. In a study in Guatemala, reduction in the energy intake of pre-school children from 100 to 90 kcal/kg/day was accompanied by a fall in expenditure without change in N balance or weight gain (Torun, 1986). It seems, therefore, that faced with an inadequate energy intake the child preserved weight at the expense of physical activity. This behaviour contrasts with that of adults, who, in the hungry season, maintain or even increase physical activity at the expense of their body weight (Ferro-Luzzi, 1990). The view is widely held, though without objective confirmation, that in young children physical activity plays a key role in psychological and social development. There is also some evidence that it influences the rate of linear growth (Torun, 1986). If so, expenditure on activity should be the key criterion of the adequacy of energy intake at this age, particularly since more activity may be demanded of Third World children than in more affluent countries.

Conclusion

The results in Table 15.10 indicate an average energy requirement at two to three years of 85 kcal/kg/day, which is some 15 per cent lower than the requirement proposed in the Rome report (WHO, 1985).

So far in this chapter it has been assumed that we are dealing with normal children and all estimates of requirements have been related to body weight. The requirements for catch-up by children whose actual weight is below their expected weight is considered at the end of this chapter. A further point was raised in Chapter 2. The BMR is the main component of energy expenditure in young children, and there is some evidence that the BMR/kg is inversely related to length or height. J. M. Walker *et al.* (1990) found that in short so-called normal children, with an SD score for height of −2, the BMR/kg lean body mass was about 30 per cent greater than in control children at the 50th centile of height (Fig. 15.3). This may explain the surprising finding of S. P. Walker *et al.* (1990) in Jamaica, that stunted children had a 33 per cent greater energy intake per kg than non-stunted children in the same environment. If these findings are confirmed, it may be advisable that in populations with a high prevalence of stunting, estimates of average energy requirements should be increased, quite apart from extra needs for catch-up. It would be difficult without more information to assess how great the increase should be.

The calculations that have been made in this section give an impression of precision that may be misleading. Long ago Widdowson (1962) pointed out

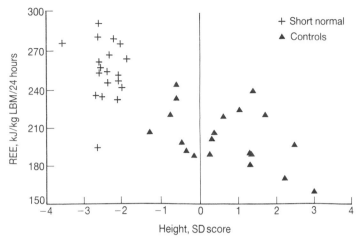

Fig. 15.3   Relation between resting energy expenditure per kg lean body mass and SD score for height in 'normal' growth-retarded children. Reproduced by permission from J. M. Walker *et al.* (1990).

that in a group of normal children, there may be a two-fold range of energy intake per kg body weight. More recent figures for both intake and expenditure show a coefficient of variation between subjects of 10 to 20 per cent. This variability has to be borne in mind when the estimates of energy requirements are being put to practical use. However, it seems justified to conclude that the mean energy requirement of young children in a healthy environment is lower than that previously proposed.

Protein requirements

All calculations of protein requirements relate to a situation in which the energy requirements are met. If they are not, the requirement for protein, as protein, becomes meaningless because part of it is oxidized to provide energy. There is ample evidence cited in the Rome report (WHO, 1985) from animal experiments and from studies in children and adults that satisfactory nitrogen balances cannot be achieved if energy intakes are inadequate. In fact, as Table 15.11 shows, N balance can be used as a measure of the fulfilment of energy needs.

For protein, as for energy, there are two approaches to estimating requirements: observed intakes and physiological measurements.

Protein (nitrogen) requirements up to four months

Intakes

The Rome report based the protein requirements of healthy infants up to four months on the intake of nitrogen in breast milk, on the assumption that up to this age it is natural for babies to be exclusively breast-fed. The protein content of milk was taken as N x 6.25. This is not strictly correct, as will be discussed below. The Rome figures are shown in Table 15.12. It is assumed

Table 15.12 Average intake of protein from breast milk by infants aged from birth to four months

Age (months)	Breast milk volume[a] (ml)	Average protein intake[b] (g/kg/day)
Boys		
0–1	720	2.46
1–2	795	1.93
2–3	850	1.74
3–4	820	1.49
Girls		
0–1	660	2.39
1–2	730	1.93
2–3	780	1.78
3–4	755	1.53

[a] Breast milk volumes from Wallgren (1944) and Whitehead and Paul (1981). Intakes of girls taken as 8 per cent less than of boys.
[b] Median NCHS weight at mid-point of month. From WHO (1985), Table 29.

that breast milk provided the ideal balance between protein and energy, so that an amount of milk that satisfies an infant's energy needs will also meet the needs for protein. There is some variation in the protein:energy (P/E) ratio of milks from different mothers, although there is surprisingly little information about the extent of this variation. The assumption that human milk is a 'gold standard' for the infant's protein requirements is based on the average composition of mother's milk.

When babies are no longer exclusively fed on breast milk, the intake cannot be used as a measure of requirement; supplementary foods may be either too high in protein, e.g. cow's milk, or too low, e.g. cereal gruels. At this stage it has been customary to resort to factorial estimates of protein requirement.

Factorial estimates

Table 15.13 shows the calculations produced by the FAO/WHO/UNU group (WHO, 1985). The amounts are expressed in the first instance as mg N/kg/day, rather than as protein, because the actual measurements are made in terms of nitrogen.

Table 15.13 Factorial estimates of average protein requirement at three to four months and at one year. Values are expressed in terms of nitrogen.

	Requirement, mg N/kg/day	
Factor	3–4 months[a]	1 year
N increment for growth	55	24
N increment × 1.5	81	36
Corrected for 70% efficiency	116	51
N for maintenance	120	120
Sum	236	171
In terms of protein, g/kg/day	1.47	1.07

[a] Adapted from WHO (1985)

Maintenance requirement

The maintenance requirement is the amount needed to maintain constant body N, and has been estimated by measurements of N balance (Fig. 15.4). At the point M on the *x*-axis the intake just balances the obligatory losses in urine and faeces and from the skin which would be observed if the protein intake were zero (B on the *y*-axis). The slope of the line AB represents the efficiency of utilization of food, N. The Rome report estimated the maintenance requirement as 120 mg N/kg/day, decreasing slightly with age to a value of 100 mg N/kg/day in adults, and proposed 70 per cent as a reasonable value for the efficiency. These estimates were based largely on studies by Huang *et al.* (1980). Balance studies reported by Fomon (1986) give rather different values: 84 mg N/kg/day for maintenance and 62 per cent for efficiency. It is important, therefore, to realize that current estimates are derived from limited data and cannot be regarded as very firm.

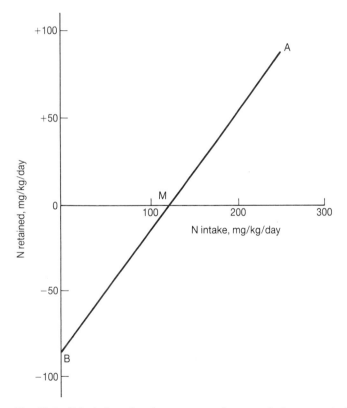

Fig. 15.4 Calculation of maintenance requirement of nitrogen and efficiency of utilization from balance measurements. The maintenance requirement (M) is the intercept on the *x*-axis, at zero N retention. The efficiency is the slope (70 per cent retained per 100 mg intake).

There seem to be two reasons for the inefficiency with which N is used, even after it has been absorbed and even when, as in human or cow's milk, the amino acid composition of the protein is considered to be optimal. The first is that in human milk about 30 per cent of the total N is non-protein N, of which a large part is urea. Calculating the protein content as total N x 6.25, leading to an average 'protein' content of about 11 g/l, is therefore incorrect. The 'true' protein content is about 8 g/l, and some authors have claimed that this value, rather than that based on total N, should be used for estimating the protein requirements of breast-fed infants. This argument assumes that the non-protein N is not available. Moreover, although the end result may be converted to protein, as in Table 15.12, actual measurements are always made in terms of nitrogen. Fomon, on the basis of studies with ^{15}N-labelled urea, claimed that only a small part of the urea can be utilized (Fomon *et al.*, 1988). On the other hand, Jackson (1989) found that in children recovering from malnutrition on low protein intakes some 50 per cent of labelled urea N was retained and presumably entered synthetic pathways (see Chapter 6). An explanation for inefficiency based on the unavailability of urea N would not apply to cow's milk, which contains a much smaller proportion of urea, and Waterlow *et al.* (1960) found that the efficiency of utilization of human and cow's milk N was virtually the same.

The other explanation for inefficiency is more basic: that amino acids entering the body cannot entirely escape oxidation. This is what Millward and Rivers (1988) have called the 'oxidative drive'. Amino acids are oxidized by a series of enzymes, ending with those of the urea cycle. Apparently the activity of these enzymes cannot normally be reduced below a certain minimal level. However, Chan and Waterlow (1966) found that in young children recovering from malnutrition the N of milk was utilized with almost 100 per cent efficiency. This might be regarded as an adaptation to protein depletion. Whether or not this is correct, it would clearly be unrealistic to suppose that there is a single unalterable value for the efficiency of N utilization, even when allowance has been made for the quality of the protein (see below).

Nitrogen requirement for growth

As the child grows there is an increase not only in the amount of tissues that contain protein, but also in the concentration of protein per kg tissue, at the expense of extracellular water. Fomon *et al.* (1982) have calculated from measurements of body water the increments of N from birth to ten years, taking account of both these processes. The Rome report assumed that the inefficiency factor discussed above applied to the deposition of protein as well as to maintenance, although from a metabolic point of view this assumption is not logical. In the report, therefore, the growth requirement at each age was calculated as 100/70 x (the increments estimated by Fomon). Infants do not, however, grow regularly from day to day, nor even over longer periods. Figure 15.5 illustrates this point very vividly from day-by-day measurements of low birth-weight infants, in whom, because growth is fast, differences in velocity are magnified. A day of poor growth may be followed by a day of catch-up growth, which requires more food.

Black and Cole (1983) found that in the first six months of life the within-subject coefficient of variation of food intake from day to day was of the order of 10 per cent. Dewey and Lönnerdal (1983) observed that 'the wide range in breast milk volume in well-nourished populations is due more to variations in infant demand than to inadequacy of milk production'. It seemed reasonable in the preparation of the Rome report to take some account of

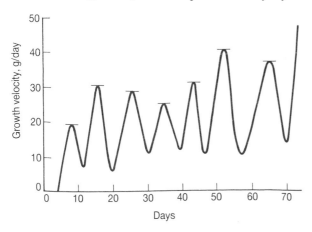

Fig. 15.5   Variability of weight velocity in premature infants.
Reproduced by permission from Greco *et al*. (1990).

this variability of demand and of intake, but by how much? The problem was tackled empirically: if the estimated requirement for growth was increased by 50 per cent, it brought the factorial estimate of average N requirement at four months into line with the average N intake from breast milk in healthy children at that age. However, this agreement is not as satisfactory as it seems; it is a contrived result because the 50 per cent increase in requirement for growth was fixed at that level precisely in order to produce agreement. A more important difficulty is that when figures for protein requirements are applied in practice, the *average* requirement has to be converted into a *safe level* of intake which takes account of the variability of requirements between individuals. The level that would cover the needs of virtually all members of a group is the mean + 2 SD, in this case the mean x 1.25. The concept has been fully described in the Rome report. However, it makes no sense to recommend that a group of healthy breast-fed infants, in order to be 'safe', *ought* to have intakes greater than they actually have.

Beaton and Chery (1988) have examined this problem statistically. We have to consider two separate distributions, that of intake and that of require-ments. In Fig. 15.6, curve I represents the observed distribution of intakes in healthy breast-fed children, and being based on actual data, is fixed. The question then is: what must be the position of the requirements curve R, so that virtually no children are at risk of a deficient intake? The conclusion from Beaton and Chery's calculations, which assume a correlation of about 0.3 between intake and requirement in an individual child, is that for virtually all members of a group of breast-fed infants to be 'safe', their *average* protein requirement must be about 1.1 g/kg/day, which is about 20 per cent less than their average intake at four months. It would follow from this that breast milk normally provides a margin of safety, and many children would get more protein than they need. If we talk in terms of Nature's provisions, this seems not unreasonable. Fomon (1986), on the other hand, has put the opposite point of view: since formula-fed infants, with a higher protein intake than those who are breast-fed, gain more lean body mass, perhaps intakes from

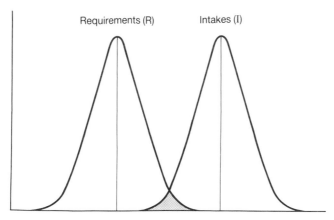

Fig. 15.6 Theoretical distributions of protein intakes and requirements. Curve I represents the distribution of intakes, with a mean at 1.4 g protein/kg/day, and a coefficient of variation (CV) of 20 per cent (arbitrary). Curve R is the distribution of requirements, with a CV of 12.5 per cent.

R has to be located to the left of I, in such a way that the area of overlap is minimal. The shaded area represents the number of children who may have intakes less than their requirements.

breast milk are suboptimal and represent a compromise between the needs of the baby and the needs of the lactating mother.

Protein (nitrogen) requirement at about one year

Between four months and one year two new factors have to be taken into account. The growth rate decreases rapidly and the child is very often consuming other foods as well as breast milk, often starchy gruels low in protein.

The factorial calculation in Table 15.13 indicates that because of the lower growth rate the requirement at one year is about three-quarters of that at four months. The factor is not very sensitive to uncertainties about the exact values for maintenance and efficiency. When other foods are introduced, the effectiveness of their proteins in meeting the child's requirement depends on their digestibility and their quality, the latter being determined by the amino acid composition of the mixed proteins. A great deal of work has been devoted to assessing the requirements for individual essential amino acids, summarized in WHO (1985). The pattern of amino acid requirements can then be used as a yardstick, against which the pattern of food proteins is compared, to give an amino acid score. Alternatively, the reference pattern can be constructed from the amino acid concentrations in milk or egg protein, which are accepted as being of high quality. However, at the present time there is renewed uncertainty and controversy about the validity of these procedures (Millward and Rivers, 1988; Millward *et al.*, 1989). Moreover, Jackson (1989) has pointed out that some amino acids normally regarded as non-essential, i.e. capable of being synthesized in the body, may become limiting under conditions of high demand, such as rapid growth. It is accepted that the quality of food proteins is not the same for young children as for adults, but the extent of the difference is not clear.

Table 15.14   Relative nitrogen absorption and retention of some vegetable protein sources, compared with casein

| Protein source | % of value for casein | | Reference |
	Absorption	Retention	
Rice	77	69	MacLean *et al.* (1978)
Black beans	75	28	Graham *et al.* (1979)
Maize	78	41	Graham *et al.* (1980)
Sorghum	57	43	MacLean *et al.* (1981)
Maize + amaranth	84	76	Morales *et al.* (1988)

From balance studies on children 10–30 months old, fed diets providing 100–125 kcal/kg, with P/E = 6.2. The retention gives a measure of the net protein utilization, compared with that of casein.

One approach to this problem is to determine protein quality by measurements of nitrogen balance in young children. This is a difficult procedure and few such studies have been done. The work along these lines by Graham and his colleagues in Peru is summarized in Table 15.14. In these studies the standard was casein, but in digestibility and quality cow's milk protein is very close to human milk (Barness *et al.*, 1957; Waterlow *et al.*, 1960; Fomon, 1974). It was an important feature of this work that all the foods were fed at a level of protein close to the maintenance requirement. This ensures that differences in quality will be clearly defined. The values for retention give a measure of overall quality compared with that of casein. The drawback of these measurements is that for the most part they were done with single protein sources rather than with mixtures, as in natural diets, where the proteins may complement each other. However, they do illustrate the low protein quality of the cereals used in many weaning diets.

From the calculations of WHO (1985) the mixed proteins of a typical Third World weaning diet might have a digestibility of 85 per cent of that of milk protein and a quality or biological value of 75 per cent (WHO, 1985). The net protein utilization (NPU) relative to that of milk is the product of these two, and would therefore be 64 per cent (0.85 x 0.75 x 100). This relative NPU is the figure used to correct for protein quality.

Use of the protein-energy ratio

A different approach to the problem (Waterlow, 1990) gets away from the concept of absolute requirements and asks the practical question: what must be the protein content of the child's food to meet its needs, provided that it eats enough to satisfy its energy requirement? The ratio of protein to energy in food (P/E) is usually expressed in terms of energy:

$$\frac{\text{crude protein (g N} \times 6.25)/100 \text{ g} \times 4 \text{ kcal/g}}{\text{total energy (kcal/100 g)}}$$

This is the *gross* P/E.

The way in which I have proposed to use the P/E ratio (Waterlow, 1990) is based on two assumptions: first, the usual one that enough of the diet is eaten to satisfy the needs for energy; secondly, that breast milk, with P/E about 7.2, supplies enough protein in amount and quality to meet the needs of practically all young children, provided again that their energy requirements are met, i.e. breast milk provides a 'safe' level of protein intake, according to the usual definition of 'safe'. This assumption can hardly be challenged (Beaton and Chery, 1988). Thus all calculations are relative to breast milk as a reference. Multiplying the gross P/E of a diet by its NPU gives a *corrected* P/E, which is a measure of the quality of the diet relative to breast milk.

As an example, a Third World diet with gross P/E 9.0 and NPU 64 would have a corrected P/E of 5.76. As estimated above (p. 246), the required P/E at one year, in terms of breast milk, would be about three-quarters of that at four months, i.e. 7.2 x 0.75 = 5.4. It could be concluded that at one year the Third World diet will just about meet the safe level. Table 15.15 shows the gross P/E ratios of some diets on one- to two-year old children and their values corrected on the assumption of NPU = 64 per cent. Clearly some of these diets would be only marginally adequate in protein.

Table 15.15   P/E ratios of some typical diets of one- to two-year old children (not breast-fed)

	Gross P/E ratio	Corrected[a] for quality
Ghana	9.2	5.9
Guatemala	10.0	6.4
India	8.4	5.4
Jamaica	11.8	7.6
Polynesia	12.6	8.1
Thailand	7.9	5.1
Uganda	12.5	8.0
Safe P/E at 1 year, based on breast milk		5.4

[a] Assuming that all diets have a net protein utilization 64 per cent of that of milk
From Waterlow and Rutishauser (1974)

Figure 15.7 shows the distribution of P/E ratios, corrected to the quality of milk protein, in the diets of young children in The Gambia and Uganda (Whitehead *et al.*, 1977). Whereas the Gambian diets are fairly uniform, with a P/E that is generally satisfactory, in Uganda a substantial proportion of children were consuming diets with a P/E so low that, on the present estimates, many would be unable to meet their protein requirements, and indeed some did develop 'subclinical' signs of malnutrition.

It should be noted that these judgements of adequacy are based on comparison with breast milk as a gold standard. The P/E of breast milk is calculated from its total N and it is of no importance in the calculation whether all the N, including that of urea, is utilized. In no food, including breast milk, is the nitrogen utilized with 100 per cent efficiency. What is important in practice is the relative efficiency.

The idea of using the P/E of diets for estimating their adequacy is not new. The original approach was to establish a 'safe' P/E as the ratio of safe level of protein intake/energy requirement (see critique by Beaton and Swiss, 1974; Payne, 1975). Quite complex statistical problems arose because of the need to take account, at the same time, of individual variability in both energy

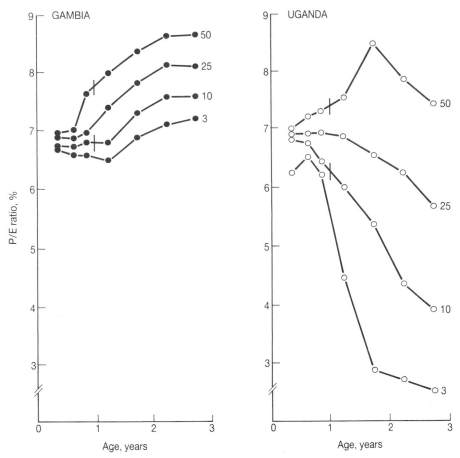

Fig. 15.7 Centiles of P/E ratios, corrected in terms of milk protein, in the diets of Gambian and Ugandan pre-school children. Reproduced by permission from Whitehead *et al.* (1977).

and protein requirements (e.g. WHO, 1985, Annex 9). Here the problem is approached from the other end: it is assumed that the P/E of human milk is 'safe', and we work back from there.

As emphasized above, the assumption that a diet will provide a safe amount of protein depends on the condition that a child eats enough of it to satisfy his energy needs. Most surveys of the intakes of pre-school children (e.g. Waterlow and Rutishauser, 1974; Landman and Jackson, 1980) have concluded that energy was more likely to be limiting than protein. That conclusion was based on the estimates of an earlier UN report (WHO, 1973) in which the requirements of children for energy were set rather higher, and those for protein rather lower, than in the 1985 report. If energy requirements are really as low as recent work suggests (see previous section p. 238), then the prevalence of inadequate energy intakes will be lower than used to be thought, and the prevalence of inadequate protein intakes may be higher.

The estimate made above of the quality of a typical Third World weaning diet led to a value of 8.4 (uncorrected) for the safe P/E of diets of children at one year. It is not suggested that such a number is more than an operational tool, directing attention to regions or groups where inadequate protein intake could be a problem for some children. Annegers (1973) showed that in West Africa, as one proceeds from north to south, P/E in the prevailing diets of the population as a whole, and not specifically of children, fell from 14 – 16 in the Sahel to 6.4 – 9.9 on the coast. He pointed out that frank kwashiorkor occurred with increasing frequency in regions where the diet had a low P/E. In Gopalan's prospective study of the development of kwashiorkor and marasmus, the average crude P/E of the diet was 8.6 and the corrected P/E 5.5.

This is very close to the value calculated above for the safe P/E of a diet with NPU 64 per cent of that of milk. Any reduction in the quality of the diet, which might well happen in individual cases, would produce a risk of inadequate protein intake. It is apparent from Table 15.14 that in some regions the average P/E of the diet was below the level that we have calculated as safe.

Conclusion

In contrast to the conclusions of the discussion on energy requirements, I have broken away from the approach adopted by WHO (1985) and have not come up with estimates of the protein requirements of children in terms of grams per day. The reasons are the difficulty introduced by the concept of safe level when applied to breast-fed infants, and the uncertainties about all the components of the factorial calculation—the requirements for mainten- ance and growth and the efficiency of utilization. It has seemed more realistic from a practical point of view not to ask: what are a child's requirements? but rather: what qualities must the food have to keep a child healthy? This, after all, is the question actually faced by mothers, policy makers and food manufacturers. In this approach the debate inevitably focuses on the values of the protein: energy ratio of foods.

I conclude, contrary to much that has been published in recent years, that some weaning diets in Third World countries contain marginal amounts of protein even when consumed in quantities that satisfy the child's energy needs. A marginal diet means one that is likely to satisfy the needs of many, perhaps most children, but not all. Any group of children, as of adults, appears to have a range of protein requirements; the data of Torun *et al.* (1984) show a coefficient of variation of 15 per cent. On a marginal intake children at the upper end of the range will be at risk. This conclusion does not conflict with Gopalan's finding (1968) that there was no difference, quanti- tative or qualitative, between the diets of children who developed kwashi- orkor or marasmus. If kwashiorkor is related to protein deficiency (Chapter 11), that is precisely what one would expect in a group of children on a diet marginally inadequate in both energy and protein. A further factor is infection, which increases the demand for protein compared with that for energy (see below).

Finally, it is important to re-emphasize that conventional estimates of pro- tein requirements are based on the needs for normal gain in weight. We should take account of the possibility that there may be special needs for particular components of growth. For example, skeletal growth may require extra amounts of sulphur amino acids for proteoglycase synthesis in cartilage. Another essential feature of linear growth is the deposition of collagen, which has a very high content of the interconvertible amino acids glycine and serine. As Jackson (1989) has pointed out, breast milk contains only a fraction of the amount that is needed for collagen formation in the young infant; the rest has to be provided by *de novo* synthesis, which may become limiting. Lastly, even so-called healthy children have infections which, as discussed in Chapters 6 and 17, will put an extra strain on protein requirements because of the need to synthesize acute phase proteins.

Energy and protein requirements for catch-up growth

Catch-up for weight usually refers to restoration of normal weight for height in the child who is malnourished or has had episodes of infection and anorexia. Catch-up in height can certainly occur (Chapter 13), but it is a much slower process and the extra daily requirement for energy and protein will be small. Although our concern here is with energy and protein it is obvious that growth cannot occur unless all the components of the tissue laid down are available, such as potassium, magnesium, phosphorus, zinc, probably other trace elements and vitamins of the B complex. For haemopoietic tissue iron and folic acid are needed, for bone vitamin D as well as calcium and phosphorus. Figure 9.1 was an example of catch-up growth being limited by an inadequate zinc content of the diet. It may happen that when growth is stimulated by the provision of food, a micronutrient becomes limiting and deficiency states develop which were not apparent before. Thus both rickets and folic acid deficiency have been observed in children recovering from PEM.

The requirements for catch-up growth have excited a good deal of interest in recent years. A publication of the United Nations University (UNU, 1979) provides an excellent overview of the subject. Other reviews and relevant articles are by Waterlow *et al.* (1976), Ashworth and Millward (1986), Roberts and Young (1988), Fjeld *et al.* (1989) and Jackson and Wootton (1990). There are some differences between the various authors in their estimates of the requirements for catch-up. The energy requirement is dictated largely by the fat content of the tissue laid down. The crucial difference, which determines the necessary P/E ratio of the food, is the value used for the protein content. Nitrogen balance studies in Jamaica on children recovering from malnutrition showed that the weight gained contained on average 17 per cent (Waterlow *et al.*, 1976), which is considerably higher than the 13.5 per cent in the reference child of Fomon *et al.* (1982). It was calculated that the protein of the food (milk) was utilized for growth with an efficiency of approximately 75 per cent. It follows that on average the protein requirement for depositing new tissue would be 0.17/0.75 = 0.23 g per g weight gained. However, as Jackson *et al.* (1977) pointed out, there is a good deal of variability in the composition of the tissue laid down. They showed an inverse correlation, as would be expected theoretically, between the energy cost of growth and the increase in muscle mass.

There is some evidence, supported by animal experiments (Allison, 1951) that malnourished subjects can utilize food protein more efficiently than those who are normally nourished. In the balance studies of Chan and Waterlow (1966) the efficiency of utilization appeared to be almost 100 per cent, although in those of Ashworth (1969) it appeared to be rather lower. This is a subject that needs further study. For the time being, to be on the safe side, we assume an efficiency of 70 per cent.

The most detailed study to date of the composition of weight gained in catch-up is that of Fjeld *et al.* (1989) in Peru. Their results are summarized in Table 15.16, and are in general agreement with our own earlier estimates. It is interesting that rapid gain is accompanied by an increase in the thermic effect of food, which presumably reflects the high rate of protein synthesis.

Table 15.16   Rate of catch-up and composition of weight gain in children recovering from severe PEM

	Moderate gain	Rapid gain
Intake, per kg/day		
metabolizable energy, kcal	116	148
protein, g	2–3	4–5
Weight gain, g/kg/day	5.7	11.8
Total daily energy expenditure,		
kcal/kg/day	92[a]	95
Energy stored, kcal/g gain	5.4[b]	4.6
Composition of gain, g/g		
protein	0.20[c]	0.14
fat	0.45[d]	0.40

Children were divided into two groups, 11 in each, which received different levels of energy and protein. Balance measurements were made at two points of time during recovery. The figures reproduced here represent the early phase.
[a] Measured with doubly labelled water; [b] calculated as ME intake − TDEE; [c] from N balance; [d] calculated as energy stored − protein energy stored
Data from Fjeld *et al.* (1989)

In the hospital setting, in which the studies quoted so far were made, it is clearly important that catch-up to normal weight for height should be achieved as quickly as possible, to minimize exposure to infection and family deprivation and to release beds for other children. The energy and protein requirements for various rates of gain are shown in Table 15.17. Rates of gain up to 20 g/kg/day are perfectly possible (Chapter 12, and Ashworth, 1969). It was not appreciated until the 1960s that in practice the limiting factor is likely to be the energy supply, which cannot be brought to the levels needed for rapid growth unless the energy density is increased by adding fat to the food.

The estimate of protein requirement takes account only of gains in tissue protein and neglects the need for restoring other proteins that may be depleted, of which the most important quantitatively is probably albumin. Table 15.18 suggests that restoration of the albumin mass might add about 5 per cent to the protein requirement for catch-up. That is too small an amount to be important in these very approximate calculations.

In the community it would be unrealistic to expect children to achieve the very rapid gains that can be attained in hospital. In a community study in Jamaica in the three months after faltering as a result of infection, 27 per cent of children gained weight at more than twice and 8 per cent at more

Table 15.17   Requirements for energy and protein at different rates of weight gain

Rate of gain (g/kg/day)	Energy (kcal/kg/day)	Protein (g/kg/day)	P/E (%)	Time needed to correct deficit (weeks)
0	75	0.75	4.0	∞
1	80	1.0	5.0	52
2	85	1.25	5.9	25
5	100	2.00	8.0	10
10	125	3.25	10.4	5
20	175	5.75	13.1	2.5

Modified from Ashworth and Millward (1986)
Assumptions:
1. A child 1 year old initially weighing 7 kg; target weight is 10 kg
2. Requirements at zero gain are the estimated maintenance requirements
3. The energy cost of weight gain is taken here as the conventional figure of 5 kcal/g, rather than the lower figure of 4 kcal/g calculated earlier for normal growth
4. The protein content of tissue gained is taken as 0.175 g/g, deposited with 70 per cent efficiency (see text)

Table 15.18   Deficit in albumin mass compared with deficit in tissue mass

	Initial state	Final state
Body weight, kg	7.0	10.0
Tissue protein concentration, g/kg	175	175
Total body protein, g	1225	1750
deficit, g		525
Plasma volume, ml, at 50 ml/kg	350	500
Albumin concentration, g/dl	2.0	4.0
Total circulating albumin, g	7.0	20.0
× 2 to allow for		
extravascular albumin mass, g	14.0	40.0
Deficit, g		26
	= 5.0% of tissue protein deficit	

than three times the normal rate (UNU, 1979). It has been estimated from studies of the impact of diarrhoeal disease (Chapter 17) that one day's illness on average produces a weight deficit of 25–40 g.

Figure 15.8 shows the extra energy and protein requirements for catch-up over a period of 100 days, with varying prevalences of illness within that period. It is assumed that the extra food is only consumed during the days when the child is well. The curves rise more steeply with increasing disease prevalence, because the more days ill, the fewer days well. The figure shows that even with a rather high prevalence of infection the extra energy needed for catch-up is only a small fraction of the total requirement. The increase in protein requirement is relatively greater. In the absence of infection the required P/E of the food in terms of milk protein is 5.2. With 30 per cent prevalence, for catch-up within 100 days, it becomes 6.0, an increase of 15 per cent.

In Fig. 15.8 the target was arbitrarily set as catch-up in 100 days for a child whose weight started on the normal curve. No implication is intended that this is an optimal rate. To regain the normal weight curve in 60 days would clearly be better. If a child were infected for 20 days, to regain the deficit in

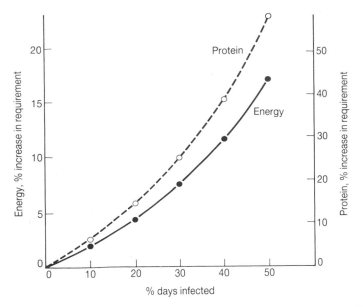

Fig. 15.8 Percentage increases in energy and protein requirements to allow for catch-up in 100 days at different prevalences of infection. It is assumed that one day infected produces a deficit of 30 g in weight gain.

the next 40 days would require an increase in energy of 9 per cent, in protein of 29 per cent, in the P/E of food of 18 per cent.

Although with usual prevalences of illness such as 10–20 per cent the extra requirements for catch-up are quite small, the other side of the coin is that small shortfalls of intake will over a long period of time lead to large deficits in weight. In the Third World it would be common to find a child who had a normal weight at four months but weighed only 7.5 kg at one year. This is a deficit of 2.5 kg acquired over eight months, or 10 g/day, and it could result from the child being infected for 30 per cent of the time, with no catch-up in between.

The calculations presented so far in this section have for simplicity been made for a child of a particular weight, 10 kg. However, requirements are usually expressed per kg body weight, so the question arises whether the weight used for calculating a child's requirements for catch-up should be the actual weight, the expected (reference) weight for age or the expected weight for height. FAO/WHO/UNU (WHO, 1985) recommended weight for height as the basis, and this is logical. However, there are likely to be situations when it is necessary to provide extra food without every single child being weighed and measured. In such a case it would be reasonable to base food supplies for each age-group on the reference weight for age. Even if this is generous at first for severely underweight children, it will allow for more rapid catch-up. It is true that children who are stunted but not wasted need only small amounts of extra food. Unless they are to become obese, catch-up in height, which is relatively slow, must determine the proper rate of increase in weight. However, experience shows that when children recovering from malnutrition have regained their expected weight for height, even if they are still somewhat stunted, their appetite, food intake and rate of weight gain fall off (Chapter 12). In a few this regulatory mechanism apparently does not operate and they do become obese.

The conclusion is that except in extreme situations, such as young children with very high prevalences of infection, an increase of 5–10 per cent in the intakes of both energy and protein, above the requirement of healthy children, should generally cover the needs for catch-up. However, if the basic diet is inadequate or marginal, even these modest increases may not be met. Energy intake may be limited by low energy density of the food (see Chapter 16); weaning diets that contain little or no milk or animal protein may be unable to provide the small extra requirement of protein. On the other hand, our calculations provide no justification for advocating special weaning foods containing some 20 per cent of the protein, on which a great deal of time and money was spent in the 1960s and 1970s (McLaren, 1975).

We return to the subject of catch-up from the stand-point of what happens in the field, in the chapter on infection (Chapter 17).

References

Allison, J. B. (1951). Interpretation of nitrogen balance data. *Federation Proceedings* **10:** 676–683.

Annegers, J. F. (1973). The protein-calorie ratio of West African diets and their relationship to protein-calorie malnutrition. *Ecology of Food and Nutrition* **2:** 225–235.

Ashworth, A. (1969). Growth rates in children recovering from protein-calorie malnutrition. *British Journal of Nutrition* **23:** 835–845.

Ashworth, A., Millward, D. J. (1986). Catch-up growth in children. *Nutrition Reviews* **44:** 157–163.

Barness, L. A., Baker, D. *et al.* (1957). Nitrogen metabolism of infants fed human and cow's milk. *Journal of Pediatrics* **51:** 29–39.

Beaton, G. H., Chery, A. (1988). Protein requirements of infants: a re-examination of approaches. *American Journal of Clinical Nutrition* **48:** 1403–1412.

Beaton, G. H., Swiss, L. D. (1974). Evaluation of the nutritional quality of food supplied: prediction of 'desirable' or 'safe' protein-calorie ratios. *American Journal of Clinical Nutrition* **27:** 485–504.

Black, A. E., Cole, T. J. (1983). Daily variations in food intake of infants from 2 to 18 months. *Human Nutrition:Applied Nutrition* **37A:** 448–458.

Blaxter, K. L. (1989). *Energy metabolism in animals and man.* Cambridge University Press.

Brooke, O. G., Alvear, J., Arnold, M. (1979). Energy retention, energy expenditure and growth in healthy immature infants. *Pediatric Research* **13:** 215–220.

Butte, N. F., Garza, C. *et al.* (1984). Human milk intake and growth in exclusively breast-fed infants. *Journal of Pediatrics* **104:** 187–195.

Butte, N. F., O'Brian Smith, E., Garza, G. (1990). Energy utilization of breast-fed and formula-fed infants. *American Journal of Clinical Nutrition* **51:** 350–358.

Chan, H., Waterlow, J. C. (1966). The protein requirement of infants at the age of about 1 year. *British Journal of Nutrition* **20:** 775–782.

Chavez, A., Martinez, C. (1984). Behavioral measurements of activity in children and their relation to food intake in a poor community. In Pollitt, E., Amante, P. (eds) *Energy intake and activity.* Alan R. Liss, New York, pp. 303–321.

Coward, W. A. (1988). The doubly-labelled-water ($^2H_2^{18}O$) method: principles and practice. *Proceedings of the Nutrition Society* **47**: 209–218.

Davies, P. S. W., Livingstone, M. B. E. *et al.* (1991). Total energy expenditure during childhood and adolescence. *Proceedings of the Nutrition Society* **50**: 14A.

Dewey, K. G., Lönnerdal, B. (1983). Milk and nutrient intake of breastfed infants from 1 to 6 months: relation to growth and fatness. *Journal of Pediatrics, Gastroenterology and Nutrition* **2**: 497–506.

Duggan, M. B., Milner, R. D. G. (1986). The maintenance energy requirement for children: an estimate based on a study of children with infection associated underfeeding. *American Journal of Clinical Nutrition* **43**: 870–878.

Ferro-Luzzi, A. (1990). Seasonal energy stress in marginally malnourished rural women: interpretation and integrated conclusions of a multicentre study in three developing countries. *European Journal of Clinical Nutrition* **44**: Suppl.1, 41–46.

Fjeld, C. R., Schoeller, D. A., Brown, K. H. (1988). Energy expenditure of malnourished children during catch-up growth. *Proceedings of the Nutrition Society* **47**: 227–231.

Fjeld, C. R., Schoeller, D., Brown, K. H. (1989). Body composition of children recovering from severe protein-energy malnutrition at two rates of catch-up growth. *American Journal of Clinical Nutrition* **50**: 1266–1275.

Fomon, S. J. (1960). Comparative study of adequacy of protein from human milk and cow's milk in promoting nitrogen retention by normal full-term infants. *Pediatrics* **26**: 51–56.

Fomon, S. J. (1967). *Infant nutrition*, 1st edn. W. B. Saunders Co., Philadelphia.

Fomon, S. J. (1974). *Infant nutrition*, 2nd edn. W. B. Saunders Co., Philadelphia.

Fomon, S. J. (1986). Protein requirements of term infants. In Fomon, S. J., Heird, W. C. (eds) *Energy and protein needs during infancy*. Academic Press, New York, pp. 55–68.

Fomon, S. J., Bier, D. M. *et al.* (1988). Bioavailability of dietary urea nitrogen in the breastfed infant. *Journal of Pediatrics* **113**: 515–517.

Fomon, S. J., Haschke, F. *et al.* (1982). Body composition of reference children from birth to age 10 years. *American Journal of Clinical Nutrition* **35**: 1169–1175.

Food and Agriculture Organization (1980). *Report on the informal gathering of investigators to review the collaborative research programme on protein requirements and energy intake*. Document ESN/Misc/80/3. FAO, Rome.

Gopalan, C. (1968). Kwashiorkor and marasmus: evolution and distinguishing features. In McCance, R. W., Widdowson, E. M. (eds) *Calorie deficiencies and protein deficiencies*. Churchill, London, pp. 49–58.

Graham, G. G., Morales, E. *et al.* (1979). Nutritive value of brown and black beans for infants and small children. *American Journal of Clinical Nutrition* **32**: 2362–2366.

Graham, G. G., Glover, D. V. *et al.* (1980). Nutritional value of normal, opaque-2 and sugary-2 opaque-2 maize hybrids for infants and children. *Journal of Nutrition* **110**: 1061–1069.

Greco, I., Capasso, A. *et al.* (1990). Pulsatile weight increases in very low birthweight babies appropriate for gestational age. *Archives of Disease in Childhood* **65**: 373–376.

Haggarty, P., McGaw, B. A. *et al.* (1991). The effect on the doubly- and triply-labelled water methods of water hydrogen incorporation into body fat of growing pigs. *Proceedings of the Nutrition Society* **50**: 30A.

Huang, P. C., Lin, C. P., Hsu, J. Y. (1980). Protein requirements of normal infants at the age of about 1 year: maintenance nitrogen requirements and obligatory nitrogen losses. *Journal of Nutrition* **110**: 1727–1735.

Jackson, A. A. (1989). Optimizing amino acid and protein supply and utilization in the newborn. *Proceedings of the Nutrition Society* **48**: 293–301.

Jackson, A. A., Wootton, S. A. (1990). The energy requirements of growth and catch-up growth. In Schürch, B., Scrimshaw, N. S. (eds) *Activity, energy expenditure and energy requirements of infants and children*. Nestlé Foundation, Lausanne, pp. 185–214.

Jackson, A. A., Picou, D., Reeds, P. J. (1977). The energy cost of repleting tissue deficits during recovery from protein-energy malnutrition. *American Journal of Clinical Nutrition* **30:** 1514–1517.

Jackson, A. A., Golden, M. H. N. *et al.* (1983). Whole body protein turnover and nitrogen balance in young children at intakes of protein and energy in the region of maintenance. *Human Nutrition:Clinical Nutrition* **37C:** 433–446.

James, W. P. T., Haggarty, P., McGaw, B. A. (1988). Recent progress in studies on energy expenditure: are the new methods providing answers to the old questions? *Proceedings of the Nutrition Society* **47:** 195–208.

Kennedy, N., Badaloo, A. V., Jackson, A. A. (1990). Adaptation to a marginal intake of energy in young children. *British Journal of Nutrition* **63:** 145–154.

Landman, J., Jackson, A. A. (1980). The role of protein deficiency in the aetiology of kwashiorkor. *West Indian Medical Journal* **29:** 229–238.

Lawrence, M., Lawrence, F. *et al.* (1991). A comparison of physical activity in Gambian and UK children aged 6–18 months. *European Journal of Clinical Nutrition* **45:** 243–252.

Lifson, N. (1966). Theory of use of the turnover rates of body water for measuring energy and material balance. *Journal of Theoretical Biology* **12:** 46–74.

Lucas, A., Ewing, G. *et al.* (1987). How much energy does the breast-fed infant consume and expend? *British Medical Journal* **295:** 75–77.

McLaren, D. S. (1975). The protein fiasco. *Lancet* **2:** 93–96.

MacLean, W. C., Klein, G. L. *et al.* (1978). Protein quality of conventional and high protein rice and digestibility of glutinous and non-glutinous rice by preschool children. *Journal of Nutrition* **108:** 1740–1747.

MacLean, W. C., De Romana, G. L. *et al.* (1981). Protein quantity and digestibility of sorghum in pre-school children: balance studies and plasma free amino acids. *Journal of Nutrition* **111:** 1928–1936.

Meeks-Gardner, J. M., Grantham-McGregor, S. M. *et al.* (1990). Dietary intake and observed activity of stunted and non-stunted children in Kingston, Jamaica. Part II: observed activity. *European Journal of Clinical Nutrition* **44:** 585–594.

Millward, D. J., Rivers, J. W. P. (1988). The nutritional role of indispensable amino acids and the metabolic basis for their requirements. *European Journal of Clinical Nutrition* **42:** 367–394.

Millward, D. J., Jackson, A. A. *et al.* (1989). Human amino acid and protein requirements: current dilemmas and uncertainties. *Nutrition Research Reviews* **2:** 109–132.

Morales, E., Lembcke, J., Graham, G. G. (1988). Nutritional value for young children of grain-amaranth and maize amaranth mixtures: effect of processing. *Journal of Nutrition* **118:** 78–85.

Paul, A. A., Black, A. E., Whitehead, R. G. (1988). Follow-up of energy intake and growth of children initially breast-fed. *Proceedings of the Nutrition Society* **47:** 92A.

Payne, P. R. (1975). Safe protein-calorie ratios in diets. The relative importance of protein and energy intake as causal factors in malnutrition. *American Journal of Clinical Nutrition* **28:** 281–286.

Payne, P. R., Waterlow, J. C. (1971). Relative energy requirements for maintenance, growth and physical activity. *Lancet* **2:** 210–211.

Prentice, A. M., Lucas, A. *et al.* (1988). Are current dietary guidelines for young children a prescription for overfeeding? *Lancet* **2:** 1066–1069.

Roberts, S. B., Young, V. R. (1988). Energy costs of fat and protein deposition in the human infant. *American Journal of Clinical Nutrition* **48:** 951–955.

Rutishauser, I. H. E., Whitehead, R. G. (1972). Energy intake and expenditure in 1–3 year old Ugandan children living in a rural environment. *British Journal of Nutrition* **28:** 145–152.

Schoeller, D. A., Ravussion, E. *et al.* (1986). Energy expenditure by doubly labelled water: validation in humans and proposed calculation. *American Journal of Physiology* **50**: R823–R830.

Schofield, W. N., Schofield, C., James, W. P. T. (1985). Basal metabolic rate—review and prediction, together with an annotated bibliography of source material. *Human Nutrition:Clinical Nutrition* **39C**: Suppl.1, 1–96.

Southgate, D. T., Barrett, I. M. (1966). The intake and excretion of calorific constituents of milk by babies. *British Journal of Nutrition* **20**: 363–372.

Spady, D. W., Payne, P. R. *et al.* (1976). Energy balance during recovery from malnutrition. *American Journal of Clinical Nutrition* **29**: 1073–1088.

Torun, B. (1986). Role of energy metabolism in regulation of protein requirements. In Taylor, T. G., Jenkins, N. K. (eds) *Proceedings of the XIIIth International Congress of Nutrition*. John Libbey, London, pp. 414–418.

Torun, B., Chew, F., Mendoza, R.D. (1983). Energy costs of activities of pre-school children. *Nutrition Research* **3**: 401–406.

Torun, B., Cabrera-Santiago, M. I., Viteri, F. E. (1984). Protein requirements of pre-school children: milk and soy-bean protein isolate. In Rand, W. M., Uauy, R., Scrimshaw, N. S. (eds) *Protein-energy requirement studies in developing countries: results of international research*. United Nations University, Tokyo, pp. 182–191.

United Nations University (1979). Protein-calorie requirements under conditions prevailing in developing countries: current knowledge and research needs. *Food and Nutrition Bulletin*, Suppl.1.

Vasquez-Velasquez, L. (1988). Energy expenditure and physical activity of malnourished Gambian infants. *Proceedings of the Nutrition Society* **47**: 233–239.

Walker, J. M., Bond, S. A. *et al.* (1990). Treatment of short normal children with growth hormone—a cautionary tale? *Lancet* **336**: 1331–1334.

Walker, S. P., Powell, C. A., Grantham-McGregor, S. M. (1990). Dietary intakes and activity levels of stunted and non-stunted children in Jamaica. Part 1. Dietary intakes. *European Journal of Clinical Nutrition* **44**: 527–534.

Wallgren, A. (1944–45). Breast milk consumption of healthy full-term infants. *Acta Paediatrica Scandinavica* **32**: 778–790.

Waterlow, J. C. (1990). Protein requirements of infants: an operational assessment. *Proceedings of the Nutrition Society* **49**: 27–34.

Waterlow, J. C., Millward, D. J. (1989). Energy cost of turnover of protein and other cellular constituents. In Wieser, W., Gnaiger, E. (eds) *Energy transformations in cells and organisms*. Georg Thieme, Stuttgart, pp. 277–282.

Waterlow, J. C., Rutishauser, I. H. E. (1974). Malnutrition in man. In Cravioto, J., Hambraeus, L., Vahlquist, B. (eds). *Early malnutrition and mental development*. Almqvist and Wiksell, Uppsala, pp. 13–26.

Waterlow, J. C., Ashworth, A., Griffiths, M. (1980). Faltering in infant growth in less developed countries. *Lancet* **2**: 1176–1177.

Waterlow, J. C., Ashworth-Hill, A., Spady, D. W. (1976). Energy costs and protein requirements for catch-up growth in children. In Williamson, A. W. (ed) *Early nutrition and later development*. Pitman, Tunbridge Wells.

Waterlow, J. C., Wills, V. G., Gyorgy, P. (1960). Balance studies in malnourished Jamaican infants. 2. Comparison of absorption and retention of nitrogen and phosphorus from human milk and a cow's milk mixture. *British Journal of Nutrition* **14**: 199–205.

Whitehead, R. G., Paul, A. A. (1981). Infant growth and human milk requirements. *Lancet* **2**: 161–163.

Whitehead, R. G., Paul, A. A. (1984). Growth charts and the assessment of infant feeding practices in the western world and in developing countries. *Early Human Development* **9**: 187–207.

Whitehead, R. G., Paul, A. A., Cole, T. J. (1981). A critical analysis of measured food energy intakes during infancy and early childhood in comparison with current recommendations. *Journal of Human Nutrition* **35**: 339–348.

Whitehead, R. G., Coward, W. A. *et al.* (1977). A comparison of the pathogenesis of PEM in Uganda and The Gambia. *Transactions of the Royal Society of Tropical Medicine and Hygiene* **71**: 189–195.

Widdowson, E. M. (1962). Nutritional individuality. *Proceedings of the Nutrition Society* **21**: 121–128.

Wong, W. W., Butte, N. F. *et al.* (1990). Comparison of energy expenditure estimated in healthy infants using doubly labelled water and energy balance methods. *European Journal of Clinical Nutrition* **44**: 175–184.

World Health Organization (1973). *Energy and protein requirements*. Report of a joint FAO/WHO Expert Committee. WHO Technical Report Series No. 522. WHO, Geneva.

World Health Organization (1983). *Measuring changes in nutritional status: Annex 3. Reference data for the weight and height of children*. WHO, Geneva.

World Health Organization (1985). *Energy and protein requirements*. Report of a joint FAO/WHO/UNU Expert Consultation. Technical Report Series No. 724. WHO, Geneva.

16

Breast feeding and weaning

Introduction

Most of us, implicitly or explicitly, regard breast feeding as the ideal source of both food and protection for the infant in an adverse environment. Not everyone agrees. Fomon (personal communication) writes that to 'argue that the lactation process has been modified by evolutionary forces so that the milk of each species is ideally suited to meeting the nutritional needs of its young . . . is a romantic notion that is at variance with the evidence'. Be that as it may, the promotion of breast feeding is the order of the day. In Western countries an increasing number of mothers, particularly of the upper classes, are breast feeding their babies, at least for a time. It has not always been so: in 1978 Davis began a review of the Jelliffes' book *Human milk in the modern world* (Jelliffe and Jelliffe, 1978) with the words: 'In the early fifties a talk advocating breast-feeding given by an Englishman in Boston was received with the polite incredulity that a seminar on bow-and-arrow warfare would have aroused in the Pentagon . . . the world has moved on since then.' Nevertheless, there is much concern that the world has not moved far enough or fast enough, and that there is an increasing trend away from breast feeding, particularly in the urban slums of the Third World (King and Ashworth, 1987). Any attempts to promote this trend by the infant formula industry are banned by the WHO/UNICEF Code of Practice for Marketing, but even if the code is adhered to, that does not solve the problem. There are many other pressures on women not to start breast feeding or to stop it after only a short time.

A question that has been much discussed is the time for which exclusive breast feeding can meet an infant's needs. The previous chapter was concerned with the demand, this chapter with the supply. Since the subject of this book is protein-energy malnutrition, only those two components are considered here. The WHO Collaborative Breast-feeding Study contains a well-referenced summary of the other nutrients in human milk (WHO, 1985).

Volume of breast milk

Methods of measuring milk intake

The traditional method of measuring breast milk intake by test weighing seems to be reasonably accurate when done under well-controlled conditions by experienced staff (Brown *et al.*, 1982), although a comparison in bottle-fed infants between test-weighing and direct measurement showed that test-weighing underestimated intakes by an average of 9 per cent (Borschel *et al.*, 1986). A useful increase in the accuracy of test weighing can be achieved by using modern electronic balances, which have a smaller measurement error and which damp the effect of the baby's movements (Coward, 1984). The method, however, is time-consuming, it interferes with the mother's normal activities and it cannot be used when the baby sleeps with the mother and is fed on demand many times during the night.

Estimates of 24-hour intake from day-time measurements only are not very reliable (Brown *et al.*, 1982). To get over this problem, Woolridge *et al.* (1987), working in Thailand, have proposed a method in which mother and baby are weighed before and after a night's sleep, with no interruptions in between. The method involves an estimate of the evaporative water loss from both baby and mother. Comparison with direct test-weighing gave satisfactory agreement. In a new approach being developed by Baum and his colleagues the baby sucks on a plastic nipple shield attached to the breast. The shield incorporates a flow-meter and a sampling device. According to the results published so far (Jackson *et al.*, 1987), the rate of milk flow was underestimated by 20–30 per cent, and not all mothers and babies accepted the device. The method is useful for sampling (see below); whether the measurement of volume can be improved remains to be seen.

An important recent advance is the measurement of milk intake by isotope dilution, using water labelled with deuterium, the stable isotope of hydrogen (Coward *et al.*, 1979). There are two variants of the method. In the first and simplest a small dose of labelled water is given to the baby and measurements of deuterium concentration in saliva or urine are made at intervals for some seven days. The zero-time intercept of the slope gives the deuterium space, V, and the slope, k, gives the fractional rate of water turnover in the baby. If it is assumed that there is no change in the baby's body water over the period of measurement, the total water intake is kV. This will include any water given to the baby in addition to breast milk, which therefore has to be measured separately. In bottle-fed infants the labelled water method gave reasonably satisfactory agreement with direct measurement of intake (Vio *et al.*, 1986; Lucas *et al.*, 1987), but there were rather large differences when the comparison was made with test-weighing (Coward *et al.*, 1979; Butte *et al.*, 1983, 1991).

In the second variant of the method labelled water is given to the mother and deuterium concentrations in the mother's milk and the infant's saliva are measured at intervals for about 14 days. This allows calculation at the same time of the baby's intake of breast milk and of its intake of water from other sources. The method was first developed by Coward, who has described the mathematical theory and the details of the calculation (Coward *et al.*, 1982; Coward, 1984), and it has been applied in the field in The Gambia (Coward *et al.*, 1982) and in Papua-New Guinea (Orr-Ewing *et al.*, 1986).

The dose-to-mother method appears to be more accurate than the dose-to-baby; a comparison with test-weighing showed good agreement (Butte *et al.*, 1988*b*).

The labelled water method has two great advantages: it gives an integrated estimate of the infant's milk intake over 10–14 days, thus reducing the effect of day-to-day fluctuations (see below); and it involves minimal disturbance of the mother and baby. Orr-Ewing *et al.* (1986) commented that in Papua-New Guinea their estimates of milk output were greater than those previously reported by test-weighing, probably because the technique 'allowed normal feeding patterns to continue in a setting in which conventional test-weighing procedures cause considerable disruption'.

The disadvantage is that the measurements of labelled water have to be made in a mass spectrometer, which is an expensive and complex instrument; however, since deuterated water is completely stable there is no problem about storing the samples and transporting them to a laboratory where the measurements can be made. Since in theory the dose-to-mother labelled water method should be the 'gold standard', it is to be hoped that through international co-operation it will come to be used more widely.

Amounts of breast milk ingested

Table 16.1 shows average amounts of breast milk consumed by exclusively breast-fed infants in the four studies in industrialized countries quoted in the previous chapter (Table 15.1). These intakes were all obtained by test-weighing over at least two days. Where figures are given separately for the two sexes, girls consumed about 10 per cent less than boys. It is not possible to say that the results are representative, since in these countries mothers who agree to breast-feed exclusively for six months or more are probably exceptionally dedicated. Some authors have recorded even greater amounts, of more than a litre a day, e.g. Tarjan *et al.* in Hungary (WHO, 1985*a*) and Rattigan *et al.* (1981) in Australia. There seems no doubt, from the intakes

Table 16.1 Some estimates of intakes by exclusively breast-fed children in developed countries

Age, months		1	2	3	4	5	6
Sweden[a]	boys	645	750	800	820	–	820
	girls	580	700	730	750	–	740
UK[b]	boys	–	790	820	830	790	920
	girls	–	680	740	775	815	840
USA[c]		670	755	780	810	805	895
USA[d]		750	725	720	740	–	–

References: [a] Wallgren (1945); [b] Whitehead and Paul (1981); [c] Dewey and Lönnerdal (1986); [d] Butte *et al.* (1984*a*)
All intakes measured by test weighing.
There is some uncertainty about the ages, since some authors report data at 1 month, etc.; others at 1–2 months, etc.
Further data are listed by Butte and Garza (1985).

of twins and the old accounts of wet-nursing, that healthy well-fed and well-motivated women are physiologically capable of producing very large amounts of milk for at least a year, but here we are concerned with the usual rather than the exceptional.

It has generally been supposed that in the Third World undernutrition of mothers would reduce their capacity for lactation. Jelliffe and Jelliffe (1978) reviewed the older data. Representative outputs from their paper would be:

1 – 6 months: 600 ml milk
6 – 12 months: 490 ml milk
12 – 24 months: 415 ml milk

The Jelliffes warn that the numbers can only be regarded as approximate because of differences in the methods of collection. There were indeed very wide variations between the ten or more different studies that they summarized. Ashworh and Feachem (1985) believed that poor maternal nutrition may lead to a deterioration in milk output and stated: 'it is generally agreed that breast milk output is usually somewhat less in poorly nourished communities.' However, Fig. 16.1 perhaps suggests a more encouraging picture. At

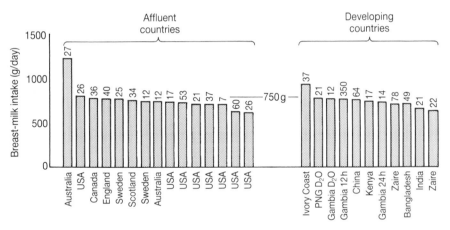

Fig. 16.1 Average breast milk intake at two to three months from 16 studies in affluent and 11 in developing countries. A. M. Prentice, personal communication.

the critical age of three months there is little difference in the intakes from mothers in affluent and developing countries. The results of some recent studies, illustrated in Table 16.2, show that in three out of the five countries volumes of 700 ml or more were maintained well into the second six months of life and in some cases longer, in spite of the fact that in most cases the babies were given some supplementary food, often from a very early age. We cannot unfortunately tell whether the exceptionally high intakes reported from Papua-New Guinea are an artefact of the labelled water method; the results from the other three countries, where mothers persisted with breast feeding into the second six months, were obtained by test-weighing and may well be too low (Borschel *et al.*, 1986). It seems reasonable to conclude that

Table 16.2   Some recent estimates of breast-milk intakes in Third World countries

Age (months)	Intake, g (to nearest 10 g)				
	Papua[†a] New Guinea	The Gambia[b]	Indonesia[c]	Bangladesh[d]	Myanmar[e]
0–2	610	680	840	570	450
2–4	770	680	750	660	580
4–6	860	640	730	730	700
6–9	900	610	700	730	–
9–12	850	590	670*	–	–

† By doubly labelled water method; all others by test weighing.
* Some supplements added
References: [a] Orr-Ewing *et al.* (1986); [b] Prentice *et al.* (1986); [c] van Steenbergen *et al.* (1991); [d] Brown *et al.* (1986); Khin-Maung-Naing and Tin-Tin-Oo (1991).

a clear difference between breast-milk intakes in Western and Third World countries has not been established.

All these intakes which have been quoted are averages; the variability has always been found to be very large. Figure 16.2 is a good example. All authors are agreed that there is much greater variability between mothers than in the day-to-day outputs of a single mother (Black *et al.*, 1983; Neville *et al.*, 1984; Stuff *et al.*, 1986). Figure 16.3 shows an example of both sources of variation. Approximate values would be 20 per cent for the coefficient of variation between mothers and 10 per cent for that within mothers.

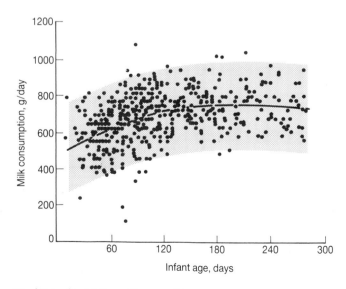

Fig. 16.2   Variability of breast milk consumption of infants in Bangladesh. Reproduced by permission from Brown *et al.* (1986).

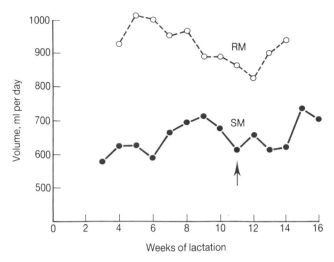

Fig. 16.3 Within- and between-infant variation in weekly milk intake of two infants RM and SM. Each point is the mean of seven 24-hour measurements. The arrow represents the introduction of supplementary foods. Drawn from data of Wheeler (1973).

Energy and protein content of breast milk

Sampling

To determine an infant's daily intake of energy and nutrients it is necessary to have samples that are representative of the milk produced over 24 hours. This is particularly important in relation to energy, because of the variability of the fat content of human milk. There is a large literature on the subject of sampling (see, for example, Ferris and Jensen, 1984; Garza and Butte, 1986). There are three basic approaches: expression of all the milk from one breast for one or more feeds or throughout the 24 hours, the milk that is not used for analysis being fed back to the baby by bottle; collection of small aliquots at specified times during a feed; or continuous sampling from a nipple shield (Williams *et al.*, 1985). The first approach should give representative results, but involves a good deal of interference with the mother and baby.

Energy content

As mentioned in the previous chapter, if the energy content of milk is measured by bomb calorimetry, it has to be converted to metabolizable energy to allow for incomplete absorption of fat and incomplete oxidation of protein, the factor generally used being 0.92 (Southgate and Barrett, 1966). In many papers it is not clearly stated exactly what was done. Alternatively, the protein, carbohydrate and fat content can be measured and the usual

Atwater factors applied (4, 4 and 9 kcal/g) (Garza and Butte, 1985). A simple method—the creamatocrit—has been introduced for estimating the fat content in very small samples by centrifuging in capillaries and measuring the length of the fat layer (Lucas *et al.*, 1978).

More than 50 per cent of the energy of breast milk is derived from fat, and the fat content is particularly variable, both over the course of a day (Garza and Butte, 1986; Jackson *et al.*, 1988) and, as is well known, over the course of a feed (Hytten, 1954). The hind-milk may contain almost twice as much fat as fore-milk. A recent study showed the fat content increasing from 30 to 50 g/l in the course of feeds lasting seven minutes (Woodward *et al.*, 1989). This is why the question of sampling is so important and so difficult. By contrast, the concentrations of lactose and of protein are more constant (Butte *et al.*, 1988*a*).

When comparable methods of sampling are used, it appears that the greater part of the variation in energy content, as in volume, results from differences between mothers rather than from day-to-day variation in the milk from the same mother (Prentice *et al.*, 1981*a*; Butte *et al.*, 1988*a*).

In trying to derive average values we therefore have to bear in mind that the overall coefficient of variation is at least 20 per cent. A rounded-off value commonly used for the energy content of human milk in affluent countries is 670–700 kcal/l. The figure for Sweden in Table 16.3, from the WHO Collaborative Study in Breast-feeding (WHO, 1985*a*), is unusually high. The table shows that the energy content was lower in the milks from developing countries. However, it is difficult to have much confidence in comparisons between different countries because of probable differences in methods of sampling and analysis. Calculation from the values tabulated by Jelliffe and Jelliffe (1978) gives a mean of 730 kcal/l for industrialized countries and 630 kcal/l for the 13 Third World countries that they list. The results obtained by Brown *et al.* (1986) in Bangladesh are in this range, the energy content decreasing from 640 kcal/l in the first month to 570 at nine months. Thus it has been

Table 16.3 Mean energy values in different countries of breast milk at 3 and 6 months after delivery

	Energy, kcal/l	
	3 months	6 months
Hungary	600	650
Sweden	790	810
Guatemala		
well-to-do	560	–
urban poor	600	590
rural	560	570
Philippines		
well-to-do	610	560
urban poor	640	580
rural	610	600
Zaïre		
urban poor	570	610
rural	630	610

Values rounded to nearest 10 kcal.
The coefficients of variation of the different series averaged 18 per cent (range 10–27).
Data from WHO (1985)

generally supposed that the energy content of breast milk is lower in malnourished than in well-nourished mothers, but this is not borne out by the findings in Table 16.3, where within each country there is no significant difference between the rich and poor groups. A comparison in Brazil (Marín *et al.*, 1984) showed that the mean energy content of milk from well-nourished mothers was 695 kcal/l while that from mothers considered to be malnourished was 770 kcal/l.

Protein content

It has been common practice to calculate the protein content of human milk as total nitrogen x 6.25, as in the FAO/WHO/UNU report (WHO, 1985*b*). This gives what in the previous chapter was called the crude protein content. Technically, such a calculation is incorrect, because some 30 per cent of the total N in human milk is non-protein N. Thus if the crude protein content by the conventional calculation is 11–12 g/l, the true content is 8–9 g/l. About 50 per cent of the non-protein N is urea. The remainder consists mainly of free amino acids, amino sugars and their derivatives. The function of these compounds in the child's development is not well understood. The amino sugars are components of gangliosides of the brain and perhaps the immature infant is limited in his capacity to synthesize them. It would surely be going too far to dismiss all the non-protein nitrogen of human milk as 'unavailable' (see Chapter 7).

The N content of human milk is much less variable than the fat content. Nevertheless, there appear to be consistent differences between subjects that are not negligible, for example from 1.4 to 1.8 g/l in the five subjects reported by Butte *et al.* (1988*a*). In Wheeler's longitudinal study (Fig. 16.3) the total N of milk between four and 24 weeks ranged from 2.2 to 1.4 g/l for one infant and from 2.3 to 1.6 g/l in the other. The FAO/WHO/UNU report (WHO, 1985*b*) suggests an average value for mature milk, based on a number of compilations, of 1.85 g N/l, giving a crude protein content (N x 6.25) of 11.5 g/l. Lönnerdal (1986) concluded that 'malnourished' mothers do not have lower protein concentrations in their milk.

Minerals and trace elements

Intakes of minerals and trace elements of breast-fed children are touched on in Chapters 4 and 9. The papers of Butte *et al.* (1987) and Karra *et al.* (1988) provide useful information on the amounts of these elements in human milk.

Factors affecting the volume and composition of breast milk

Maternal nutritional status

Since pregnancy, and even more lactation, impose increased requirements for energy and protein, one might expect that if a mother starts her reproductive career in a marginal state of nutrition, her condition would deteriorate with each successive pregnancy. Merchant and Martorell (1988) concluded tentatively that maternal nutritional depletion does occur as a result of a demanding reproductive history. On the other hand both Briend (1985) in Senegal and Prentice *et al.* (1981*b*) in The Gambia observed no difference in the body weights of mothers with one or many children.

Even if a mother in the Third World can maintain a perhaps precarious steady state, the frequency of low birth weight (Chapter 18) suggests that she cannot fully meet the demands made on her. If this applies to the outcome of pregnancy it should surely apply also to the greater demands of lactation. In the longitudinal study of Brown *et al.* (1986) in Bangladesh, milk production averaged about 700 g/day from four to ten months; considering the low body weight of the mothers (average BMI* = 18), this seems a very satisfactory performance. However, fat and energy concentrations in milk were significantly related to maternal fat stores, as measured by skinfold thickness. Some mothers gained body weight and fat during the course of lactation; these gains were associated with increases in the amount and energy concentration of their milk. The authors concluded that 'despite their remarkably good lactational capacity, the mothers' milk production was limited to some extent by their nutritional status and may therefore be further increased with nutritional improvement'.

There were seasonal changes in milk output in Bangladesh, which have also been documented in The Gambia (Prentice *et al.*, 1986). During the wet season, when an increase in work load coincided with a decrease in food intake, the body weight of the mothers fell by 10 per cent, and so did the average milk volume. This fall particularly affected children over six months of age. The similarity of the findings in Bangladesh and The Gambia is interesting, since the Gambian women started at a better level of nutrition (mean BMI = 20.6).

Parity

Another factor that has been examined is maternal parity. In The Gambia parity had no effect on the volume of breast milk below a parity of 9 (Prentice, 1985*a*). However, many authors have found that the milk of primiparae has a higher fat concentration than that of multiparae. In The Gambia the fat content of milk from mothers of parity 3 was only 82 per cent of that of milk from primiparae (Prentice, 1985*b*).

Supplementary feeding of the mother

If it is true that in the Third World a mother's milk production may be limited by her food intake, then the slogan 'feed the nursing mother, thereby the infant' would make sense. A number of trials have been set up to test this hypothesis, going back to the early work of Gopalan (1958) over 30 years ago. In most cases there has been no effect on milk production, and when there was an effect it was small in relation to the extra food given. In Indonesia a supplement of 400 kcal and 6–7 g protein had no effect on milk intake, even though the mothers had very low pre-pregnancy weights (BMI 18.5)

* BMI = body mass index: $Wt(kg)/Ht^2(m^2)$.

(Van Steenbergen *et al.*, 1989). In The Gambia an even larger supplement produced no change in milk output (Prentice *et al.*, 1983). These mothers were adequately nourished (BMI 20.6). In a study in Myanmar a daily supplement of 900 kcal and 40 g protein led to an increase in milk intake of about 100 g/day (Khin-Maung-Naing and Tin-Tin-Oo, 1987). Although this increase would not be negligible in terms of the infants' requirements, the cost of such a programme would be prohibitive. In many of the trials there is no guarantee that the mother does herself eat all the extra food. Ashworth and Feachem (1986) have critically reviewed these interventions and conclude: 'attempts to improve lactation by maternal supplementation have not achieved any sizeable increase in milk output, though some improvement in milk quality has been observed'.

Experimentally, short-term reduction in the energy intake of well-nourished mothers, by 30 per cent, had no effect on milk volume (Strode *et al.*, 1986). In the USA Butte *et al.* (1984*b*) concluded that successful lactation was compatible with gradual weight reduction and attainable with energy intakes less than current recommendations.

Infant demand

Hippocrates observed 'Children who are naturally well-nourished do not suck milk in proportion to their fleshiness' and 'Children with voracious appetites and who suck much milk do not put on flesh in proportion' (Jones, 1923). We would probably describe these children less vividly, as efficient and inefficient utilizers of food. It may be that the wide variations in milk intake that were discussed earlier result not so much from differences in women's physiological capacity for lactation but from differences in infant demand.

Ounsted and Sleigh (1975) observed that small-for-dates babies consumed much more milk per kg body weight than large-for-dates babies and gained weight much faster. This represented a move towards the mean, which was more marked in breast-fed than in bottle-fed babies. They concluded that there is a powerful self-regulatory control of the infant's intake. Hall (1975) suggested that within a feed the baby regulates its intake in response to the increasing fat content of the milk.

Prentice *et al.* (1986) made a detailed statistical analysis of maternal and infant factors affecting milk intake in The Gambia. In comparisons between children the factors that came through most strongly were the baby's weight, its rate of weight gain, and the feeding frequency. Prentice inclines to the view that a baby's appetite and activity in suckling are determined by its requirements and that the correlation between milk intake and weight velocity is caused 'by fast-growing babies demanding and receiving more milk rather than by the babies of inherently good lactators growing faster'. These ideas have an important bearing on the question of requirements (Chapter 15); given the observed range of intakes, the strength of the correlation between intake and requirement is a crucial factor in arriving at estimates that can be applied to groups, such as the safe level of protein intake.

There is some experimental evidence to support the concept that the driving force is the infant's demand. Dewey and Lönnerdal (1986) produced an increase in milk output by expression of the breasts. The babies took more milk for a time but quickly returned to their basal level of intake.

In animals, as in humans, the frequency of milk removal is an important determinant of the volume of milk secreted. One mechanism is that sucking stimulates the release of hormones that stimulate milk production. Another mechanism recently proposed is that of local feedback control. Human milk has been found to contain a factor that inhibits the synthesis of milk components in the mammary gland, specifically casein and lactose (Prentice *et al.*, 1989*a*). An increased frequency of breast feeding leads to a more effective removal of this locally active inhibitor.

Protective factors in breast milk

Breast milk contains both soluble immunoglobulins and a variety of immunologically active cells (for reviews see Mata, 1982, and Hayward, 1983). Quantitatively, the most important of the immunoglobulins are lactoferrin and IgA, but a variety of other components such as lysozyme, complement and lactoperoxidase may be functionally important although present in much smaller amounts. The concentrations in colostrum are very high, but rapidly fall in the first weeks after birth.

At one to two months human milk contains about 1 g/l of secretory IgA (Table 16.4) and 2 g/l of lactoferrin, so that if the true protein content of human milk is 9 g/l, these two immunoglobulins account for one-third of it, or even more, according to McClelland *et al.* (1978). Prentice *et al.* (1987) found that, at six weeks, only 1 per cent of the lactoferrin ingested and 17 per cent of the IgA appeared in the faeces, so these components of milk protein must be to a very large extent nutritionally available. As lactation proceeds the concentrations of both lactoferrin and sIgA tend to decline, although Mata (1982) reports very high concentrations of sIgA in the milk of Guatemalan women (about 2 g/l) after one year of lactation.

Table 16.4 Secretory IgA content of human milk at one to two months of lactation

Country	sIgA, g/l
Sweden[a]	0.83
UK[b]	0.95
USA[c]	0.85
Ethiopia[a]	
well-to-do	0.61
poor	0.43
Guatemala[a]	
well-to-do	0.84
poor	1.02
The Gambia[b]	0.80

References: [a] Cruz *et al.* (1982); [b] Prentice *et al.* (1989*b*); [c] Butte *et al.* (1984*c*)

The table does not give any consistent indication that sIgA concentrations are lower in poor than in better-off women. One would expect them to be higher, since the mothers are likely to be more exposed to infection. It is unlikely that the capacity to synthesize 1 g/day of sIgA protein would be compromised by poor nutritional status of the mother, since this amount is a very small fraction of whole-body protein synthesis.

Secretory IgA must have an important protective function, particularly in the period immediately after birth, before the infant's own immunological defences are properly established. It contains a wide range of antibodies, with activities against rotavirus and bacterial enterotoxins, antibodies that block attachment of bacteria to the intestinal mucosa and antibodies to food proteins (Welsh and May, 1979; Mata, 1986). Ibrahim (1985) has suggested that human milk may be useful in the treatment of protracted diarrhoea, presumably through local effects in the gut. More generally, the ability of the mother to secrete antibodies directed against specific antigens in her environment imparts to human milk an environmental specificity with significant protective potential (Garza and Hopkinson, 1988). Prentice *et al.* (1987, 1989*b*) have considered the question of how the protective activity of sIgA could be maintained in spite of the fact that the greater part of it is digested and destroyed in the gastrointestinal tract. They found a correlation between the frequency of stools and the amount of immune protein excreted and suggested that perhaps a substantial part of the digestion of sIgA, which is relatively resistant to proteolytic activity, occurs in the large intestine. Another possibility is that fragments of sIgA produced in the course of digestion may retain antimicrobial activity.

The role of lactoferrin, which is present in even larger amounts in human milk, is still rather obscure. *In vitro* lactoferrin has been shown to inhibit the growth of a number of bacteria, but there is no firm evidence that it exerts this effect *in vivo*. Structurally, lactoferrin resembles transferrin, but it binds iron more tightly (Brock, 1980). It does not seem to have any action in preventing the absorption of iron, and Brock suggests that it may even facilitate iron excretion, particularly in the immediate post-natal period when the infant's iron stores are high. By removing free iron and thus preventing bacterial proliferation and free radical generation (Chapter 10) lactoferrin could in fact have a protective effect. It is interesting that the two species which have a high concentration of lactoferrin in their milk, man and the guinea-pig, are both slow-growing and therefore do not need a large supply of iron to support haemopoiesis during growth.

Breast milk also contains relatively large numbers of cells, mainly macrophages and lymphocytes. The latter produce lymphokynes and other growth factors which stimulate proliferation and differentiation in lymphoid tissue and its capacity to react to antigens (Stephens, 1986). The cells in breast milk may therefore play an important role in the infant's transition from passive to active immunity.

The list of protective factors does not end with cells and immunoglobulins. Thirty years ago Gyorgy isolated a small molecular weight factor from human milk that stimulated the growth of *Lactobacillus bifidus*, which is present in large numbers in the stools of breast-fed infants but not in those fed cow's milk (Gyorgy, 1958). He speculated that this micro-organism, which generates acid, might play an important protective role. The bifidus factor, as Gyorgy called it, which is present in human milk in a concentration 40 times greater than in cow's milk, is an amino sugar and contains N-acetyl neuraminic acid (Gyorgy, 1971), a substance that has a very wide biological role.

Protective effect of breast feeding— the epidemiological evidence

There is an enormous literature on this subject, which has been well summarized up to 1984 by Jason *et al.* (1984). They tabulate in some detail the results of 30 studies made in the Third World, with comments on study design. Various outcomes are considered in this review, not only death but hospitalization and episodes of infectious disease, mainly diarrhoea. When exclusive bottle feeding is compared with exclusive breast feeding the risk ratio ranged in different studies from 1.7 to 50. In these comparisons there are many confounding variables which have not always been taken into account. However, the conclusions of Jason *et al.*, though cautious, are clear: 'The weight of the evidence from less-developed countries strongly supports an inverse association between breast-feeding and overall mortality, between breast-feeding and diarrhoea-related morbidity and mortality, and between breast-feeding and morbidity and mortality in the high-risk newborn.' The question of the relation of nutritional state to morbidity and mortality is discussed in Chapters 17 and 18.

One question that is not yet clear is the relative importance of contamination of food and feeding utensils compared with other sources of exposure. A study of Habicht *et al.* (1988) in Malaysia illustrates the importance of the total environment (Table 16.5). In breast-fed children the lack of sanitary

Table 16.5   Interaction of feeding pattern and sanitation on infant mortality (7 days–1 year)

	Adjusted mortality rate	
	Toilet and piped water	
	Present	Not present
Breast-fed	0.019	0.037
Not breast-fed	0.047	0.190

From Habicht *et al.* (1988)

facilities doubled the mortality, whereas in those not breast-fed it was increased four-fold. In such a case the exact route of infection is not just an academic question; if it were known it might be possible to mitigate the effect of unsanitary conditions. In a further analysis of the Malaysian data Habicht *et al.* (1986) showed that the younger the infant and the longer the exclusive breast feeding, the greater the benefit in terms of deaths averted. The difference in morbidity and mortality between breast- and bottle-fed babies is greatly reduced when environmental conditions are not so bad. It could be argued that if children are getting enough food to maintain a satisfactory nutritional status, they will be able to resist the effects of infection (Chapter 17). Thus in Jamaica bottle-fed children were ingesting milk that was highly contaminated with faecal bacteria, but it had no effect on their growth (Hibbert and Golden, 1981).

However, in more severe conditions breast is clearly better than bottle. Two questions then follow: for how long is exclusive breast feeding adequate before supplements need to be introduced? and what are the risks of supplementation?

Adequacy of exclusive breast feeding

It is the official policy of WHO and UNICEF that exclusive breast feeding should be adequate to fulfil a baby's needs for four to six months. The fact that weight gain in Third World countries begins to fall off as early as two to three months (Waterlow *et al.*, 1980) and in rich countries at four to six months (Whitehead and Paul, 1981; Salmenperä *et al.*, 1985) has been taken to indicate that the reference is inappropriate. Seward and Serdula (1984) pointed out, very reasonably, that the growth faltering occurring between three and six months, even if it is the beginning of a downward trend, is dwarfed by the severe faltering that occurs after six months. Be that as it may, breast feeding alone cannot be adequate for ever, and the question 'for how long is it adequate?' remains a valid one.

In theory it should be possible to answer the question from our knowledge of the infant's requirements for energy and protein, as we attempted to do some years ago (Waterlow and Thomson, 1979). If the average energy requirement at four to six months is 90 kcal/kg/day and weight is to follow the reference median, the energy requirement at six months would be 700 kcal/day and about a litre of milk would be needed to fulfil it. Whitehead and Paul (1981), on the basis of their findings in children in Cambridge, reached an almost identical figure—980 ml for a child at six months to grow along the 50th centile. From the results already summarized (Table 16.1), this is probably beyond the capacity of most mothers. However, things are not so simple, because both the mother's milk production and the infant's requirement have a range of variation. If a baby had a high requirement of 100 kcal/kg/day and a mother who could only produce 600 ml of milk/day, the baby's energy supply would become inadequate by the second month. Conversely, a baby with a low requirement of 75 kcal/kg/day and a mother who could produce 900 ml of milk/day would be adequately fed on the breast alone for nearly seven months. We do not know whether these are realistic situations. The question whether demand and supply are related is clearly crucial. There is some evidence, discussed above, that they may be, but the strength of the correlation is unknown. Moreover, we do not know whether having a high or low requirement is a permanent characteristic or whether it is a transient state, a temporary position within a normal range of variation. In this situation the only solution seems to lie in observations in the field to see what actually happens to a cohort of exclusively breast-fed infants.

Several studies in developing countries have examined this question, e.g. Rowland (1986) in The Gambia, Hijazi *et al.* (1989) in Jordan and Zumrawi *et al.* (1987a) in the Sudan. No attempt was made to measure breast-milk output; the natural criterion of adequacy was growth. The principal objective of the work in The Gambia was to compare the growth of exclusively breast-fed and supplemented children (see below). The objective in Jordan and Khartoum was to try to identify the time when exclusively breast-fed children began to falter in weight gain, the idea being that weight gain would be a more sensitive criterion than attained weight.

A child was described as 'faltering' if its weight gain over four weeks was less than −2 SD of that expected from the reference data of Fomon (1974) and of Tanner *et al.* (1966). Probably most paediatricians would regard such a small gain as unsatisfactory. Figure 16.4 shows the cumulative incidence of faltering in the Jordan cohort. According to this definition, 15 – 20 per cent of children faltered by four months and nearly 50 per cent by six months. The Khartoum study showed a very similar picture.

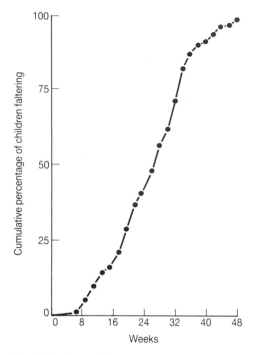

Fig. 16.4 Proportion of children faltering after different durations of exclusive breast feeding. Faltering is defined as weight gain below −2 SD of the reference for two consecutive two-week periods (see text). Data from Jordan study, reproduced by permission from Hijazi *et al.* (1989).

One difficulty in the analysis of the results was that in both cohorts mothers began to introduce supplements at varying times from about one month onwards, so that the number of exclusively breast-fed (EBF) children was steadily reduced. Another difficulty was that in both EBF and supplemented children many periods of faltering were triggered by or accompanied by an episode of respiratory infection or diarrhoea, so that it is not possible to conclude that faltering resulted simply from an inadequate intake of food from the breast. On the other hand, what is important in practice is the performance of exclusively breast-fed children under the conditions of real life. A further problem in interpreting these studies is that faltering did not have a lasting effect. Clearly there was catch-up, since at six months the mean weights of the cohorts in both Jordan and Khartoum were close to the WHO median.

It was therefore not possible with this design to give an unequivocal answer to what seemed at first to be a simple question. Those children who were maintained exclusively on the breast for six months grew well, but they were a minority, which may have been in some way biologically selected. The majority of children in both cohorts were supplemented before six months, and we cannot tell how they would have fared if they had not been given extra food.

Supplementary feeding

The other side of the question: for how long is exclusive breast feeding adequate? is: when should supplementary food be introduced?* Figure 16.5 illustrates what has been called the 'weanling's dilemma' (Rowland, 1986) or the 'suckling's dilemma' (Waterlow, 1981). The word 'wean' means 'to accustom to food other than milk' (OED). Rowland (1986) and Milla (1986) use 'weaning' to describe the whole period from the time when the child is first given some supplementary food until it is completely removed from the breast. Another terminology is to call it 'weaning on' when supplementary foods are first introduced and 'weaning off' when breast feeding ceases completely. It is the suckling who has to face the dilemma before weaning on starts; afterwards he has no choice.

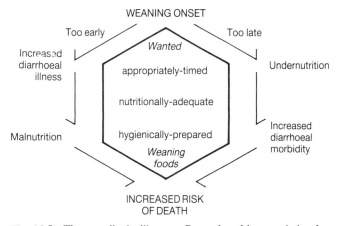

Fig. 16.5   The weanling's dilemma. Reproduced by permission from Rowland (1986).

Underwood and Hofvander (1982), in a well-balanced report prepared for WHO, have discussed in detail the pros and cons of early supplementation. The arguments against it are: the increased danger of infection; the possibility that decreased frequency of suckling will reduce the stimulus to milk production and hence lead to an ever-increasing demand for supplementary food; and the possibility that supplements will delay the maturation of the gut that is stimulated by breast milk and is important for the development of immune function and for preventing the entry of macromolecular allergens.

---

* In the older paediatric literature 'complementary' referred to food given at the end of a breast-feed, 'supplementary' to food given instead of a breast-feed, i.e. at a different time. With breast feeding on demand, many times in 24 hours, the distinction ceases to be useful, and the term 'supplement' is used here to indicate any addition to breast milk.

The only advantage of early supplementation is to prevent growth faltering, but it may be questioned whether mild or moderate faltering matters. Some paediatricians think not; the opinion of the Swedish Academy of Paediatrics, quoted by Underwood and Hofvander, was 'no added calories are better than dirty calories'. Personally, I am not so sure.

How important is the extra risk of infection? Some figures have already been given for the comparison between exclusive breast feeding (EBF) and exclusive bottle feeding. Here we are concerned with partial breast feeding (PBF). In the Malaysian study mentioned above, compared with infants who were not breast-fed, PBF reduced the infant mortality rate by 3.2 per 1000 born per month of breast feeding, and EBF reduced it by 6.8 per month (Habicht *et al.*, 1986). When it comes to morbidity, the advantage of EBF over PBF is less clear. Table 16.6 summarizes data from various Third World countries (Feachem and Koblinsky, 1984). Overall, the EBF children had an advantage, particularly before six months, but except in Ethiopia it was small. In a study in north-east Brazil, PBF children were ill with diarrhoea for 8 per cent of the time, compared with 1.4 per cent for EBF children. In the study of Zumrawi *et al.* (1987*b*) in Khartoum, in the cohort as a whole supplementation had no significant effect on the prevalence of infection.

Table 16.6   Relative risk of diarrhoea morbidity in partially breast-fed compared with exclusively breast-fed children of lower socio-economic groups in Third World countries

Country	Relative risk	
	Below 6 months	6–12 months
Colombia	2.37	2.37
Costa Rica, 0–2 months	1.37	–
3–5 months	3.31	–
Guatemala, 3–5 months	0.85	1.23
India, Punjab	1.33	1.36
Delhi	1.39	1.05
[a]Tamil Nadu	1.09	–
Ethiopia	6.19	0.34
Uganda	1.71	0.64
[a]Sudan	–	1.42

[a] Data from Feachem and Koblinsky (1984) except for Sudan (Zumrawi *et al.*, 1987*b*) and Tamil Nadu (A. Joseph, unpublished observations).

Underwood and Hofvander (1982) conclude that, in general, supplements 'should not be introduced to exclusively breast-fed infants before 4 months nor delayed beyond the age of 6 months. When growth falters, however, appropriate remedial steps should be taken regardless of age.'

In real life practice varies widely in different parts of the world (Table 16.7) and does not always conform to these recommendations. In many communities it is traditional for supplementary food to be given from an early age even from birth (e.g. Brown, 1978; King and Ashworth, 1987). Figure 16.6 illustrates the average pattern of feeding observed in two cohorts of rural children, in India and Kenya. In general urban mothers start supplements earlier than rural mothers. The reasons for the choice of different feeding

Table 16.7 Proportion of infants regularly given food in addition to breast milk at two ages

Country		2–3 months	6–7 months
Chile	urban	59	100
	rural	56	96
Guatemala	urban	52	87
	rural	12	62
Nigeria	urban	64	90
	rural	35	86
Zaïre	urban	32	83
	rural	35	72
Philippines	urban	23	82
	rural	29	77
India	urban	6	19
	rural	2	12

From Underwood and Hofvander (1982).

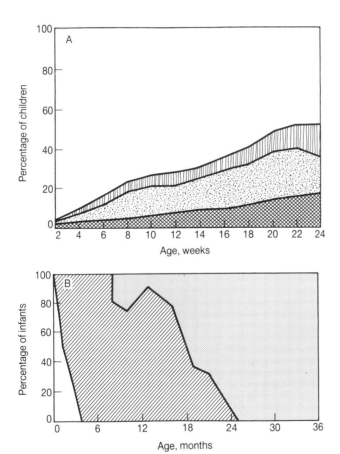

Fig. 16.6 Patterns of infant feeding. A. India, Tamil Nadu: ☐, exclusively breast-fed; ▦, supplements < 10 per cent of energy intake; ▒, supplements 10–25 per cent; ▨, supplements > 25 per cent. Data from A. Joseph, unpublished. B. Kenya, Machakos district: ☐, exclusively breast-fed; ▨, breast + supplements; ▒, fully weaned. From Van Steenbergen *et al.* (1978).

patterns in Third World countries have been reviewed in detail by Forman (1984).

In many cultures there is a wide range of variation in the age at which mothers start to give supplementary food. In surveys in Mexico, Kenya and Malaysia the majority of mothers, rural as well as urban, gave as their reason for starting supplements that the baby was hungry and their milk supply in-adequate (Dimond and Ashworth, 1987). In The Gambia babies who were supplemented before three months of age were underweight compared with those who were not supplemented, but after three months the difference disappeared (Rowland, 1986). In the Khartoum study already referred to (Zumrawi *et al.*, 1987*a*), there was no objective evidence that mothers began to give supplements because the child was not gaining weight satisfactorily.

Weight gain is the natural criterion of the benefits and drawbacks of early supplementation. Figure 16.7, from rural India, shows that PBF children did rather worse than those who were exclusively breast-fed. In rural Indian communities early supplementation is the exception (Table 16.7), so that the PBF children may represent a special sub-group. In another study in India PBF children were slightly heavier than EBF, in spite of a higher prevalence of infections (Ramachandran, 1989). In the Gambian and Khartoum studies there was no significant difference in attained weight at six months between EBF and PBF children (Zumrawi *et al.*, 1987*a*).

It is dangerous to generalize from a few examples, but there is surely some discrepancy between theory and practice. Kimati (1986), in a paper with the provocative title 'Who is ignorant? Rural women who feed their well-nourished children, or the nutrition experts? The Tanzania story', has attacked the attempt to impose Western ideas on a culture that is assumed to be ignorant. However, he notes that a substantial number of children in

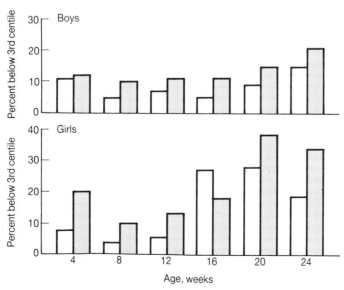

Fig. 16.7 Percentage of children in a sample from rural Tamil Nadu below the third NCHS centile for weight at different ages. ☐, exclusively breast-fed; ▨, supplemented. Data from A. Joseph, unpublished.

Tanzania do die of PEM, so that there is room for improvement. Dimond and Ashworth (1987) point out that interventions aimed at prolonging exclusive breast feeding have often not been successful. In Zaïre, for example, the main constraint was the widespread practice of mothers resuming farm-work within six weeks of delivery. They suggest that it may be more sensible to concentrate on improving the nutritional and hygienic quality of the supplements. Methods for achieving this have been discussed by Rowland (1986).

The problem takes on an extra dimension in urban communities where many women have to go to work and cannot take their babies with them. Here, perhaps, the emphasis should be on providing facilities that enable the mothers to continue some breast feeding, even if supplementary feeds have to be given in between.

Duration of partial breast feeding

When infants pass six months of age the nature of the problem changes. The question is no longer whether they should be supplemented, but rather the length of time for which partial breast feeding should be continued.

In many communities it is traditional for the mother to go on giving the breast throughout the second year and even for three years. This practice is probably of great benefit to the child as a source of extra nutrients and of extra protection. The foods that are given to a child in the second year are very often porridges or paps made from plantains, cassava, yams, cornmeal, etc., with a low energy density and a low content of protein and micronutrients. Even small quantities of breast milk could be quite important. In fact, some of the studies already cited indicate that some women continue to produce substantial amounts of breast milk, 500 ml or more per day, between 18 and 24 months.

Briend and Bari (1989) in Bangladesh have shown that continuation of breast feeding had an important effect on mortality between 12 and 36 months. For children aged 12–17 months the relative risk of death was six times as great in those who were fully weaned as in those who were still partially breast-fed, falling to three times between 30 and 36 months. The protection provided by partial breast feeding was particularly important in children who were already undernourished (Fig. 16.8).

There are two other advantages of continued breast feeding. The incidence of diarrhoeal disease is greatest in the last part of the first year and in the second year. These children usually have anorexia (Chapter 17). Dickin *et al.* (1990) observed that the intake of breast milk was maintained even when other foods were refused, so that the decrease in energy intake during diarrhoea was much less in children who were still receiving breast milk.

The other advantage is that sucking stimulates the production of the hormone prolactin, which suppresses ovulation. The endocrine mechanism has been described by Glasier and McNeilly (1990). The risk of ovulation is influenced by the frequency of breast feeds, their duration and the extent of supplementary feeding (Gray *et al.*, 1990). The continuation of partial breast feeding helps to prolong lactational amenorrhoea beyond six months postpartum, and to increase the birth interval (Fig. 16.9). (Delvoye *et al.*, 1976; Delgado *et al.*, 1978; Lunn *et al.*, 1980; Shatrugna *et al.*, 1982; Anderson *et*

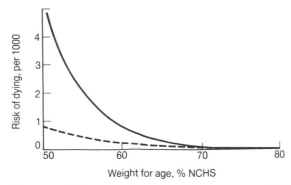

Fig. 16.8 Risk of dying in relation to weight for age (% NCHS) in breast-fed (− − − −) and non-breast-fed (———) children between 12 and 36 months old in Matlab, Bangladesh.
Reproduced by permission from Briend and Bari (1989).

al., 1984). This is extremely important for the prevention of PEM (see Chapter 20). It has been proposed that 'lactational amenorrhoea should be regarded as an appropriate method of fertility control for many women'. This strategy should be incorporated into family planning programmes (Consensus Statement, 1988).

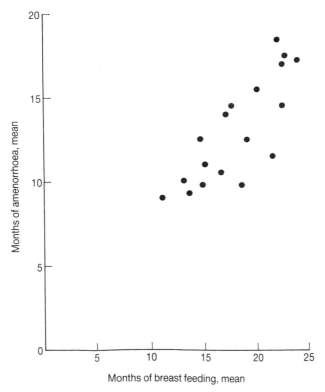

Fig. 16.9 Relation between duration of breast feeding and duration of amenorrhoea in various populations. Reproduced by permission from McCann *et al.* (1981).

Diet at and after weaning

The natural progression for a child after it ceases to be exclusively breast-fed is first to receive some supplementary foods; then, when it is fully weaned from the breast, some kind of food specially prepared to be suitable for a young child; and finally to share in the family meals (Fig. 16.6). It is with the second stage that we are concerned in this section; the 'specially prepared food' is referred to as 'weaning food'. The subject has been reviewed by Cameron and Hofvander (1983) and more recently by Walker (1990).

This intermediate stage, particularly if it starts rather early, e.g. in the second year, presents particular difficulties for the mother and dangers for the child. For the mother the preparation of special food in addition to the family diet requires time and fuel for cooking. If it is prepared in a batch to last for a day, there is danger of bacterial contamination (Rowland *et al.*, 1978; Black *et al.*, 1981, 1989). For women in towns who have to work away from home, commercial weaning foods are expensive. Nevertheless, in three countries in an intermediate stage of development, Kenya, Mexico and Malaysia, a high proportion of mothers, rural as well as urban, were giving 'branded', i.e. commercially produced cereals from three months onwards (Dimond and Ashworth, 1987).

Village-scale preparation represents a half-way house between production in the home and on the industrial scale. The Royal Tropical Institute, Amsterdam, has issued guidelines, quoted by Walker (1990) on 'an appropriate intermediate technology which is adapted to local conditions, for the small-scale batch manufacture of locally acceptable weaning foods'. A project that is being pursued experimentally in some parts of the world is the production at the village level of a protein concentrate from green leaves (Pirie, 1978). The protein in the juice pressed out of the leaves is precipitated by heat and brings down with it β-carotene and iron, so that the product should be nutritionally very useful. It remains to be seen whether this and other village-level preparations are economically viable.

From the point of view of the child, some weaning diets have an adequate P/E ratio (Chapter 15, Table 15.14), but others, based on staples with a low protein content, such as cassava and plantain, or containing protein of low biological value, such as maize, are marginal or inadequate. Nevertheless, the first objective is to secure an adequate energy intake, so that what protein there is can be fully utilized.

The nature of the gruels or paps that are the main basis of the foods fed at weaning makes it difficult for the child to fulfil his energy requirement, even with a good appetite. Cereal grains, such as wheat, barley, maize, sorghum and rice contain starch granules, which swell irreversibly on cooking, binding water. This leads to a 'thick' consistency or high viscosity (Mellander and Svanberg, 1984). The viscosity rises steeply with increasing concentration of cereal. Different cereals and even different varieties of the same cereal differ in their consistency (viscosity) at a given concentration. To achieve a consistency that is acceptable, water has to be added to dilute the paste, resulting in a low energy density. The problem is particularly serious when children are ill, because they prefer more liquid foods. Because the child's energy requirement is high in relation to the size of his stomach, it becomes difficult for him to eat enough unless food is given frequently.

Rutishauser and Frood (1973) found that young children in Uganda could eat enough of the traditional weaning food in which the staple was plantain to satisfy their energy requirement if they were fed five times a day, but such frequent feeding is not always possible. Rutishauser (1974) concluded that energy density was the decisive factor in limiting energy intake.

One way of improving the cereal paps is by the addition of fat, preferably as a vegetable oil. This not only increases the energy density but also decreases the viscosity (Hellstrom *et al.*, 1981). In northern Uganda a groundnut and sesame paste is used in the traditional weaning diet. The sesame contains an antioxidant which prevents the oil in the food becoming rancid.

Another approach traditionally used in some communities is to malt the cereal before it is used (Brandtzaeg *et al.*, 1981). The grain is soaked in water for one or more days until it begins to sprout and is then dried, pounded and cooked. The enzyme α-amylase is synthesized during germination and by splitting the starch reduces the water-binding.

The effects of germination have been studied with gruels based on wheat (Gopaldas *et al.*, 1988), barley (Hansen *et al.*, 1989), maize (Hellstrom *et al.*, 1981), rice (Gopaldas *et al.*, 1986) and sorghum (Mellander and Svanberg, 1984). Table 16.8 shows the remarkable effect of the addition of even a small amount of germinated meal in increasing energy density and decreasing the volume and number of feeds needed to fulfil the energy requirement. The concentrations of cereal have been adjusted to maintain an acceptable viscosity.

Table 16.8 Concentrations of barley needed to satisfy 60 per cent of the daily energy requirement of a one-year old child

	Concentration[a] (% dry matter)	Energy density (kcal/g)	Volume[b] needed (ml)	Number of daily meals[c]
Normal barley, refined	6	0.20	2770	11
High lysine barley, ungerminated				
wholemeal	16	0.65	1000	4
refined	10	0.35	1730	7
High lysine barley, ungerminated + 1% germinated				
wholemeal	23	0.90	720	3
refined	24	0.90	700	3

[a] Maximum concentration for acceptable viscosity: 400 BU.
[b] Volume needed to provide 60 per cent of daily energy requirement.
[c] Number of meals of 250 ml each to provide indicated volume.
From Hansen *et al.* (1989)

Other traditional processes that are used in the preparation of weaning foods in different parts of the world are fermentation and souring (Rowland, 1986), but their effect on energy density seems to have been little investigated. Recent studies in Ghana (Mensah *et al.*, 1990) have shown that fermentation of porridge used for the preparation of weaning food caused a highly significant reduction in the growth of gram-negative bacilli during storage (Fig. 16.10). A preliminary study has shown that yogurt, prepared by fermenting milk with a culture of *Streptococcus haemophilus* and *Lactobacillus bulgaricus* had a beneficial effect, compared with unfermented milk, in the treatment of persistent diarrhoea (Boudraa *et al.*, 1990).

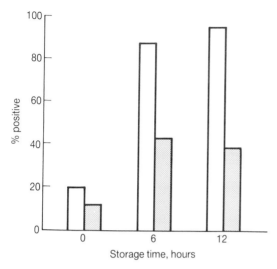

Fig. 16.10   Effect of fermentation of porridge on growth of gram negative bacilli during storage.▨, fermented;☐, unfermented. Reproduced by permission from Mensah *et al.* (1990).

We need to know more about the extent to which these various processes are traditionally used in different parts of the world, and whether, as Church and Doughty (1976) suggested, they have any effect on the incidence of PEM. Sserunjogi and Tomkins (1990) have described how different kinds of staples (sorghum, millet, cassava, plantains) are processed at the village level in Uganda, and they have tried to find out why different processes are accepted and used by some groups but not by others.

It seems, then, that simple technologies for increasing energy density are available; the problem is how to get them accepted and more widely used. The extra time and work that women have to put in may well be the limiting factor.

References

Anderson, J. E., Marks, J. S., Park K-T. (1984). Breast-feeding, birth interval and infant death. *Pediatrics* **74**: Suppl. 695–701.
Ashworth, A., Feachem, R. G. (1985). Interventions for the control of diarrhoeal diseases among young children: improving lactation. Document CDD/85.2. World Health Organization, Geneva.
Black, A. E., Cole, T. J. *et al.* (1983). Daily variation in food intake of infants from 2 to 18 months. *Human Nutrition:Applied Nutrition* **37A**: 448–458.
Black, R. E., Brown, K. H. *et al.* (1981). Contamination of weaning foods and

transmission of enterotoxigenic Escherichia coli diarrhea in children in rural Bangladesh. *Transactions of the Royal Society of Tropical Medicine and Hygiene* **76**: 259–264.

Black, R. E., de Romana, G. L. *et al.* (1989). Incidence and etiology of infantile diarrhea and major routes of transmission in Huascar, Peru. *American Journal of Epidemiology* **129**: 785–799.

Borschel, M. W., Kirksey, A., Hannemans, R. E. (1986). Evaluation of test-weighing for the assessment of milk volume intake of formula-fed infants and its application to breast-fed infants. *American Journal of Clinical Nutrition* **43**: 367–373.

Boudraa, G., Touhami, M. *et al.* (1990). Effect of feeding yogurt versus milk in children with persistent diarrhoea. *Journal of Pediatric Gastroenterology and Nutrition* **11**: 509–512.

Brandtzaeg, B., Malleshi, N. G. *et al.* (1981). Dietary bulk as a limiting factor for nutrient intake, with special reference to the feeding of pre-school children. III. Studies of malted flour from ragi, sorghum and green gram. *Journal of Tropical Pediatrics* **27**: 184–189.

Briend, A. (1985). Normal fetal growth regulation: nutritional aspects. In Gracey, M., Falkner, F. (eds) *Nutritional needs and assessment of normal growth*. Nestlé Nutrition Workshop No. 7. Nestlé Nutrition, Vevey/Raven Press, New York, pp. 1–21.

Briend, A., Bari, A. (1989). Breastfeeding improves survival, but not nutritional status, of 12–35 months old children in rural Bangladesh. *European Journal of Clinical Nutrition* **43**: 603–608.

Brock, J. H. (1980). Lactoferrin in human milk: its role in iron absorption and protection against enteric infection in new-born infants. *Archives of Disease in Childhood* **55**: 417–421.

Brown, R. E. (1978). Weaning foods in developing countries. *American Journal of Clinical Nutrition* **31**: 2066–2072.

Brown, K. H., Black, R. E. *et al.* (1982). Clinical and field studies of human lactation: methodological and field considerations. *American Journal of Clinical Nutrition* **35**: 745–756.

Brown, K. H., Akhtar, N. A. *et al.* (1986). Lactational capacity of marginally malnourished mothers: relationships between maternal nutritional status and quantity and proximate composition of milk. *Pediatrics* **78**: 909–919.

Butte, N., Garza, C. F. (1985). Energy and protein intakes of exclusively breast fed infants during the first four months of life. In Gracey, M., Falkner, F. (eds) *Nutritional needs and assessment of normal growth*. Nestlé Nutrition Workshop No. 7. Nestlé Nutrition, Vevey/Raven Press, New York, pp. 63–84.

Butte, N. F., Garza, C., Smith, E. O. (1988a). Variability of macronutrient concentrations in human milk. *European Journal of Clinical Nutrition* **42**: 345–349.

Butte, N. F., Garza, C. *et al.* (1983). Evaluation of the deuterium dilution technique against the test-weighing procedure for determination of breast milk intake. *American Journal of Clinical Nutrition* **37**: 996–1003.

Butte, N. F., Garza, C. *et al.* (1984a). Human milk intake and growth in exclusively breast-fed infants. *Journal of Pediatrics* **104**: 187–195.

Butte, N. F., Garza, C. *et al.* (1984b). Effect of maternal diet and body composition on lactational performance. *American Journal of Clinical Nutrition* **39**: 296–306.

Butte, N. F., Goldblum, R. M. *et al.* (1984c). Daily ingestion of immunologic components in human milk during the first four months of life. *Acta Paediatrica Scandinavica* **73**: 296–301.

Butte, N. F., Garza, C. *et al.* (1987). Macro- and trace-mineral intakes of exclusively breast-fed infants. *American Journal of Clinical Nutrition* **45**: 42–48.

Butte, N. F., Wong, W. W. *et al.* (1988b). Human milk intake measured by administration of ^2H_2O to the mother: a comparison with the test-weighing technique. *American Journal of Clinical Nutrition* **47**: 815–821.

Butte, N. F., Wong, W. W. *et al.* (1991). Measurement of milk intake: tracer-to-infant deuterium dilution method. *British Journal of Nutrition* **65**: 3–14.

Cameron, M., Hofvander, Y. (1983). *Manual on feeding infants and young children*, 2nd edn. Oxford University Press.

Church, M. A., Doughty, J. (1976). Value of traditional food practices in nutrition education. *Journal of Human Nutrition* **30**: 9–12.

Consensus Statement (1988). Breast feeding as a family planning method. *Lancet* **2**: 1204–1205.

Coward, W. A. (1984). Measuring milk intake in breast-fed babies. *Journal of Pediatric Gastroenterology and Nutrition* **3**: 275–279.

Coward, W. A., Cole, T. J. *et al.* (1982). Breast-milk intake measurement in mixed-fed infants by administration of deuterium oxide to their mothers. *Human Nutrition:Clinical Nutrition* **36C**: 141–148.

Coward, W. A., Whitehead, R. G. *et al.* (1979). New method for measuring milk intakes in breast-fed babies. *Lancet* **2**: 13–14.

Cruz, J. R., Carlsson, B. *et al.* (1982). Studies on human milk. III. Secretory IgA quantity and antibody levels against *Escherichia coli* in colostrum and milk from underprivileged and privileged mothers. *Pediatric Research* **16**: 272–276.

Davis, J. (1978). Case for breast-feeding. *Lancet* **2**: 201–202.

Delgado, H., Lechtig, A. *et al.* (1978). Nutrition, lactation and post-partum amenorrhoea. A review article. *American Journal of Clinical Nutrition* **31**: 322–327.

Delvoye, P., Delogne-Desnoek, J., Robyin, C. (1976). Serum prolactin in long-lasting lactation amenorrhoea. *Lancet* **2**: 288–289.

Dewey, K. G., Lönnerdal, B. (1986). Infant self-regulation of breast milk intake. *Acta Paediatrica Scandinavica* **75**: 893–898.

Dickin, K. L., Brown, K. H. *et al.* (1990). Effect of diarrhoea on dietary intake by infants and young children in rural villages of Kwara state, Nigeria. *European Journal of Clinical Nutrition* **44**: 307–317.

Dimond, H. J., Ashworth, A. (1987). Infant feeding practices in Kenya, Mexico and Malaysia: the rarity of the exclusively breast-fed infant. *Human Nutrition: Applied Nutrition* **41A**: 51–64.

Feachem, R. G., Koblinsky, M. A. (1984). Interventions for the control of diarrhoeal diseases among young children: promotion of breast-feeding. *Bulletin of the World Health Organization* **62**: 271–291.

Ferris, A. M., Jensen, R. G. (1984). Lipids in human milk: a review. 1. Sampling, determination and content. *Journal of Pediatric Gastroenterology and Nutrition* **3**: 108–122.

Fomon, S. J. (1974). *Infant nutrition*, 2nd edn. W. B. Saunders and Co., Philadelphia, pp. 118–151.

Forman, M. R. (1984). Review of research on the factors associated with choice and duration of infant feeding in less developed countries. *Pediatrics* **74**: Suppl. 667–694.

Garza, C., Butte, N. F. (1985). Determination of the energy content of human milk. In Jensen, R. G., Neville, M. C. (eds) *Human lactation: milk components and methodologies*. Plenum Press, New York, pp. 121–126.

Garza, C., Butte, N. F. (1986). Energy concentration of human milk estimated from 24h pools and various abbreviated sampling schemes. *Journal of Pediatric Gastroenterology and Nutrition* **5**: 943–948.

Garza, C., Hopkinson, J. M. (1988). Physiology of lactation. In Tsang, R. C., Nichols, B. L. (eds) *Nutrition during infancy*. Hanley and Belfus, Philadelphia, pp. 20–34.

Glasier, A., McNeilly, A. S. (1990). Physiology of lactation. In Franks, S. (ed) *Endocrinology of pregnancy: Baillière's clinical endocrinology and metabolism*. Baillière Tindall, London, pp. 379–395.

Gopalan, C. (1958). Studies on lactation in poor Indian communities. *Journal of Tropical Pediatrics* **4**: 87–95.

Gopaldas, T., Deshpande, S., John, C. (1988). Studies on a wheat-amylase-rich food (ARF). *Food and Nutrition Bulletin (UNU)* **10**: 50–54.

Gopaldas, T., Mehta, P. *et al.* (1986). Studies on reduction of viscosity of thick rice gruels with small quantities of an amylase-rich malt. *Food and Nutrition Bulletin (UNU)* **8**: 42–47.

Gray, R. H., Campbell, O. M. *et al.* (1990). Risk of ovulation during lactation. *Lancet* **1**: 25–29.

György, P. (1958). N-containing saccharides in human milk. In Wolstenholm, G. E. W., O'Connor, C. M. (eds) *CIBA Foundation symposium on the chemistry and biology of mucopolysaccharides*. CIBA Foundation, London, pp. 140–154.

György, P. (1971). Uniqueness of human milk: biochemical aspects. *American Journal of Clinical Nutrition* **24**: 970–975.

Habicht J-P., DaVanzo, J., Butz, W. P. (1986). Does breastfeeding really save lives, or are the apparent benefits due to biases? *American Journal of Epidemiology* **123**: 279–290.

Habicht J-P., DaVanzo, J., Butz, W. P. (1988). Mother's milk and sewage: their interactive effects on infant mortality. *Pediatrics* **81**: 456–461.

Hall, B. (1975). Changing composition of human milk and early development of an appetite control, *Lancet* **1**: 779–782.

Hansen, M., Pedersen, B. *et al.* (1989). Weaning foods with improved energy and nutrient density prepared from germinated cereals. 1. Preparation and dietary bulk of gruels based on barley. *Food and Nutrition Bulletin* (UNU) **11**: 40–45.

Hayward, A. R. (1983). The immunology of breast milk. In Neville, M. C., Neifert, M. R. (eds) *Lactation: physiology, nutrition and breast-feeding*. Plenum Press, New York, pp. 249–270.

Hellstrom, A., Hennansson A-M. *et al.* (1981). Dietary bulk. II. Consistency as related to dietary bulk: a model study. *Journal of Tropical Pediatrics* **27**: 127–136.

Hibbert, J. M., Golden, M. H. N. (1981). What is the weanling's dilemma? *Journal of Tropical Pediatrics* **27**: 255–258.

Hijazi, S. S., Abulaban, A., Waterlow, J. C. (1989). The duration for which exclusive breast-feeding is adequate. *Acta Paediatrica Scandinavica* **78**: 23–28.

Hytten, F. E. (1954). Clinical and chemical studies in human lactation. II. Variation in major constituents during a feeding. *British Medical Journal* **1**: 176–179.

Ibrahim, G. J. (1985). Breast milk and the absorption process. *Journal of Tropical Pediatrics* **31**: 2–3.

Jackson, D. A., Woolridge, M. W. *et al.* (1987). The automatic sampling shield: a device for sampling suckled breast milk. *Early Human Development* **15**: 295–306.

Jackson, D. A., Imong, S. M. *et al.* (1988). Infant weight in relation to nutritional intake and morbidity in Northern Thailand. *European Journal of Clinical Nutrition* **42**: 725–739.

Jason, J. M., Nieburg, P., Marks, J. S. (1984). Mortality and infectious disease associated with infant-feeding practices in developing countries. *Pediatrics* **74**: Suppl. 702–727.

Jelliffe, D. B., Jelliffe, E. F. P. (1978). The volume and composition of human milk in poorly nourished communities. A review. *American Journal of Clinical Nutrition* **31**: 492–515.

Jelliffe, D. B., Jelliffe, E. F. P. (1978). *Human milk in the modern world: psychosocial, nutritional and economic significance*. Oxford University Press.

Jones, W. H. S. (trans) (1923). *Hippocrates*, Vol. III. Loeb edition, Heinemann, London, p. 323.

Karra, M. V., Kirksey, A. *et al.* (1988). Zinc, calcium and magnesium concentrations in milk from American and Egyptian women throughout the first 6 months of lactation. *American Journal of Clinical Nutrition* **47**: 642–648.

Khin-Maung-Naing, Tin-Tin-Oo (1987). Effect of dietary supplementation on lactation performance of undernourished Burmese mothers. *Food and Nutrition Bulletin* **9:** 59–61.

Khin-Maung-Naing, Tin-Tin-Oo (1991). Growth and milk intake of exclusively breast-fed Myanmar infants from birth to five months. *European Journal of Clinical Nutrition* **45:** 203–207.

Kimati V. P. (1986). Who is ignorant? Rural mothers who feed their well-nourished children or the nutrition experts? The Tanzania story. *Journal of Tropical Pediatrics* **32:** 130–136.

King, J., Ashworth, A. (1987). Historical review of the changing pattern of infant feeding in developing countries: the case of Malaysia, the Caribbean, Nigeria and Zaïre. *Social Science Medicine* **25:** 1307–1320.

Lönnerdal, B. (1986). Effects of maternal dietary intake on human milk composition. *Journal of Nutrition* **116:** 499–513.

Lucas, A., Gibbs, J. A. H. *et al.* (1978). Creamatocrit: simple clinical technique for estimating fat concentrations and energy values of human milk. *British Medical Journal* **1:** 1018–1020.

Lucas, A., Ewing, G. *et al.* (1987). Measurement of milk intake by deuterium dilution. *Archives of Disease in Childhood* **62:** 796–800.

Lunn, P. G., Austin, S. *et al.* (1980). Influence of maternal diet on plasma prolactin levels during lactation. *Lancet* **1:** 623–625.

McCann, M. F., Liskin, L. S. *et al.* (1981). Breastfeeding, fertility and family planning. *Population Reports* [J] **24:** J525–J576.

McClelland, D. B. L., McGrath, J., Samson, R. R. (1978). Antimicrobial factors in human milk. Studies of concentration and transfer in human milk. Studies of transfer to the infant during the early stages of lactation. *Acta Paediatrica Scandinavica* **67:** Suppl. **271,** 1–20.

Marín, P. C., Aranjo, G. *et al.* (1984). Energy content of breast milk of poor Brazilian mothers. *Lancet* **1:** 232–233.

Mata, L. J. (1982). Breast feeding, diarrheal disease and malnutrition in less developed countries. In Lifshitz, F. (ed) *Pediatric nutrition. Infant feedings—deficiencies—diseases.* Marcel Dekker, New York, pp. 355–372.

Mata, L. (1986). Breast-feeding and host defense. *Frontiers in Gastrointestinal Research* **13:** 119–133.

Mellander, O., Svanberg, U. (1984). Compact calories, malting and young child feeding. In Jelliffe, D. B., Jelliffe, E. F. P. (eds) *Advances in international maternal and child health Vol. 4.* Oxford University Press, pp. 84–94.

Mensah, P. P. A., Tomkins, A. M. (1990). Fermentation of cereals for reduction of bacterial contamination of weaning foods in Ghana. *Lancet* **336:** 140–143.

Merchant, K., Martorell, R. (1988). Frequent reproductive cycling: does it lead to nutritional depletion of mothers? *Progress in Food and Nutrition Science* **12:** 339–369.

Milla, P. J. (1986). The weanling's gut. *Acta Paediatrica Scandinavica* Suppl. **323:** 5–13.

Neville, M. C., Keller, R. P. *et al.* (1984). Studies on human lactation. I. Within feed and between breast variation in selected components of human milk. *American Journal of Clinical Nutrition* **40:** 635–646.

Orr-Ewing, A. K., Heywood, P. F., Coward, W. A. (1986). Longitudinal measurements of breast milk output by ^2H_2O technique in rural Papua New Guinean women. *Human Nutrition: Clinical Nutrition* **40C:** 451–468.

Ounsted, M., Sleigh, R. (1975). The infant's self-regulation of food intake and weight gain. *Lancet* **1:** 1393–1397.

Pirie, N. W. (1978). *Leaf protein and its by-products in human and animal nutrition.* 2nd edn. Cambridge University Press.

Prentice, A. (1985*a*). The effect of maternal parity on lactational performance in a rural African community. In Hamosh, M., Goldman, A. S. (eds) *Human lactation 2*. Plenum Press, New York, pp. 165–173.

Prentice, A. (1985b). The influence of maternal parity on breast-milk composition. In Schaub, J. (ed) *Composition and physiological properties of human milk*. Elsevier, Amsterdam, pp. 309–319.

Prentice, A., Addey, C. V. P., Wilde, C. J. (1989a). Evidence for local feedback control of human milk secretion. *Biochemical Society Transactions* **17**: 122–123.

Prentice, A., Prentice, A. M., Whitehead, R. G. (1981a). Breast milk fat concentrations of rural African women. 1. Short-term variation within individuals. *British Journal of Nutrition* **45**: 483–494.

Prentice, A., Ewing, G. *et al*. (1987). The nutritional role of breast-milk IgA and lactoferrin. *Acta Paediatrica Scandinavica* **76**: 592–598.

Prentice, A., MacCarthy, A. *et al*. (1989b). Breast-milk IgA and lactoferrin survival in the gastro-intestinal tract—a study in rural Gambian children. *Acta Paediatrica Scandinavica* **78**: 505–512.

Prentice, A. M., Paul, A. *et al*. (1986). Cross-cultural differences in lactational performance. In Hamosh, M., Goldman, A. S. (eds) *Human lactation 2*. Plenum Press, New York, pp. 13–44.

Prentice, A. M., Roberts, S. B. *et al*. (1983). Dietary supplementation of lactating Gambian women. I. Effect on breast-milk volume and quality. *Human Nutrition: Clinical Nutrition* **37C**: 53–64.

Prentice, A. M., Whitehead, R. G. *et al*. (1981b). Long-term energy balance in child-bearing Gambian women. *American Journal of Clinical Nutrition* **34**: 2790–2799.

Ramachandran, P. (1989). Lactation – nutrition – fertility interactions. In Gopalan, C., Kaur, S. (eds) *Women and nutrition in India*. Nutrition Foundation of India, Special Publications Series No. 5, New Delhi, pp. 194–223.

Rattigan, S., Ghisalberti, A. V., Hartmann, P. E. (1981). Breast milk production in Australian women. *British Journal of Nutrition* **45**: 243–249.

Rowland, M. G. M. (1986). The weanling's dilemma: are we making progress? *Acta Paediatrica Scandinavica* **323**: 33–42.

Rowland, M. G. M., Barrell, R. A. E., Whitehead, R. G. (1978). Bacterial contamination in traditional Gambian weaning foods. *Lancet* **1**: 136–138.

Rutishauser, I. H. E. (1974). Factors affecting the intakes of energy and protein by Ugandan pre-school children. *Ecology of Food and Nutrition* **3**: 213–222.

Rutishauser, I. H. E., Frood, J. D. L. (1973). The effect of a traditional low-fat diet on energy and protein intake, serum albumin concentration and body-weight in Ugandan preschool children. *British Journal of Nutrition* **29**: 261–268.

Salmenperä L., Perheentupe, J., Sumes, M. A. (1985). Exclusively breastfed healthy infants grow slower than reference infants. *Pediatric Research* **19**: 307–312.

Seward, J. F., Serdula, M. K. (1984). Infant feeding and infant growth. *Pediatrics* **74**: (Suppl.) 728–762.

Shatrugna, V., Raghuramulu, N., Prema, K. (1982). Serum prolactin levels in undernourished Indian lactating women. *British Journal of Nutrition* **48**: 193–199.

Southgate, D. A. T., Barrett, I. M. (1966). Intake and excretion of calorific constituents of milk by babies. *British Journal of Nutrition* **20**: 363–372.

Sserunjogi, L., Tomkins, A. (1990). The use of fermented and germinated cereals and tubers for improved feeding of Ugandan infants and children. *Transactions of the Royal Society of Tropical Medicine and Hygiene* **84**: 443–446.

Stephens, A. (1986). Development of secretory immunity in breast fed and bottle fed infants. *Archives of Disease in Childhood* **61**: 263–269.

Strode, M. A., Dewey, K. G., Lönnerdal, B. (1986). Effects of short-term calorie restriction on lactational performance of well-nourished women. *Acta Paediatrica Scandinavica* **75**: 222–229.

Stuff, J. E., Garza, C. *et al*. (1986). Sources of variance in milk and caloric intakes in breast-fed infants: implications for lactation study design and interpretation. *American Journal of Clinical Nutrition* **43:** 361–366.

Tanner, J. M., Whitehouse, R. H., Takaishi, M. (1966). Standards from birth to maturity for height, weight, height velocity and weight velocity. British children, 1963, part II. *Archives of Disease in Childhood* **41:** 613–635.

Underwood, B. A., Hofvander, Y. (1982). Appropriate timing for complementary feeding of the breast fed infant. *Acta Paediatrica Scandinavica* Suppl. **294:** 5–32.

Van Steenbergen, W. M., Kusin, J. A. *et al.* (1978). Food intake, feeding habits and nutritional state of the Akamba infant and toddler. *Tropical Geographical Medicine* **30:** 505–522.

Van Steenbergen, W. M., Kusin, J. A. *et al* . (1989). Energy supplementation in the last trimester of pregnancy in East Java, Indonesia: effect on breast-milk output. *American Journal of Clinical Nutrition* **50:** 274–279.

Van Steenbergen, W. M., Kusin, J. A. *et al.* (1991). Nutritional transition in infancy in East Java, Indonesia. 1. A longitudinal study of feeding pattern, breast milk intake and the consumption of additional foods. *European Journal of Clinical Nutrition* **45:** 67–75.

Vio, F. R., Infante, C. B. *et al.* (1986). Validation of the deuterium dilution technique for the measurement of fluid intake in infants. *Human Nutrition: Clinical Nutrition* **40C:** 327–332.

Walker, A. F. (1990). The contribution of weaning foods to protein-energy malnutrition. *Nutrition Research Reviews* **3:** 25–48.

Wallgren, A. (1945). Breast milk consumption of healthy full-term infants. *Acta Paediatrica Scandinavica* **32:** 778–790.

Waterlow, J. C. (1981). Observations on the suckling's dilemma—a personal view. *Journal of Human Nutrition* **35:** 85–98.

Waterlow, J. C., Thomson, A. M. (1979). Observations on the adequacy of breast-feeding. *Lancet* **2:** 238–242.

Waterlow, J. C., Ashworth, A., Griffiths, M. (1980). Faltering in infant growth in less developed countries. *Lancet* **2:** 1176–1178.

Welsh, J. K., May, J. T. (1979). Anti-infective properties of breast milk. *Journal of Pediatrics* **94:** 1–9.

Wheeler, E. F. (1973). Food intake and rate of weight gain in two healthy breast-fed infants. *American Journal of Clinical Nutrition* **26:** 631–639.

Whitehead, R. G., Paul, A. A. (1981). Infant growth and human milk requirements. *Lancet* **2:** 161–163.

Williams, A. F., Akinbuge, F. M., Baum, J. D. (1985). A comparison of two methods of milk sampling for calculating the fat intake of breast-fed babies. *Human Nutrition: Clinical Nutrition* **39C:** 193–202.

Woodward, D. R., Rees, B., Boon, J. A. (1989). Human milk fat content: within-feed variation. *Early Human Development* **19:** 39–46.

Woolridge, M. W., Jackson, D. A. *et al.* (1987). Indirect test weighing: a non-intrusive technique for estimating night-time breast milk intake. *Human Nutrition: Clinical Nutrition* **41C:** 347–362.

World Health Organization (1985*a*). *The quantity and quality of breast milk*. Report on the WHO Collaborative Study on Breast-feeding. WHO, Geneva.

World Health Organization (1985*b*). *Energy and protein requirements*. Report of a Joint FAO/WHO/UNU Expert Consultation. Technical Report Series No. 724. WHO, Geneva.

Zumrawi, F. Y., Dimond, H., Waterlow, J. C. (1987*a*). Faltering in infant growth in Khartoum Province, Sudan. *Human Nutrition: Clinical Nutrition* **41C:** 383–395.

Zumrawi, F. Y., Dimond, H., Waterlow, J. C. (1987*b*). Effects of infection on growth in Sudanese children. *Human Nutrition: Clinical Nutrition* **41C:** 453–461.

17

Nutrition and infection
in collaboration with
A. M. Tomkins

Outline of the problem

The monograph by Scrimshaw *et al.* (1968) played a seminal part in stimulating interest in the relationships of nutrition and infection. It came just at a time when attention was shifting from established PEM as seen in hospitals to the environment in which malnutrition occurs. Recent reviews are by Martorell and Ho (1984), Keusch and Farthing (1986), Tomkins (1986, 1991) and Ulijaszek (1990). A summary of clinical and epidemiological studies has been compiled by Tomkins and Watson (1989).

The relationships are both close and complex. On the one hand resistance to infection is reduced if nutritional status is poor. Examples range from the susceptibility of malnourished patients in hospital to develop wound infection and pneumonia to that of malnourished children and adults to die from infectious disease under famine conditions. On the other hand, infection may have profound influences on nutritional state. This is seen in individuals with severe infections such as AIDS, who lose a great deal of weight. Infections may also precipitate widespread weight loss throughout a community, as happens in children during a severe epidemic of measles.

These relationships have attracted the attention of a spectrum of research workers ranging from the molecular biologist to the social scientist. In the context of the malnourished child in a poor environment, it is always necessary to recognize the influence of the social environment on the malnutrition/infection relationship. For instance, two children of similar age and nutritional status in the same village may both suffer a severe attack of rotavirus diarrhoea. If the first child is nursed and encouraged to feed by his mother, who is able to provide a range of tempting food and drink, it is likely that the nutritional status will be relatively unchanged. However, if the mother of the second child has to work away from the home for many hours and is unable to spare the cash or the time to nurse her child through the infection, the nutritional impact of diarrhoea on growth will be considerable, or the child may even die.

Similarly, when the incidence, duration, or severity of infection are being analysed in relation to nutritional indicators, it is important to consider whether the poor social and environmental conditions that caused the malnutrition in the first place may be responsible for the increased risk. For instance, children with poorer nutritional status in a village community may have increased attack rates for respiratory infection or diarrhoea. However, they may come from poorer homes with more crowding and lower standards of hygiene and sanitation, in which case malnutrition might be regarded as a marker of a disadvantaged child rather than a biologically active risk factor. In any appraisal of the strength or causes of the malnutrition/infection relationship it is important to control for such confounding variables.

Many attempts have been made to analyse the risk of infection according to defined levels of nutritional deficiency (see below). In some communities the association between anthropometric indices and subsequent risk of infection or death is linear, in others there is a threshold of nutritional status below which the risk increases sharply (Tomkins, 1986). In others again there may be much weaker associations between malnutrition and infection. Thus the predictive value of anthropometric indices, widely proclaimed as essential for monitoring child health, may vary considerably between countries. Notwithstanding these important differences, which usually relate to children with mild and moderate malnutrition, there is overwhelming evidence that the child with severe malnutrition is seriously at risk of infection in any community.

Although the subject of this book is protein-energy malnutrition, it must also be recognized that deficiencies of some micronutrients, particularly vitamin A, riboflavin, iron and zinc, which are often associated with PEM, can have a profound influence on the host's response to infection as well as on rates of microbial proliferation. The strength and nature of the relationships vary according to the level of micronutrient deficiency, environmental exposure and social factors. The prevalence of infections such as malaria and measles may also cause differences in the response to nutritional rehabilitation. Mortality rates and catch-up growth rates are very different in Nutrition Centres in regions where infection is common compared with regions which have effective immunization programmes against measles, where there is no malaria and early recognition and treatment of tuberculosis.

A simplified model of these relationships is shown in Fig. 17.1. It demon-

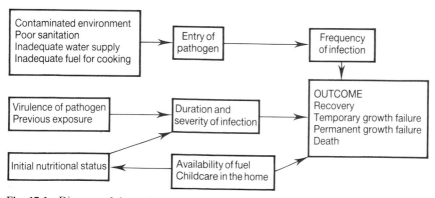

Fig. 17.1 Diagram of the main interrelationships between infection and nutrition.

strates the various factors which contribute to the malnutrition/infection complex and emphasizes that for maximal reduction of the prevalence of this complex in children a range of changes in the physical and social environment is necessary. However, the diagram also identifies specific interventions that are useful in themselves.

General mechanisms of response to infection and their effect on nutritional state

The main elements of the body's response to infection are listed in Table 17.1. The relationship is in both directions: some responses are modified by the nutritional state, others have an adverse effect on it. It seems that sometimes nutrition has to be sacrificed in the interests of host defence, but if a child is already malnourished when it becomes infected its capacity for defence is likely to be compromised.

Table 17.1   Components of the response to infection

Production of cytokines, particularly interleukin-1
Anorexia
Pyrexia
Catabolic losses
Malabsorption
Production of acute phase proteins
Decreased circulating concentrations of micronutrients
Impairment of immune response, particularly of cell-mediated immunity

The host's nutritional state is also important for the infective agent. Thus the growth of most pathogens, especially parasites and bacteria, is influenced both *in vitro* and *in vivo* by levels of nutrients, and a reduction of protein or micronutrient concentrations may protect the host against infection. For example, experiments on rats infected with malaria showed that a low protein diet reduced parasitaemia and mortality (Edirisinghe *et al.*, 1981).

Research in recent years has shown that most of the responses listed in Table 17.1 are mediated by cytokines, a group of polypeptides or low molecular weight proteins which are released by macrophages and are active in minute amounts. Of these the most important is interleukin-1 (for reviews see Dinarello, 1984; Keusch and Farthing, 1986; Grimble, 1989, 1990). Bhaskaram and Sivakumar (1986) have shown that monocytes from malnourished children have a reduced production of interleukin-1. In children with vitamin A deficiency a large dose of vitamin A potentiated production of the cytokine by macrophages (Bhaskaram *et al.*, 1989).

Anorexia

Anorexia is a classical symptom of infection in children and undoubtedly plays a major role in producing secondary malnutrition (Mata *et al.*, 1977; Martorell *et al.*, 1980; Pereira and Begum, 1987). Energy intake may be reduced by some 20 per cent. The mechanism by which appetite is suppressed has not been clearly defined, but it probably involves interleukin-1, since when *E.coli* endotoxin is injected into animals there is a striking reduction in food intake. In children the appetite for solids is reduced more than for liquids; breast milk is particularly well tolerated, so the maintenance of breast feeding is important for nutritional support (Hoyle *et al.*, 1980; Dickin *et al.*, 1990). A study in The Gambia showed that decrease in food intake was quantitatively three times more important than malabsorption in accounting for weight faltering during infection (Tomkins, 1983).

The functional value of a reduction in food intake is difficult to assess. It may be that it limits bacterial and parasitic growth, but it cannot be maintained for long without detriment to the host's nutritional state and the practice of 'starving a fever', popular in many communities, is not to be encouraged. Attention to local causes of anorexia, such as dehydration, painful buccal lesions from monilia infection and pain are all important in the management of infection-induced anorexia.

Fever

There is presumably some advantage to the host in a rise in body temperature through increased efficiency of the immune response, but there is also a cost, since in well-nourished subjects energy expenditure increases by 10–15 per cent for each 1°C rise in body temperature. As mentioned earlier (Chapter 6), children with severe PEM are unable to produce a fever or to increase their metabolic rates in response to infection, which may therefore easily remain undiagnosed. In a study of children with acute measles in Kenya even a moderate degree of malnutrition (mean weight for height Z-score, −1.6) was enough to prevent a rise of BMR in the presence of fever (Duggan and Milner, 1986*a*, *b*). The children were nevertheless in negative energy balance because of a fall in their intake.

Metabolic effects

It has long been recognized that infection and trauma produce a negative nitrogen balance. This results from an increase in protein breakdown, probably mainly in muscle (Waterlow, 1984). Tomkins *et al.* (1983) showed that in children with measles the rise in protein breakdown, the consequent negative nitrogen balance and the increase in 3-methyl histidine output were much less pronounced in those who were also malnourished. The effect on muscle is probably mediated by an increase in cortisol, which is a catabolic hormone for muscle (Chapter 9).

Infections, at least if severe, are accompanied by changes in the pattern of substrate oxidation. Goldstein and Elwyn (1989) concluded that septic patients oxidize less glucose, convert less glucose to fat and oxidize more fat than normal subjects. The reduction in glucose oxidation occurs in spite of raised plasma insulin levels, because of peripheral insulin resistance.

There are important changes in the synthesis of circulating proteins. Albumin synthesis is reduced, so that the plasma concentration falls. At the same time, stimulated by interleukin-1, there is an increased production of acute phase proteins such as fibrinogen, C-reactive protein, and α_1-antitrypsin

(Fleck *et al.*, 1985; Fleck, 1989). It is of interest that these proteins are all glycoproteins; one function attributed to vitamin A is the promotion of glycosylation (De Luca, 1977), so that if the vitamin is deficient the production of these presumably protective proteins may be reduced.

In infection there are also increases in the plasma concentrations of metal-binding proteins: lactoferrin, derived from leucocytes, rises, causing a reduction in the plasma concentration of free iron; metallothionein and caeruloplasmin levels increase, indicating increased binding of plasma zinc and copper. Plasma concentrations of riboflavin, retinol and ascorbic acid decrease during infection. These features of the metabolic response to infection appear to be remarkably consistent for a range of experimental and clinical infections (Srinavas *et al.*, 1988). There are several putative advantages in terms of host protection (see below).

Intestinal function

In children diarrhoea is often a feature of systemic infections such as malaria or localized infections such as otitis media. There have been some studies showing malabsorption during acute respiratory infection (Cook, 1971), and there is evidence of changes in gut permeability in children with measles (Behrens *et al.*, 1987). Naturally the digestion and absorption of food are particularly affected by intestinal infections, especially those which cause damage to the jejunal mucosa with loss of microvilli (Tomkins, 1981). The impact of diarrhoea on intestinal absorption has been well defined physiologically at the luminal, brush border and intracellular level. Most attention has been concentrated on the absorption of water and electrolytes, but malabsorption of macronutrients cannot be ignored (Torun and Chew, 1991). Reductions in intestinal enzyme activity may reduce the absorption of carbohydrate and protein. If there is impairment of mixed micelle formation there may be significant malabsorption of fats.

In healthy children in a Third World community on a typical high fibre diet the intestine absorbs 95 per cent of fat, 90 per cent of nitrogen and more than 90 per cent of dietary carbohydrate. In acute diarrhoea these figures may drop by 10 – 20 per cent. Table 17.2 shows results of studies in Guatemala. In Bangladeshi children with acute diarrhoea, absorption of carbohydrate was 74 per cent in rotavirus patients, 92 per cent in diarrhoea caused by enterotoxin-producing *E. coli* (ETEC) and 77 per cent in *Shigella* diarrhoeas (Molla, 1983).

Many children with diarrhoea also lose endogenous nutrients. In Bangla-

Table 17.2 Absorption of macronutrients in the acute phase of diarrhoea

	Apparent absorption, % of intake	
	Milk diet	Vegetable diet
Energy	73	71
Fat	76	58
Protein	65	44

From Torun and Chew (1991)

deshi children with diarrhoea there were raised levels of α_1-antitrypsin in the faeces, a marker for loss of protein. The highest losses were observed in cases due to shigellosis complicating measles (Sarker *et al.*, 1986). The quantitative significance of these losses was discussed in Chapter 6.

Micronutrients are not well absorbed during diarrhoea. This is particularly true of vitamin A, the absorption of which is affected by the reduction of mixed micelles and more rapid intestinal transit. Absorption of iron and zinc is also likely to be impaired; even minor general infections cause a dramatic reduction in the absorption of iron (Beresford *et al.*, 1971). Malabsorption of folic acid and vitamin B_{12} are well described in adults, and may contribute to the folate deficiency that is not infrequent in malnourished children (Chapter 12).

All these effects are more serious in children in whom gastrointestinal function and structure are already impaired by malnutrition (Chapter 5), leading to the familiar vicious cycle.

Immune responses

It has sometimes been suggested that increased production of immunoglobulins and leucocytes in infection represents a drain on protein resources that will compromise the host's protein nutrition. Perhaps these responses underlie, at least in part, the increase in whole-body protein synthesis that is observed in infection and trauma (Waterlow, 1984), but their quantitative importance from the point of view of protein metabolism has not been defined. Of more significance is the extent to which immune responses are modified or inhibited by malnutrition (Table 17.3). This subject has been discussed in detail in numerous reviews, e.g. Suskind (1977), Chandra (1980, 1983, 1988*a*, *b*).

It appears that the humoral immune response is only affected in acute and severe PEM and is rapidly restored as the child recovers. As a consequence, even moderately malnourished children are still able to respond to routine immunization procedures.

It has long been recognized that cell-mediated immunity (CMI) is undoubtedly impaired in malnutrition (Bhaskaram and Reddy, 1974; Kielmann *et al.*, 1976). Many years ago it was shown that children with PEM have a reduced response to tuberculin testing (Harland, 1965). This kind of observation has been repeatedly confirmed. Chandra (1988*b*) has shown a beautiful relationship between the size of the skin response and serum albu-

Table 17.3 Effects of malnutrition on the immune response

Atrophy of lymphoid tissues
Depression of delayed cutaneous hypersensitivity
Reduced thymidine uptake by T-cells
Impaired maturation of T-lymphocytes
Reduction in the ratio of helper to suppressor T-cells
Reduction of secretory IgA levels in serum and of sIgA response to viral vaccines
Impaired killing of bacteria by leucocytes
Reduction of complement component C_3
Serum levels of IgG and IgM normal or high, and humoral response to antigens not reduced
    except in severe PEM

From Chandra (1972, 1988*b*)

min concentration (Fig. 17.2). A reduction in the size of the thymus was also noted (Smythe *et al.*, 1971), which has been attributed by Golden *et al.* (1977) to zinc deficiency. A decrease in plasma thymulin, a zinc-protein produced by the thymus, has been described in PEM (Wade *et al.*, 1988). The basic defect in CMI is a reduced production of T-lymphocytes and helper cells. The response of lymphocytes *in vitro* to mitogens is also suppressed. These effects appear to be more severe in wasted than in stunted children, but quantitative relationships to the degree of nutritional deficit have not been defined, nor has the functional significance of the impairment in CMI. In the words of McMurray *et al.* (1981), 'no-one has titrated the impaired CMI response to determine the minimal ability to prevent disease'. This statement seems still to be true ten years later.

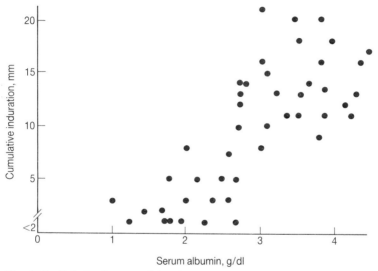

Fig. 17.2 Relation between delayed cutaneous hypersensitivity response and serum albumin concentration. Reproduced by permission from Chandra (1988*b*).

The bactericidal activity of polymorphonuclear leucocytes, which depends on the production of hydrogen peroxide, is strikingly reduced (Selvaraj and Bhat, 1972).

After this brief description of the general responses to infection and the way in which they interact with nutritional state, we come to the effect of specific infections and pathological conditions.

Effects of specific infections and pathological states

Diarrhoea

Acute diarrhoea is the commonest of all the illnesses in Third World children, who for the most part live in a contaminated environment. Its prevalence is highest towards the end of the first year and in the second year of life (Fig.

17.3), when 10–20 per cent of children may have diarrhoea on any one day (Martorell *et al.*, 1975). The main organisms responsible for diarrhoea are shown in Table 17.4, but very often no pathogens are isolated.

The mechanisms by which these organisms produce their effects are well recognized and have been reviewed elsewhere (Tomkins and Hussey, 1989). In general, the small intestinal diarrhoea can be caused by tissue destruction (by rotavirus, for instance) or by stimulation of the adenylate cyclase system within the mucosal cells by the production of toxins (heat-stable or heat-labile). The secretory responses, with faecal losses of fluids and electrolytes, are highest in the severely malnourished. This is probably explained by the

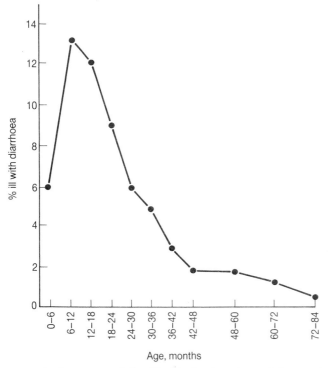

Fig. 17.3 Percentage of time ill with diarrhoea in rural Guatemalan children at different ages. Reproduced by permission from Martorell (1989).

Table 17.4 The main organisms producing diarrhoea in Third World children

Diarrhoea originating in the jejunum	Diarrhoea originating in the colon
Rotavirus	*Shigella sp.*
Enterotoxigenic *E. coli* (ETEC)	*Salmonella sp.*
Enteropathogenic *E. coli* (EPEC)	Enteroinvasive *E. coli* (EIEC)
Vibrio cholerae	*Campylobacter*
Campylobacter sp.	*Entamoeba histolytica*
Giardia lamblia	
[a]*Aeromonas sp.*	
[a]*Klebsiella sp.*	

[a] May produce enterotoxins capable of stimulating secretion of fluid and electrolytes from the jejunal mucosa.

changes in villus morphology that occur in malnutrition (Chapter 5). Zinc deficiency contributes to the additional fluid losses in PEM (Roy *et al.*, 1990).

Children with severe malnutrition have achlorhydria, so that colonization of the upper intestine by gut pathogens is relatively easy (Gracey *et al.*, 1977). Considering how frequently the child's food is contaminated by bacteria, it is perhaps surprising that malnourished children do not have diarrhoea all the time. Recent studies suggest that it may be only certain bacterial strains that cause diarrhoea. Strains of *E.coli* that have the plasmid for adhesion to the enterocytes are of particular interest (enteroadhesive *E.coli*).

In addition to the specific gut pathogens already mentioned, most severely malnourished children have large numbers of bacteria in the upper intestine, ranging from 10^4 to 10^9 organisms per ml of intestinal fluid. This 'soup' of organisms may have several effects. Firstly, there may be metabolic products which are toxic to the jejunal mucosa. Bile acids produced by the bacterial overgrowth may be responsible for damage to enterocytes. It is of interest that the jejunal mucosa of subjects with severe protein deficiency states living in a clean environment (e.g. nephrotic syndrome) is of normal structure, suggesting that the blunting of the villi found almost universally in malnourished children is not due to malnutrition alone.

Secondly, extracts of the bacterial soup have produced increased fluid secretion when perfused into experimental animals, suggesting that there may be a secretory effect. Thirdly, the presence of certain bacteria capable of deconjugating bile salts (e.g. *Bacteroides, Clostridia, Veilonella* and certain strains of *E.coli*) causes a reduction of the concentration of bile salts below that required for the efficient formation of mixed micelles. Effective absorption of fat is therefore reduced.

The establishment of the bacterial soup is possible because of the failure of a combination of gut immune defence systems, including gastric acidity, secretory IgA and cellular immunity. Antibiotics may disturb the normal balance of the autochthonous flora, which is usually made up of lactobacilli and streptococci. Several studies show that a significant proportion of cases of persistent diarrhoea (see below) have received antibiotics in the preceding month (Roy *et al.*, 1983).

Persistent diarrhoea syndrome (PDS)

For epidemiological purposes 'diarrhoea' is defined as the presence of three or more liquid stools in a day. Most episodes of diarrhoea last from three to seven days. Diarrhoea is arbitrarily described as persistent if it is continuous for 14 days or more (WHO, 1988). According to WHO, 3–20 per cent of diarrhoeal episodes become persistent, the incidence varying in different countries. In an Indian study 15 per cent of children between birth and three years experienced persistent diarrhoea during one year of surveillance. It has been estimated that PDS accounts for about 50 per cent of diarrhoea-related deaths (WHO, 1988). The clinical features of PDS have been described in detail by Lo and Walker (1983) and by McNeish (1986). PDS is commoner in younger children and in those with poor nutritional status.

There appear to be many causal factors. Enteroadhesive *E.coli* and *Shigella sp.* are especially important. In some cases the PDS is due to a prolonged infection with a gut pathogen as a result of depression of the immune clearance system. However, in many cases no particular pathogens have been isolated. Some of these children may have gut damage as part of a systemic illness. PDS is well described in measles, where there is evidence of damage to individual enterocytes and also to the entire mucosa, causing changes in intestinal permeability and loss of endogenous nutrients. Reduction in pancreatic exocrine secretion is found in severe malnutrition (Chapter 5), but its contribution compared with the other causes of PDS is probably minimal. PDS also occurs in malnourished children with tuberculosis. Early improvement in the diarrhoea following chemotherapy has been noted clinically, but the mechanism of PDS in tuberculosis is unclear.

Dietary allergens are an important cause of PDS in many communities. Allergy to cow's milk protein is the best described, but a range of dietary proteins, including vegetable protein such as soya bean, have also been incriminated. There is a series of immunological reactions by the lymphocytes in the jejunal mucosa whereby lymphokines are released. These have toxic effects, resulting in villus damage. Withdrawal of the offending antigen from the diet leads to improvement of the villus structure and on re-introduction, as a test challenge, the mucosa becomes blunted again. To identify precisely which dietary allergen is responsible it is necessary to investigate intensively, including by biopsy, before and after dietary challenge. The introduction of the lactulose/mannitol permeability test (Chapter 5) (Behrens *et al.*, 1987), in which the selectivity of absorption of sugars is used as a marker of mucosal damage, is a useful advance. Recently Lunn *et al.* (1991*a*) have shown that in children with PDS in The Gambia the lactulose: mannitol ratio was seven times as high as in normal children and more than twice as high as in those with acute diarrhoea, indicating severe mucosal damage. In some children this damage persisted for many months, and there was a significant negative relationship between the lactulose: mannitol ratio and rates of growth in weight and length (Lunn *et al.*, 1991 *b*).

A high proportion of cases of PDS occur in infants who were small at birth. A range of immunological deficiencies has been described in such children, rendering them more susceptible to infection. The age at which dietary antigens are introduced into the infant's diet appears to affect the subsequent response. Thus, an infant with low birth-weight who is fed contaminated weaning foods from an early age is at especially high risk of developing PDS.

Carbohydrate intolerance is a variable contributor to PDS, according to the diet. Secondary lactase deficiency occurs in all population groups if the jejunal mucosa becomes blunted from any cause. When the child has primary lactase deficiency (determined by ethnic group), which is then complicated by secondary lactase deficiency, the levels of jejunal lactase may become very low. If it receives lactose in breast milk or cow's milk as repeated small feeds throughout the day, there will usually be just enough lactase to digest the dietary lactose. If the lactose is given as a large bolus there may be insufficient lactase and osmotic diarrhoea results. Individual monosaccharide intolerance may also occur transiently, and food or oral rehydration fluids containing more than 3 per cent sugar are likely to cause an osmotic diarrhoea in children with acute diarrhoea or PDS. Roy *et al.* (1990) have found that a rice-based diet was effective in promoting carbohydrate absorption in PDS. There is no justification for total parenteral nutrition (TPN) in the management of PDS. Orenstein (1986) showed that with continuous enteral feeding normal stools were restored in three weeks, whereas with TPN it took ten weeks.

Management of diarrhoea in the community

The management of diarrhoea in hospital has been described in Chapter 12. In the community, where children are likely to be less severely malnourished, episodes of acute diarrhoea are generally self-limiting, provided that two principles are adhered to: first, that dehydration is prevented, or if present adequately treated; secondly, that the child's food intake is maintained as far as possible.

Only in very severe dehydration does fluid need to be given intravenously and this lies outside the scope of community treatment. Clinical assessment of the presence and degree of dehydration is difficult, particularly in malnourished children. Golden (1989) found rather poor agreement between purely clinical assessment and estimates based on weight loss. The classical sign of dehydration is loss of skin turgor. However, in wasted children with reduced subcutaneous fat the skin has in any case lost its turgor. In children in the early stages of kwashiorkor the extracellular tissues may be full of fluid while at the same time the intravascular volume is critically reduced. Thus very careful attention has to be paid to other clinical signs. These include a rapid pulse (>120/min) with low volume, severe dryness of the buccal mucosa, sunken fontanelle, drowsiness and reduced urine output. These are indications for urgent oral rehydration. An outline of recommendations for diagnosis and management is given in Table 17.5.

Table 17.5   Scheme for home diagnosis and treatment of dehydration

	Severity of condition		
	A	B	C
ASK:			
Liquid stools/day	less than 4	4–10	more than 10
Vomiting	none or slight	some	frequent
Thirst	normal	more than normal	unable to drink
Urine	normal	scanty, dark	none for 6 hours
LOOK:			
Condition	alert	sleepy or irritable	very sleepy, floppy, fits, unconscious
Tears	present	absent	absent
Eyes	normal	sunken	very dry, sunken
Mouth	wet	dry	very dry
Breathing	normal	fast	very fast and deep
FEEL:			
Skin-pinch	goes back quickly	goes back slowly	goes back very slowly
Pulse	normal	faster than normal	very fast, weak, or cannot be felt
Fontanelle	normal	sunken	very sunken
ACT:	ORS after each loose stool: 50–100 ml for child below 2 years 100–200 ml for older child	ORS for 4–6 hours: 200–400 ml at 2–6 months 400–600 ml at 6–12 months 600–800 ml at 1–3 years	take if possible to health centre; needs intravenous or intragastric fluids

Modified from Diarrhoea Dialogue, 1984.

Oral rehydration solutions (ORS)

Oral rehydration with electrolyte solutions has been used for a long time in the treatment of mild and moderate diarrhoea, but a breakthrough came in the 1960s with the demonstration by Phillips and his colleagues, working on cholera in Bangladesh, that glucose has an important effect in promoting the absorption of water and sodium chloride (Nalin *et al.*, 1968). This finding is firmly based on the physiology of the absorption and secretion of water and electrolytes in the gastrointestinal tract (Field *et al.*, 1989). It was described in a leading article in the *Lancet* (1978) as 'potentially the most important medical advance this century'. However, the advance was not only a scientific one; of equal significance was the initiative taken by WHO and UNICEF to extend the concept of oral rehydration therapy (ORT) from the clinic to the community. This required the provision of a suitable mixture of sugar and salts that could be made available in packets, for solution in water. There was some concern that the most appropriate composition of the rehydration solution might be different for temperate climates, where hypernatraemia is common and for tropical climates, where dehydration is characteristically isotonic or hypotonic. However, Hirschhorn (1980) has argued on physiological grounds that a single poly-electrolyte solution can be used in all situations.

In addition to glucose and NaCl, potassium has to be added to restore the losses (Chapter 4), and bicarbonate, lactate or citrate to counter acidosis. The composition recommended by WHO is shown in Table 17.6.

Table 17.6 Composition of the WHO/UNICEF oral rehydration solution

	g/litre	mmol/litre
Sodium chloride	3.5	60
Tri-sodium citrate	2.9	30 (of sodium)
or		
Sodium bicarbonate	2.5	30
Potassium chloride	1.5	20
Glucose (anhydrous)	20	110

From WHO (1976)

The Na^+ concentration originally recommended of 90 mmol/l has now been reduced to 80 mmol/l, but in severely malnourished children even this may lead to Na^+ overload and attention should be given to signs of fluid retention —increased respiratory rate and peri-orbital oedema. Many clinicians therefore prefer a lower Na^+ concentration, down to 30 mmol/l. The practice of diluting the standard formula 1:1 with water is not recommended because it reduces the glucose concentration.

In spite of greatly increased production of packaged ORS in recent years it is far from universally available and its cost is not negligible. According to a recent estimate (Elliott *et al.*, 1990), it has been used in only about 20 per cent of diarrhoeal episodes. Therefore an extension of the strategy of oral rehydration therapy has been to recommend that mothers should use a home-made solution of sugar and salt (SSS). Various simple recipes have been proposed, in terms of teaspoonfuls, pinches, etc., and special spoons have been devised for measuring the amounts of sugar and salt. The various recipes result in an enormously wide range of concentrations (WHO, 1986). According to WHO, concentrations of NaCl between 30 and 80 mmol/l are acceptable; the sucrose concentration, in molar terms, should be 1–1.4 times that of salt for most effective absorption. If the SSS is too dilute it will be ineffective; if too concentrated there is the danger of making dehydration worse if the fluid in the gut is hyper-osmolar. In spite of these sources of difficulty and the fact that SSS does nothing to counteract potassium deficiency or acidosis, WHO considers that it has been quite effective in preventing dehydration, at least in mild diarrhoea.

The latest advance in the ORT story is the development in Bangladesh, India and Kenya of cereal-based rehydration solutions (Molla *et al.*, 1989). Progress so far has been summarized by Elliott *et al.* (1990). The original work was done with rice, and it was shown that, in comparison with standard ORS, the rice-based solution reduced the number and volume of stools (Fig. 17.4). Potato, millet, maize and other cereal flours have an equally good effect. A further advantage over sugar is that there is no danger of producing osmotic diarrhoea. The cereal also provides some potassium and a little protein; amino acids may have a synergistic effect with carbohydrate in promoting the absorption of water and salt, and consideration is now being given to the possibility of including some source of protein. The flour is made into a thin soup by cooking with 1 litre of water and cooking salt is then added, as with the SSS. If too much flour is used or the mixture is cooked too vigorously for too long (5–7 minutes is adequate) it becomes too gelatinous.

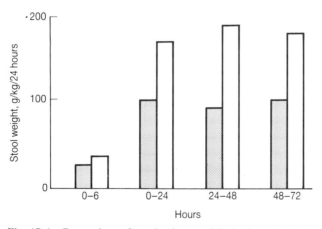

Fig. 17.4 Comparison of stool volumes with rice-based and glucose-based oral rehydration solutions. Data of Islam *et al.* (1989). ▨, rice-based ORS; ☐, glucose ORS. Reproduced by permission from Elliott *et al.* (1990), Fig. 8.

These cereal-based fluids should be ideal for rehydration in the home, since they can be made with almost any available and acceptable staple. The only disadvantages are that the cereal has to be cooked, which requires time and fuel, and it may become contaminated if it is not used immediately.

Feeding

The cereal-based ORS does not in itself provide significant amounts of food. The old paediatric tradition of 'resting' the gut in diarrhoea has long since been abandoned as unphysiological, leading to mucosal atrophy and poor weight gain, and it is now recommended that as far as possible food should be given together with oral rehydration solutions. The ideal food in this situation is breast milk; children with diarrhoea are usually anorexic, but there is evidence that they will continue to take breast milk even though they refuse solid foods (Dickin *et al.*, 1990). Breast feeding should therefore be continued for as long as possible. Indeed, a study in Myanmar showed that intestinal losses were lower if infants were breast-fed while receiving ORS (Khin-Maung-U *et al.*, 1985). If vomiting occurs the oral fluids should be given in smaller amounts and more frequently. If formula feeds are given they should be in full strength. Many studies show that the previous practice of starting with dilute feeds which progressively become more concentrated produces slower weight gain than full-strength feeds. Intolerance to lactose in human or animal milk is rare, provided that not too much is given at one time. Solid foods should be offered as soon as the child is able to eat. Indeed, good results have been reported by giving a normal diet *ad libitum* from the beginning (Torun and Chew, 1991).

In older children most studies show a reduction in intake of solids, particularly in areas where the basic diet is a thick porridge (The Gambia), or tortillas (Guatemala) (Martorell *et al.*, 1980). Here methods of reducing the viscosity of the food could be very useful (Chapter 16).

There are few indications for the use of antibiotics in the treatment of diarrhoea. If blood and mucus are present, *Shigella sp.*, enteroinvasive *E.coli* or *Entamoeba histolytica* may be suspected. Cotrimoxazole or ampicillin or halidixic acid may be used for management of these forms of dysentery. Metronidazole, preferably as syrup, is useful for the treatment of *Giardia lamblia*. Mixtures containing kaolin or pectin, traditionally used for the symptomatic treatment of diarrhoea, are not recommended (WHO, 1990).

Figure 17.5 shows an example of the effectiveness of oral rehydration

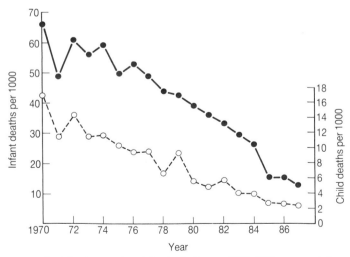

Fig. 17.5   Diarrhoea-related deaths in Egypt 1970–1987. ●——●, infants: deaths from diarrhoea per 1000 births,○---○, children aged one to four: deaths per 1000 per year. The National Control of Diarrhoeal Diseases Project was introduced in 1983. Drawn from data of El-Rafie *et al.* (1990) and reproduced by permission.

therapy and better nutritional management in contributing to the reduction of mortality from diarrhoeal disease in Egypt. The possibility of using fermented foods for preventing bacterial contamination and consequent diarrhoea was discussed in Chapter 16.

Measles

In Africa in particular measles is a major killing disease in children (see Chapter 18), and it often precipitates severe PEM (Scrimshaw *et al.*, 1968; Morley, 1969). It seems to have an especially profound effect on appetite and food intake may remain depressed for several weeks (Fig. 17.6). Fever and painful buccal lesions contribute to the anorexia, which is sometimes compounded by local cultural beliefs of withholding food during the period of acute illness. The measles virus damages the jejunal mucosa during the early stages and as the secondary complications of bronchopneumonia, shigellosis and PDS occur there may be further mucosal damage. Growth faltering has been noted during the post-measles dysentery phase in particular. Mention has already been made of the severe catabolic effects and negative energy balance found in children with measles.

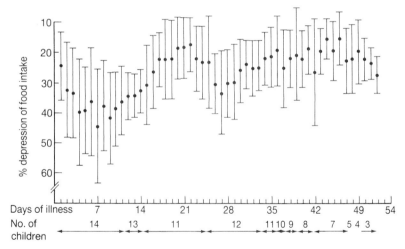

Fig. 17.6 Depression of food intake after measles in 14 children. The lower line gives the number of children whose appetite remained depressed at the corresponding time. Reproduced by permission from Pereira and Begum (1987).

Measles is particularly associated with vitamin A deficiency (see p. 309); indeed, the combination of these two is the commonest cause of blindness in children in many parts of Africa. There are several factors that affect vitamin A status as part of the general metabolic response to infection. Plasma retinol is reduced and urinary excretion of vitamin A metabolites increased; there is also a decrease in the hepatic synthesis of retinol-binding protein, the carrier protein for retinol, and a temporary reduction in vitamin A absorption. The measles virus causes local conjunctival damage, increasing the requirements of vitamin A for repair of the epithelial surface. It is likely that the role of vitamin A in glycoprotein synthesis is an important factor determining the degree of damage to conjunctiva, lungs and intestine in measles.

Bhaskaram *et al.*, (1986) investigated the effect of nutritional state, as assessed by weight for age on the course, outcome and immune status of children with measles. The duration and complications of measles were similar in well-nourished and malnourished children, and the cell-mediated immune response was low, irrespective of nutritional state. They concluded that the reportedly greater severity of measles in Africa than in India cannot be explained simply by differences in nutritional status.

Respiratory infections

Infections of the respiratory tract and of the middle ear make an important contribution to morbidity and mortality, particularly in the first year of life, second only to that of diarrhoeal disease (see Chapter 18). They have an indirect effect on nutritional status and growth through their influence on food intake and appetite. Breathless children find it difficult to eat and drink and may also have increased energy expenditure. In pertussis vomiting after eating is very common for weeks after the acute infection and it is difficult to coax a child to eat, particularly solids.

Tuberculosis

Children with tuberculosis show very poor 'catch-up' growth despite intensive feeding. This only improves when chemotherapy has been established. Whereas the diagnosis of acute respiratory infection is relatively easy, that of tuberculosis in malnourished children is extremely difficult. They may not be febrile, despite a severe clinical infection and the clinical signs of dyspnoea may not be marked. The Mantoux test is frequently, though not invariably, negative because of the depressed cellular immunity. It is very difficult to obtain sputum in children and the sample is nearly always negative for acid-fast bacilli. Laryngeal swabs or gastric washings rarely increase the yield above 10 per cent. In some cases a diagnosis can be established by a positive result on a lymph-gland aspirate. Histology and culture of liver or bone marrow specimens is often unrewarding. Finally, the chest radiographic appearances are not diagnostic; there are many causes of diffuse infiltration of the lung fields.

Therefore, in most cases the diagnosis of tuberculosis is made clinically. Classification systems of major and minor signs have been proposed, but all suffer from the defect that in the absence of an identified organism there is no 'gold standard' with which to compare them. It is important to remember tuberculosis as a cause of severe PEM and of failure to respond to nutritional management. If a severely malnourished child is failing to gain weight satisfactorily after two or three weeks following the start of nutritional rehabilitation and he really is eating 150–200 kcal/kg body weight/day, then tuberculosis chemotherapy should be seriously considered.

Chronic infections such as tuberculosis are also important contributors to anaemia in severe malnutrition. Interleukins have inhibitory effects on haemopoiesis and until systemic infections are satisfactorily treated, improvements in haematological status will lag behind improvements in growth.

Malaria

The impact of malaria on nutrition is much influenced by the species of parasite (more severe in *Plasmodium falciparum* than in *P.ovale* or *P.vivax* infection) and by the underlying malarial immunity (McGregor, 1982). Malaria has metabolic effects similar to other systemic infections. Rates of whole-body protein synthesis and breakdown are increased, with breakdown exceeding synthesis so that there is loss of body nitrogen. Prolonged infection, as occurs in endemic areas where populations have partial immunity, causes elevation of gamma globulins and a decrease in plasma albumin and transferrin. There are important effects of malaria on placental function, so that birth weight may be depressed. Malarial chemoprophylaxis or effective public health measures against malarial transmission have produced an increase in birth weight in the Solomon Islands and Thailand (Nosten *et al.*, 1991). In an investigation of Nigerian infants and children studied from birth, there was little difference in weight and height between those who received regular chloroquine and those who did not. However, the chloroquine group had a higher plasma albumin concentration, greater mid-arm circumference and higher haemoglobin level (Bradley-Moore *et al.*, 1985).

In the bone marrow malaria causes a decrease in haemopoiesis; by direct and indirect actions it increases the haemolysis of erythrocytes, leading to anaemia. Serum ferritin concentrations are raised in acute malarial fever. Malaria also has a major role as an immune suppressor, thereby increasing the prevalence and severity of infections such as diarrhoea and respiratory disease.

Intestinal parasites

Ascaris

Ascaris is one of the commonest parasites in Third World children, but it is difficult to assess the intensity of the infection. The number of eggs counted in a faecal specimen is not a reliable indicator of the number of worms. When there is a high worm load the fecundity decreases as a result of competition for intraluminal nutrients. This, together with the rather limited efficacy of certain drugs used against *Ascaris*, may explain some of the conflicting results between different studies. Improvement in growth following deworming has been noted in children with Grade II or Grade I malnutrition in India, Tanzania and Kenya (Crompton, 1986). There was no nutritional improvement in children in Brazil and Papua-New Guinea, but in both these groups they were relatively well-nourished before the antihelminthics were given. In general it seems that *Ascaris* can be a significant contributor to moderate malnutrition where the diet is poor, but its role in mild malnutrition is less clear (Stephenson *et al.*, 1980). There is increasing interest in the finding that within a community there is a group of people who have particularly high loads of *Ascaris*, so-called 'wormy people'. It would be ideal if the characteristics of this group could be identified so that anti-*Ascaris* therapy could be targeted towards them. However, as yet this has not been possible.

The situation in severe malnutrition is clearer. Several studies have shown that absorption of nitrogen and fat is increased after deworming, especially in those with heavy worm loads. In addition to the intestinal effects, *Ascaris* has a systemic phase of its life cycle during which, in the early stages of infection at least, there are immunological responses with release of lymphokines. These may account for the anorexia frequently noted in *Ascaris* infection. *Ascaris* may also cause secondary lactase deficiency.

Schistosoma

The impact of *Schistosoma* varies according to the species. *Schistosoma haematobium* infection in Nigerian boys was found to be associated with thinness (Oomen *et al.*, 1979). Treatment of Kenyan school children with metrifonate for *S.haematobium* was followed by significant improvement in a range of anthropometric indices (Stephenson *et al.*, 1980). *Schistosoma mansoni* is a more serious infection, with severe weight loss and decrease of plasma albumin in advanced cases. Chronic infections are accompanied by impairment of height gain and children are typically both short and thin.

Trichuris

Some recent studies have emphasized the importance of the *Trichuris* parasite. Although not sufficiently recognized elsewhere, it is associated with weight loss, stunting and anaemia in St Lucia (Cooper and Bundy, 1986; Cooper *et al.*, 1990) and in Malaysia. There may be finger-clubbing, probably an indicator of chronic inflammation. Substantial losses of mucus and blood may occur from rectal prolapse that is common with this infestation, and a series of systemic responses (abdominal pain, allergic features, irritability) may lead to anorexia. Intestinal malabsorption is relatively rare; colonic disease is the major problem. Oedema occurred in 18 per cent of cases seen in Malaysia.

Hookworm

The iron and protein deficiencies associated with hookworm are well known (Stephenson, 1987). Eventually oedema may occur. Like *Schistosoma* infection, it is more prevalent in older children, adolescents and adults than in young children because the parasite takes a long time to produce its severe nutritional effects. However, it is a major cause of nutritional oedema in adults in endemic areas.

Giardia

In poor environments *Giardia* is ubiquitous; judging by longitudinal studies of the parasitology of infant stools and by assays of antibodies in blood, most infants become infected with this parasite during the first year of life. It appears that for some this is a mild disease while for others it is a serious cause of acute diarrhoea and PDS. Some infants and children suffer repeated infections; others have only one episode (Farthing *et al.*, 1986). There may be differences in xymodeme patterns, differentiating between strains that cause diarrhoea and those that do not. The parasite damages villi, leading to malabsorption of most nutrients. It decreases fat absorption and allows the colonization of bacteria in the upper intestine. *Giardia* itself deconjugates bile salts, so it may contribute to impaired micelle formation in severe malnutrition. The parasite is only found in a proportion of stool samples but microscopy of the fluid from the upper intestine has shown that in some parts of the world it is present in the majority of children with severe PEM.

Cryptosporidium

Originally described in immunologically suppressed foals and more recently in patients with AIDS, *Cryptosporidium* is now recognized to cause diarrhoea in a high proportion of healthy well-nourished children who are infected for the first time. It produces a variably severe villus atrophy and malabsorption may occur. It was present in nearly half of a group of malnourished Rwandan children with post-measles diarrhoea.

Entamoeba histolytica

In adults *Entamoeba histolytica* occurs widely but it is less prevalent in children. It may, however, cause severe colitis with loss of blood and mucus. Systemic invasion to produce abscesses, particularly in the liver, can cause a profound decrease in plasma albumin and loss of body protein stores.

Treatment of intestinal parasites

There is much geographical variation in the epidemiology of intestinal parasites in children with PEM. Whenever possible, microscopy should be performed to identify specific parasites. If this cannot be done it is best to give mebendazole (for *Ascaris*, *Trichuris* and hookworm) and metranidazole, which is also an antimicrobial agent, for *Giardia*. Occasionally there may be *Strongyloides* infection. This requires thiabendazole but the drug is relatively toxic and treatment should be delayed until the child is in the catch-up phase.

AIDS

This tragic condition is likely to become increasingly important as a cause of persistent infection and malnutrition in young children. Several studies have noted that children who are born with HIV infection and then develop AIDS may show features similar to those of marasmus or kwashiorkor.

The weight loss during AIDS is the result of several mechanisms (Archer and Glinsmann, 1985). Secondary infection around the mouth, diarrhoea and fever all contribute to anorexia, which is striking. Malabsorption is well described. A few studies suggest that the virus causes villus atrophy by inhibiting multiplication of crypt cells. Parasitic infections, especially *Giardia lamblia* and *Cryptosporidium* make the villus damage even worse. The virus causes a pronounced metabolic response (Huang *et al.*, 1988).

There is preliminary evidence of increased energy expenditure in these patients, even in those without severe infection. Nutritional support is not easy because of the profound diarrhoea in many patients and the rather poor response to intravenous hyperalimentation, which has been tried in adults. In general the same principles of management are appropriate as for children with persistent diarrhoea syndrome.

Thus, consideration of the possibility of AIDS should now be routine in all assessment of the causes of malnutrition in children.

Specific nutrient deficiencies and the development and course of infections

Vitamin A deficiency

When vitamin A was discovered earlier this century it was called the 'anti-infection vitamin' because of its striking ability to prevent death from pneumonia and septicaemia in laboratory animals on a deficient diet (Green and Mellanby, 1928). Since that discovery, the effects of vitamin A deficiency on mucosae in general and on immunological function have received little attention compared to the striking features of xerophthalmia. Recently, however, the vitamin's protective properties have been re-examined (see reviews by Tomkins and Hussey, 1989 and by Thurnham, 1989). Deficiency is associated with impaired humoral and cellular immunity and with decreased activity of complement in serum and of lysozyme in leucocytes. There are profound effects on mucous membranes, which become keratinized; the production of secretory IgA is reduced, as is that of mucus, through reduction of glycoprotein synthesis. These changes impair the integrity of the membranes and their resistance to penetration by bacteria. Table 17.7 shows increased binding of bacteria to respiratory epithelial cells in children with low vitamin A status.

Table 17.7 Binding of bacteria to respiratory epithelial cells in vitamin A deficiency

	Group I[a]	Group II	Group III
Weight for height, %	87	77	74
Frequency of eye signs[b]	0	7	19
Serum retinol, μmol/l	2.2	1.1	0.4
Dietary vitamin A (retinol equivalents)	321	201	186
Bacteria per epithelial cell	4.8	7.9	10.3

[a] 10–14 children in each group; [b] some children had more than one eye sign.
From Chandra (1988c)

It was to be expected, from the function of the vitamin, that deficiency would be associated with increased susceptibility to respiratory and gastrointestinal disease. Table 17.8 shows the results of two studies which investigated the relationship between mild vitamin A deficiency and morbidity from respiratory infections and diarrhoea. In both Indonesia and India xerophthalmia was associated with an increased risk of respiratory infection, but in India there was no relation to diarrhoea. Xerophthalmia was apparently more severe in the Indonesian than in the Indian children. A critique of the results has been published by Forman (1989).

These field studies were performed in regions where there is a high prevalence of vitamin A deficiency. There is some evidence that even when this is not the case, vitamin A may reduce morbidity from respiratory infections (Tomkins and Hussey, 1989). Vitamin A deficiency may be occult and only detected by impression cytology of the conjunctiva, which shows abnormal epithelial cells and scanty or absent goblet cells (Usha *et al.*, 1990). Conversely there is an increased risk of xerophthalmia following diarrhoea and respiratory disease (Sommer *et al.*, 1987).

Table 17.8   Relationship of xerophthalmia to risk of respiratory disease and diarrhoea

Country	Age (years)	Relative risk[a]	
		Respiratory disease	Diarrhoea
Indonesia[b]			
	< 1	2.2	3.2
	1–2	2.3	3.4
	2–3	1.9	3.4
India[c]			
	< 1	0	0.5
	1–2	4.0	0.9
	2–3	2.0	1.5

[a] Risk with/without xerophthalmia
[b] From Sommer *et al.* (1984); [c] from Milton *et al.* (1987); summarized by Forman (1989)

Iron deficiency

Iron deficiency and anaemia are extremely common in Third World children. In cereal-based weaning diets virtually all the iron is in the inorganic form, which is much less well absorbed than haem iron (Layrisse *et al.*, 1969). Moreover, as mentioned earlier, even a mild infection can drastically reduce the absorption of iron, by mechanisms that are not well understood (Beresford *et al.*, 1971).

Immunological studies of subjects with iron deficiency show that humoral immunity is relatively intact, but there is a reduction in cell-mediated immunity. The disadvantages for the host's defence system may be counterbalanced by the fact that iron deficiency is associated with inhibition of the growth of many pathogenic bacteria, both *in vitro* and *in vivo*.

There have been a few studies of the effect of iron deficiency on morbidity in children. An increased malaria incidence was noted in iron-deficient subjects in Tanzania (Masawe *et al.*, 1974) and there were more episodes of respiratory illness and diarrhoea among iron-deficient subjects in Indonesia (Basta *et al.*, 1979). Respiratory infections were reported more frequently in children in New Zealand who had lower haemoglobins. Iron deficiency was found in 74 per cent of subjects with chronic muco-cutaneous candidiasis and it may contribute to bacterial colonization of the intestine because of its association with atrophic gastritis and decreased gastric acid production. However, definitive studies in children have not been performed.

Most studies of iron deficiency and morbidity show a reduction in morbidity following the introduction of low-dose oral supplements. However, there are important differences if other doses or routes of administration are used. High-dose oral iron therapy in Somalia was followed by an increase in malaria and amoebiasis. There was a higher mortality in Nigerian children receiving large doses of iron by mouth. Deaths were attributed to gram-negative septicaemia (McFarlane *et al.*, 1970). In another study in Nigeria the death rate was higher in children with PEM who were given iron supplements within three days of admission to hospital, compared with those in whom it was withheld for seven days (Smith *et al.*, 1989). A most striking finding has been the demonstration that children in Papua-New Guinea and Polynesian children in New Zealand had significantly increased morbidity, mainly respiratory, if they received intramuscular iron (Oppenheimer *et al.*, 1986). This may be another example of the toxic effects of iron according to the free radical hypothesis of tissue damage (Chapter 10), or it may be the effect of excess iron in enhancing microbial proliferation or in suppressing immunity.

Weinberg (1984) has stressed the role of iron-binding proteins at potential sites of invasion. The most important of these is lactoferrin, which is present in large amounts in human milk (Chapter 16), and also in other exocrine secretions and in the granules of polymorphonuclear leucocytes. Since lactoferrin is a glycoprotein, perhaps its synthesis is impaired in vitamin A deficiency.

Overall, the conclusion seems to be that when low-dose iron is given to iron-deficient subjects there is an increase in the immune response. If high-dose iron is given, the result depends on the environment. If there is much opportunity for microbial proliferation, then high doses of iron may increase infection. If there is not much infection the extra iron does not matter.

Zinc deficiency

Mucosal surfaces are frequently colonized by *Candida* in severe zinc deficiency states such as dermatitis enteropathica. Impaired cellular immunity in Jamaican children has been related to zinc deficiency. Although skin tests for cellular immunity showed improvement following the administration of topical zinc (Golden *et al.*, 1978), other studies have noted rather poor responses. In fact, in some studies of oral zinc supplementation there was a reduction in immune response (Chandra, 1984). It has also been suggested that zinc deficiency may be an important factor in the predisposition of malnourished children to become infected with *Trichuris*.

There is little information on the impact of zinc on susceptibility to infection. A recent study of the effect of zinc supplementation on diarrhoea in children in Bangladesh showed that those who received a course of zinc acetate experienced fewer episodes of diarrhoea in the following two months (Roy *et al.*, 1990).

Nutritional state and morbidity

There is clear evidence of increased incidence and prevalence of a range of infections in *severely* malnourished children, even in those living in relatively clean environments. This is familiar to every paediatrician who treats these cases (Chapter 12). The multiplication and invasion of pathogens is increased and case fatality rates are high. However, although the effect of severe malnutrition on morbidity and mortality is undoubted, the influence of mild or moderate PEM on the incidence, prevalence and severity of infections is much less clear. Most of the available information on this question relates to diarrhoea. Briend (1990) has reviewed the results of 15 studies in which, after an initial assessment of nutritional status, morbidity from diarrhoea was followed for periods of two months to two years. In 12 of the 15 studies there was some relation between nutritional state and morbidity. The association was absent in the studies with the longest period of follow-up (one to two years), during which time the nutritional state could have changed.

In a study in rural India in which morbidity was assessed weekly for a year, nutritional status, judged by weight for age, had no effect on the incidence or duration of diarrhoea (Mathur *et al.*, 1985). On the other hand, in The Gambia during the rainy season the prevalence of diarrhoea and fever increased steeply and significantly with decreasing weight for age and height for age (Fig. 17.7), but associations with weight for height were not significant (Tomkins *et al.*, 1989). In the dry season the trends were weaker or disappeared. There was no relationship of respiratory disease to nutritional status.

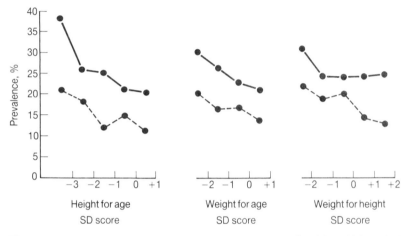

Fig. 17.7   Age-corrected prevalence of diarrhoea in young Gambian children during the rainy (————) and dry (— — — —) seasons, related to nutritional state at the beginning of each period. Reproduced by permission from Tomkins *et al.* (1989).

It is difficult to reconcile these somewhat conflicting observations. A possible hypothesis is that the incidence of diarrhoeal disease is related to the overall environmental stress, of which weight for age or height for age are appropriate indicators; on the other hand, acute malnutrition, as assessed by weight for height, is associated with increased severity and duration of diarrhoea (e.g. Black *et al.*, 1984; Bairagi *et al.*, 1987). Elimination of the pathogen, cell-mediated immunity and tissue repair are all likely to be affected by current nutritional state. Rivera *et al.* (1986) found a decreased cellular immune response in wasted but not in stunted children.

Low birth weight (small for gestational age) may also be regarded as a form of malnutrition (Chapter 18). Figure 17.8 illustrates vividly the effect of low birth weight on morbidity.

It has been suggested that discrepancies between different studies result from failure in some cases to take account of confounding variables. Pickering *et al.* (1989) examined the association between morbidity and a range of variables such as the mother's education, the style of house, water supply, sanitary facilities, etc. Some significant associations were found in the direction that one might expect. Illness and diarrhoea were reported less often in

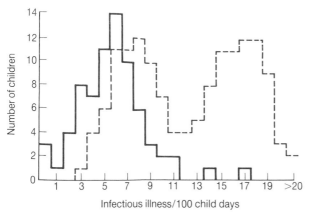

Fig. 17.8 Morbidity of healthy full-term infants (————) and of small for gestational age low birth weight infants (— — — —). Reproduced by permission from Chandra (1988).

children whose mothers had received more than primary schooling or who lived in cement-based houses rather than mud houses.

A further problem in clarifying these relationships is that a child who has an attack of diarrhoea is likely to come from a diarrhoea-prone environment and may have had a previous attack which caused it to become malnourished. This would complicate analysis of cause and effect (Chowdhury *et al.*, 1990).

In spite of the difficulties of determining the direction in which an association is working, Briend's analysis (1990) strongly suggests a real causal relationship between nutritional state and diarrhoeal morbidity. The relationship to mortality is considered in the next chapter.

Long-term effects of infection on growth

A hotly debated question is the relative importance of infection or inadequate food in producing the longer-term growth failure that is so often seen in pre-school children. The question is clearly of great importance for public health and the allocation of resources. Over the years there have been some shifts in opinion. In the 1950s the emphasis was on food and particularly protein. A change came with Gordon's work on weanling diarrhoea (1963), the WHO monograph on nutrition and infection (Scrimshaw *et al.*, 1968), and Mata's pioneering longitudinal studies in Guatemala (Mata, 1978*a*, *b*). For example, Fig. 17.9, which has been widely reproduced, shows the pattern of morbidity in relation to weight gain in a Guatemalan child. Mata and his co-workers showed that such a child has a profoundly reduced energy intake and concluded that 'there is a feeling of change from the orthodox emphasis on food to a position in which infection has greater relevance' (Mata *et al.*, 1977). In recent years there has been a tendency for the pendulum to swing the other way, perhaps because intervention measures such as improvements in sanitation, while reducing the prevalence of diarrhoea, have shown little effect on nutritional state (e.g. Briend *et al.*, 1989) (see Chapter 20).

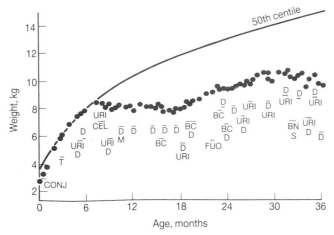

Fig. 17.9 Weight from birth to three years and episodes of infectious disease in a rural Guatemalan boy. The length of each horizontal line indicates duration of infectious disease. D, diarrhoea; URI, upper respiratory infections; BC, bronchitis; M, measles; T, oral thrush; BN, bronchopneumonia; CON, conjunctivitis; CEL, cellulitis; S, stomatitis; FUO, fever of unknown origin. Reproduced by permission of the American Society for Clinical Nutrition from Mata *et al.* (1977).

It is possible from the literature to make some quantitative estimates of the effect of infection on weight and height gain. When a child develops an infection, food intake has been observed to fall by about 20 per cent, as shown in Fig. 17.10 (Martorell *et al.*, 1980). If a child's 'normal' intake is, say, 750 kcal/day, the deficit in intake would be of the order of 150 kcal/day. If 1 g tissue corresponds to 4 – 5 kcal (Chapter 15), this implies a weight deficit of 30 – 40 g/day, which corresponds well with deficits actually observed (see below).

The end result over a period of time will depend on the proportion of days ill to days well, the weight deficit per day during illness and the weight gain per day during recovery. Figure 17.11 shows relationships between nutritional state, prevalence of infection and catch-up growth in a study in Brazil. The children had a mean age of 24 months, at which time the normal rate of gain is about 200 g/month. The better-nourished children gained almost at the normal rate in spite of very high prevalences of diarrhoea. Those who were undernourished gained at twice the normal rate so long as the diarrhoea prevalence was less than 30 per cent—a remarkable achievement!

In view of the large variability of weight gains per month even in children who are not ill (Chapter 13), it is clear that, as Briend (1990) has emphasized, any quantitative analysis of the relation between infection and growth or nutritional status must be based on observations over at least several months. The information needed is: (A) an estimate of the average per cent of the time for which a child is ill; and (B) an estimate of weight deficit per day ill, which can be obtained from regression of change in weight against duration of illness. The product A x B represents the calculated *impact* of infection in weight gain, which can be compared with actual gains.

This kind of analysis has been reported in three studies. The first was in rural Gambia (Rowland *et al*,. 1977); the second was in a suburban region of

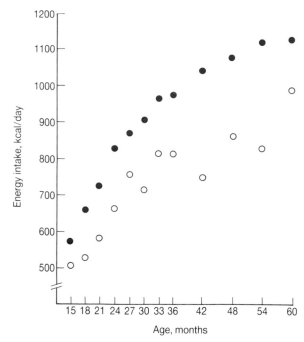

Fig. 17.10 Energy intake in the home of healthy (●) and sick (○) children in rural Guatemala. Reproduced by permission of the American Society for Clinical Nutrition from Martorell *et al.* (1980).

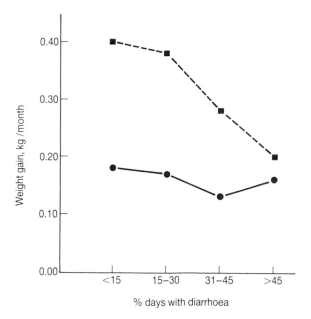

Fig. 17.11 Relation of weight gain to diarrhoea prevalence in children (average age 24 months) in North-east Brazil; – – ■ – –, children with weight for age below −3 SD; —●— , children with weight for age above −3 SD. Reproduced by permission from Schorling and Guerrant (1990).

Table 17.9   Contribution of infection to deficit in weight gain

Study	Gambia I[a]	Gambia II[b]	Khartoum[c]	
Age interval	1–2 years	6–12 months	3–6 months	6–9 months
Expected gain,[1] g	2400	2400	1630	1280
Observed gain, g	1800[2]	700[2]	1720	1020
Difference, observed–expected, g	−600	−1700	−210	−260
Calculated impact of infection	−1200[3]	−650[4]	−260[4]	−277[4]

[1] From NCHS; [2] estimated from authors' curves; [3] impact of diarrhoea only; [4] impact of diarrhoea + respiratory tract infection.
[a] From Rowland *et al.* (1977); [b] from Rowland *et al.* (1988); [c] from Zumrawi *et al.*(1987)

The Gambia (Rowland *et al.*, 1988); the third in the suburbs of Khartoum (Zumrawi *et al.*, 1987). The results are summarized in Table 17.9. In the first Gambian study the children on average had diarrhoea for 13 per cent of the time, and each day with diarrhoea produced a weight deficit of 25 g, a value similar to that derived from the study of Martorell *et al.* (1980) on food intake.

The table shows different responses in the three studies. In the first Gambian study the effect on weight gain was much less than would have been expected from the impact of infection, so that a considerable degree of catch-up had evidently been possible. In the second Gambian study the position was the opposite: the deficit in weight gain was much greater than the impact of infection, suggesting that food rather than infection was the main factor limiting growth. In Khartoum the results were intermediate: the deficit in growth could be accounted for entirely by infection, but catch-up did not occur. A somewhat different picture emerges when the Khartoum data were analysed in quartiles of attained weight at six months (Table 17.10). There was a large difference in weight gain between top and bottom quartiles, only a small part of which could be accounted for by a difference in the impact of infection, suggesting that an inadequate dietary intake played a major role

Some of the differences in responses shown in Table 17.10 could be related to the age of the children. It might be argued that children are particularly vulnerable to the effects of infection during the later months of infancy, when there is most likely to be a gap between food intake and requirements (Chap-

Table 17.10   Impact of infection on growth of children in top and bottom quartiles of attained weight at 6 months[a]

	Top quartile	Bottom quartile	Difference Top–bottom
12–24 weeks			
Weight gain, g	1770	950	+820
Impact of infection,[b] g	136	214	− 78
24–36 weeks			
Weight gain, g	1670	660	+1010
Impact of infection,[b] g	169	217	− 48

[a] The children were followed for one year, but for the purpose of other analyses, they were divided into quartiles of weight at 6 months.
[b] Diarrhoea + respiratory infection
From Zumrawi *et al.* (1987)

ter 15). Younger infants seem to fare better; in the Sudan cohort the impact of diarrhoea (g deficit in weight gain per day ill) was virtually nil in children below three months of age, with no difference between those who were exclusively or partially breast-fed. In The Gambia the impact of diarrhoea was also much less severe in the younger children; it was −6.6 g/day ill between birth and six months, compared with −15.4 g/day ill from seven to 12 months.

In a study in Peru (Lopez de Romaña *et al.*, 1989) the authors concluded that 'dietary insufficiency in the second semester may be a more important factor [than infection] in age-related decline in growth'. The energy intake of their children in the first six months of life was 90 per cent of that recommended, but it fell progressively with age to reach 75 per cent at 10–12 months.

The same kind of analysis can be applied to the effect of illness on growth in length. In the 1977 Gambian study there was a small but significant relationship between the prevalence of gastroenteritis and rate of gain in length, but illness could account for only a minor proportion of the observed deficit of growth in length between 12 and 24 months, suggesting that infection in this environment did not play an important role in the development of stunting. In the second Gambian study, in which the children were younger, there was no significant association between gain in length and any infection. Franks (1989) drew a similar conclusion from a small study on a Pacific atoll.

On the other hand, Lutter *et al.* (1989), working in Colombia, estimated that the cumulative effect of diarrhoea on length at three years of age was between 2.5 and 10 cm. The provision of supplementary food offset the effect, but even the supplemented children were 8 cm shorter than the NCHS reference. This study, therefore, still leaves us uncertain how far stunting results from infection or from deficiency of food.

Briend *et al.* (1989) have reported a study in Bangladesh which was carried out in a rather different way from those described above. Children aged six to 36 months were measured at intervals of three months. The overall prevalence of diarrhoea was 9.6 per cent. The gains over each three-month period of observation were classified in three groups, as shown in Table 17.11. The

Table 17.11 Weight and height gain in relation to the timing of diarrhoea in the previous three months before measurement

Group		No. of children	Weight gain (g/month)	Height gain (mm/month)
A.	No diarrhoea	821	155	7.8
B.	Diarrhoea in first 45 days after measurement	106	153	6.6*
C.	Diarrhoea in second 45 days after measurement	91	100*	7.6

Children aged 6–35 months were measured every three months. They were regarded as having diarrhoea only if it was present for at least 10 days.
Group B were children who had diarrhoea in the first 45 days of the three-month interval between measurements and no diarrhoea in the second 45 days;
Group C were those who had diarrhoea in the second but not the first 45 days, and therefore had less time for catch-up before being measured.
* P < 0.01 compared to children without diarrhoea.
From Briend *et al.* (1989)

deficit in weight gain related to diarrhoea was made good if a sufficient time elapsed (45 days or more) during which the child was free of diarrhoea (comparison of groups A and B). Deficit in height took longer to be established. Even without diarrhoea (group A) gains in weight were only 75 per cent and in height 80 per cent of those expected. Briend concluded that although the effects of diarrhoea were statistically significant, they were small and transient.

Some older semiquantitative studies point in the same direction. Martorell *et al.* (1977) in Guatemala calculated that over the period from birth to seven years the deficit in weight gain attributable to infection amounted to 0.49 kg, which was only 10 per cent of the total deficit in gain compared to US standards. In another study in Mexico (Condon-Paoloni *et al.*, 1977) there was very little difference in attained weights and heights at three years between children with high and low frequencies of diarrhoea.

These rather contradictory findings are precisely what one would expect if the end result is a balance between the quantitative impact of infection, the duration of anorexia and the availability of food. Both in individuals and in groups this balance will depend on many factors, including the age of the child. Cultural and social factors are clearly important, such as the time that parents can spare to coax a sick child to eat and attitudes about appropriate foods in the management of infection. It is not, perhaps, surprising that contrary judgements about the contribution of infection to growth deficit should be reached by authorities on different sides of the globe. Thus Martorell, from experience in Guatemala, states: 'A reasonable (even cautious) interpretation of the evidence is that infections are as important a cause of malnutrition as is the limited availability of food' (Martorell and Ho, 1984), whereas Briend (1990), on the basis of his studies in Bangladesh, says: 'We suggest that children in this community are malnourished mainly because they do not get enough food, outside as well as during episodes of diarrhoea'.

The studies that have been discussed above relate to relatively acute, even though repeated, episodes of illness, such as gastroenteritis or respiratory tract infections. Measles seems to be a special case, presumably because of the prolonged anorexia that it produces (Fig. 17.6). It is probably for this reason that in the Kasongo study relatively small deficits in weight and length (less than 1 SD unit) persisted for six months after the acute attack, particularly in children less than one year old (Van Lerberghe, 1990). Duggan and Milner (1986*b*) found that during the febrile stage of measles there was a negative energy balance averaging 40 kcal/kg/day, equivalent to almost half the maintenance energy requirement. The studies were repeated after varying intervals. Those children in whom the interval was longer than two months achieved an average positive balance of 38 kcal/kg/day, but with shorter periods of recovery the balances were smaller or still negative. This seems to be a situation in which, in contrast to diarrhoea, a long time has to pass before catch-up becomes possible.

Since the energy and protein requirements for catch-up growth are only a small percentage of the requirements for maintenance (Chapter 15), anorexia must be prolonged or the food supply be indeed marginal if it cannot provide this extra amount. Calloway (1982) reached a similar conclusion.

References

Archer, D. L., Glinsmann, W. H. (1985). Intestinal infection and malnutrition initiate acquired immune deficiency syndrome (AIDS). *Nutrition Research* **5:** 9–19.

Baragi, R., Chowdhury, M. K. *et al.* (1987). The association between malnutrition and diarrhoea in rural Bangladesh. *International Journal of Epidemiology* **16:** 477–481.

Basta, S. S., Soekirman *et al.* (1979). Iron deficiency anaemia and the productivity of adult males in Indonesia. *American Journal of Clinical Nutrition* **32:** 916–925.

Behrens, R. H., Lunn, P. G. *et al.* (1987). Factors affecting the integrity of the intestinal mucosa of Gambian children. *American Journal of Clinical Nutrition* **45:** 1433–1441.

Beresford, C. H., Neale, R. J., Brooke, O. G. (1971). Iron absorption and pyrexia. *Lancet* **1:** 568–572.

Bhaskaram, C., Reddy, V. (1974). Cell-mediated immunity in protein-calorie malnutrition. *Environmental Child Health* **20:** 284–286.

Bhaskaram, P., Sivakumar, B. (1986). Interleukin-1 in malnutrition. *Archives of Disease in Childhood* **61:** 182–185.

Bhaskaram, P., Madhusudhan, J. *et al.* (1986). Immune response in malnourished children with measles. *Journal of Tropical Pediatrics* **32:** 123–125.

Bhaskaram, P., Sharada, K. *et al.* (1989). Effect of iron and vitamin A deficiencies on macrophage function in children. *Nutrition Research* **9:** 35–45.

Black, R. E., Brown, K. H., Becker, S. (1984). Malnutrition is a determining factor in diarrheal duration but not incidence among young children in rural Bangladesh. *American Journal of Clinical Nutrition* **39:** 87–94.

Bradley-Moore, A. M., Greenwood, B. M. *et al.* (1985). Malaria chemoprophylaxis with chloroquine and young children: III. Its effect on nutrition. *Annals of Tropical Medicine and Parasitology* **79:** 575–584.

Briend, A. (1990). Is diarrhoea a major cause of malnutrition among under-five children in developing countries? *European Journal of Clinical Nutrition* **44:** 611–628.

Briend, A., Hasan, K. Z. *et al.* (1989). Are diarrhoea control programmes likely to reduce childhood malnutrition? Observations from rural Bangladesh. *Lancet* **2:** 319–322.

Calloway, D. H. (1982). Nutritional requirements in infectious diseases. *Review of Infectious Diseases* **4:** 891–895.

Chandra, R. K. (1972). Immunocompetence in undernutrition. *Journal of Pediatrics* **81:** 1194–1200.

Chandra, R. K. (1980). *Immunology of nutritional disorders.* Edward Arnold, London.

Chandra, R. K. (1983). Nutrition, immunity and infection: present knowledge and future directions. *Lancet* **1:** 688–691.

Chandra, R. K. (1984). Excessive intake of zinc impairs immune responses. *Journal of the American Medical Association* **252:** 1443–1446.

Chandra, R. K. (ed) (1988*a*). *Nutritional regulation of immunity.* Alan R. Liss, New York.

Chandra, R. K. (1988*b*). Nutrition, immunity and outcome: past, present and future. *Nutrition Research* **8:** 225–237.

Chandra, R. K. (1988*c*). Increased bacterial binding to respiratory epithelial cells in vitamin A deficiency. *British Medical Journal* **297:** 834–835.

Chandra, R. K., Seth, V. *et al.* (1977). Polymorphonuclear function in malnourished Indian children. In Suskind, R. M. (ed) *Malnutrition and the immune response.* Raven Press, New York, pp. 259–263.

Chowdhury, M. K., Gupta, V. M. *et al.* (1990). Does malnutrition predispose to diarrhoea during childhood? Evidence from a longitudinal study in Matlab, Bangladesh. *European Journal of Clinical Nutrition* **44:** 515–526.

Condon-Paoloni, D., Cravioto, J. *et al.* (1977). Morbidity and growth of infants and young children in a rural Mexican village. *American Journal of Public Health* **67:** 651–656.

Cook, G. C. (1971). Glucose absorption kinetics in Zambian African patients with and without systemic bacterial infections. *Gut* **12:** 1001–1006.

Cooper, E. S., Bundy, D. A. P. (1986). Trichuriasis in St. Lucia. In McNeish, A. S., Walker-Smith, J. A. (eds) *Diarrhoea and malnutrition in children.* Butterworth, London, pp. 91–96.

Cooper, E. S., Bundy, D. A. P. *et al.* (1990). Growth suppression in the *Trichuris* dysentery syndrome. *European Journal of Clinical Nutrition* **44:** 285–292.

Crompton, D. W. T. (1986). Nutritional aspects of infection. *Transactions of the Royal Society of Tropical Medicine and Hygiene* **80:** 697–705.

De Luca, L. M. (1977). The direct involvement of vitamin A in glycosyl transfer reactions of mammalian membranes. *Vitamins and Hormones* **35:** 1–57.

Diarrhoea Dialogue (1984). *Health basics: oral rehydration therapy.* Appropriate Health Resources and Technologies Action Group, 85 Marylebone High Street, London W1M 3DE, UK.

Dickin, K. L., Brown, K. H. *et al.* (1990). Effect of diarrhoea on dietary intake by infants and young children in rural villages of Kwara State, Nigeria. *European Journal of Clinical Nutrition* **44:** 307–318.

Dinarello, C. A. (1984). Interleukin-1. *Review of Infectious Diseases* **6:** 51–95.

Duggan, M. B., Milner, R. D. G. (1986*a*). Energy cost of measles infection. *Archives of Disease in Childhood* **61:** 436–439.

Duggan, M. B., Milner, R. D. G. (1986*b*). The maintenance energy requirement for children: an estimate based on a study of children with infection-associated underfeeding. *American Journal of Clinical Nutrition* **43:** 870–878.

Edirisinghe, J. S., Fern, E. B., Targett, G. A. T. (1981). Dietary suppression of rodent malaria. *Transactions of the Royal Society of Tropical Medicine and Hygiene* **75:** 591–593.

Elliott, K., Attawell, K. *et al.* (eds) (1990). *Cereal-based oral rehydration therapy for diarrhoea.* Aga Khan Foundation, Geneva and International Child Health Foundation, Columbia, Maryland, USA.

El-Rafie, M., Hassouna, W. A. *et al.* (1990). Effect of diarrhoeal disease control on infant and child mortality in Egypt. *Lancet* **1:** 334–338.

Farthing, M. J. G., Mata, L. *et al.* (1986). Natural history of *Giardia* infection of infants and children in rural Guatemala and its impact on physical growth. *American Journal of Clinical Nutrition* **43:** 395–405.

Field, M., Rao, M. C. *et al.* (1989). Intestinal electrolyte transport and diarrhoeal disease. *New England Journal of Medicine* **321:** 800–806, 879–883.

Fleck, A. (1989). Clinical and nutritional aspects of changes in acute-phase proteins during inflammation. *Proceedings of the Nutrition Society* **48:** 347–354.

Fleck, A., Colley, C. M., Myers, M. A. (1985). Liver export proteins and trauma. *British Medical Bulletin* **41:** 265–273.

Forman, M. R. (1989). Research priorities and strategies for investigating the influence of vitamin A supplementation on mortality. *Food and Nutrition Bulletin* **11:** 25–35.

Franks, A. J. (1989). Diarrhoea and malnutrition. *Lancet* **2:** 692 (letter).

Golden, M. H. N. (1989). Clinical assessment of oedema: implications for feeding the malnourished child. *European Journal of Clinical Nutrition* **43:** 581–582.

Golden, M. H. N., Jackson, A. A., Golden, B. E. (1977). Effect of zinc on thymus of recently malnourished children. *Lancet* **2:** 1057–1059.

Golden, M. H. N., Golden, B. E. *et al.* (1978). Zinc and immunocompetence in protein-energy malnutrition. *Lancet* **1:** 1226–1228.

Goldstein, S. A., Elwyn, D. H. (1989). Effects of injury and sepsis on fuel utilization. *Annual Review of Nutrition* **9:** 445–473.

Gordon, J. E., Ishwari, D. C., Wyon, J. B. (1963). Weaning diarrhoea. *American Journal of Medical Science* **245:** 345–377.

Gracey, M., Cullity, G. J., Suharjono, S. (1977). The stomach in malnutrition. *Archives of Disease in Childhood* **52:** 325–327.

Green, H. N., Mellanby, E. (1928). Vitamin A as an anti-infective agent. *British Medical Journal* **2:** 691–696.

Grimble, R. F. (1989). Cytokines: their relevance to nutrition. *European Journal of Clinical Nutrition* **43:** 217–230.

Grimble, R. F. (1990). Nutrition and cytokine action. *Nutrition Research Reviews* **3:** 193–210.

Harland, P. S. E. G. (1965). Tuberculin reactions in malnourished children. *Lancet* **2:** 719–721.

Hirschhorn, N. (1980). The treatment of acute diarrhoea in children: an historical and physiological perspective. *American Journal of Clinical Nutrition* **33:** 637–663.

Hoyle, B., Yunus, M., Chen, L. C. (1980). Breast-feeding and food intake among young children with acute diarrhoeal disease. *American Journal of Clinical Nutrition* **33:** 2365–2371.

Huang, C. M., Ruddel, M., Elin, R. J. (1988). Nutritional status of patients with acquired immunodeficiency syndrome. *Clinical Chemistry* **34:** 1957–1959.

Keusch, G. T., Farthing, M. J. G. (1986). Nutrition and infection. *Annual Review of Nutrition* **6:** 131–154.

Khin-Maung-U, Nyunt-Nyunt-Wai *et al.* (1985). Effect of breast-feeding during acute diarrhoea. *British Medical Journal* **290:** 587–589.

Kielmann, A. A., Uberoi, I. S. *et al.* (1976). The effect of nutritional studies on immune capacity and immune responses in preschool children in a rural community in India. *Bulletin of the World Health Organization* **54:** 477–483.

Lancet (1978). Water with sugar and salt. *Lancet* (editorial) **2:** 300–301.

Layrisse, M., Cook, J. D. *et al.* (1969). Food iron absorption: a comparison of vegetable and animal foods. *Blood* **33:** 430–443.

Lo, C. W., Walker, W. A. (1983). Chronic protracted diarrhoea of infancy: a nutritional disease. *Pediatrics* **72:** 786–800.

Lopez de Romaña, G., Brown, K. H. *et al.* (1989). Longitudinal studies of infectious diseases and physical growth of infants in Huascar, an underprivileged peri-urban community in Lima, Peru. *American Journal of Epidemiology* **129:** 769–784.

Lunn, P. G., Northrop-Clewes, C. A., Downes, R. M. (1991a). Chronic diarrhoea and malnutrition in The Gambia: studies on intestinal permeability. *Transactions of the Royal Society of Tropical Medicine and Hygiene* **85:** 8–11.

Lunn, P. G., Northrop-Clewes, C. A., Downes, R. M. (1991b). Intestinal permeability, mucosal injury and growth faltering in Gambian infants. *Lancet* **338:** 907–910.

Lutter, C. K., Mora, J. O. *et al.* (1989). Nutritional supplementation: effects on child stunting because of diarrhoea. *American Journal of Clinical Nutrition* **50:** 1–8.

McFarlane, G., Reddy, S. *et al.* (1970). Immunity, transferrin and survival in kwashiorkor. *British Medical Journal* **4:** 268–270.

McGregor, I. A. (1982). Malaria: nutritional implications. *Review of Infectious Diseases* **4:** 798–803.

McMurray, D. N., Watson, R. R., Reyes, M. A. (1981). Effect of renutrition on humoral and cell-mediated immunity in severely malnourished children. *American Journal of Clinical Nutrition* **34:** 2117–2126.

McNeish, A. S. (1986). The inter-relationships between chronic diarrhoea and malnutrition. In Walker-Smith, J. A., McNeish, A. S. (eds) *Diarrhoea and malnutrition in childhood*. Butterworth, London, pp. 1–6.

Martorell, R. (1989). Body size, adaptation and function. *Human Organization* **48:** 15–20.

Martorell, R., Ho, T. J. (1984). Malnutrition, morbidity and mortality. In Mosley,

H., Chen, L. (eds) *Child survival: strategies for research*. Supplement to Vol. 10 of Population and Development Review, 1984, pp. 49–68.

Martorell, R., Habicht J-P. *et al.* (1975). Acute morbidity and physical growth in rural Guatemalan children. *American Journal of Diseases of Children* **129**: 1296–1301.

Martorell, R., Lechtig, A. *et al.* (1977). Efecto de las diarreas sobre el retards en crecimiento fisico de ninos Guatemaltecos. *Archivos Latinoamericanos de Nutricion* **27**: 311–324.

Martorell, R., Yarbrough, C. *et al.* (1980). The impact of ordinary illness on the dietary intakes of malnourished children. *American Journal of Clinical Nutrition* **33**: 345–354.

Masawe, A. E. J., Muindi, J. M., Swai, G. B. R. (1974). Infections in iron deficiency and other types of anaemia in the tropics. *Lancet* **2**: 314–317.

Mata, L. J., Kromal, R. A. *et al.* (1977). Effect of infection on food intake and the nutritional state: perspectives as viewed from the village. *American Journal of Clinical Nutrition* **30**: 1215–1227.

Mata, L. J. (1978*a*). *The children of Santa Maria Cauqué: a prospective field study of health and growth*. MIT Press, Cambridge, Mass.

Mata, L. J. (1978*b*). The nature of the nutrition problem. In Joy, L. (ed) *Nutrition planning: the state of the art*. IPC Science and Technology Press, Surrey, UK, pp. 91–99.

Mathur, R., Reddy, V. *et al.* (1985). Nutritional status and diarrhoeal morbidity: a longitudinal study in rural Indian pre-school children. *Human Nutrition: Clinical Nutrition* **39C**: 447–454.

Milton, R. C., Reddy, V., Naidu, A. N. (1987). Mild vitamin A deficiency and childhood morbidity: an Indian experiment. *American Journal of Clinical Nutrition* **46**: 827–829.

Molla, A. (1983). Effects of acute diarrhoea on absorption of macronutrients during disease and after recovery. In Chen, L. C., Scrimshaw, N. S. (eds) *Diarrhoea and malnutrition: interactions, mechanisms and interventions*. Plenum Press, New York and London, pp. 143–154.

Molla, A. M., Molla, A. *et al.* (1989). Food-based oral rehydration salt solution for acute childhood diarrhoea. *Lancet* **2**: 429–431.

Morley, D. (1969). Severe measles in the tropics. *British Medical Journal* **1**: 297–300.

Nalin, D. R., Cash, R. A. *et al.* (1968). Oral maintenance therapy for cholera in adults. *Lancet* **2**: 370–373.

Nosten, F., ter Kuile, F. *et al.* (1991). Malaria during pregnancy in an area of unstable endemicity. *Transactions of the Royal Society of Tropical Medicine and Hygiene* **85**: 424–429.

Oomen, J. M. V., Meuwissen, J. H. E., Gemert, W. (1979). Differences in blood status of three ethnic groups inhabiting the same locality in northern Nigeria. Anaemia, splenomegaly and associated causes. *Tropical Geographical Medicine* **31**: 587–606.

Oppenheimer, S. J., Macfarlane, S. B. J. *et al.* (1986). Effect of iron prophylaxis on morbidity due to infectious disease: report on clinical studies in Papua-New Guinea. *Transactions of the Royal Society of Tropical Medicine and Hygiene* **80**: 596–602.

Orenstein, S. R., (1986). Enteral versus parenteral therapy for protracted diarrhoea of infancy. A prospective randomised trial. *Journal of Pediatrics* **109**: 277–286.

Pereira, S. M., Begum, A. (1987). The influence of illnesses on the food intake of young children. *International Journal of Epidemiology* **16**: 445–450.

Pickering, H., Hayes, R. J. *et al.* (1989). Alternative measures of diarrhoeal morbidity and their association with social and environmental factors in urban children in The Gambia. *Transactions of the Royal Society of Tropical Medicine and Hygiene* **81**: 853–859.

Rivera, J., Habicht J-P. *et al.* (1986). Decreased cellular immune response in wasted but not in stunted children. *Nutrition Research* **6**: 1161–1170.

Rowland, M. G. M., Cole, T. J., Whitehead, R. G. (1977). A quantitative study into the role of infection in determining nutritional status in Gambian village children. *British Journal of Nutrition* **37:** 441–450.

Rowland, M. G. M., Rowland, S. G. J. G., Cole, T. J. (1988). Impact of infection on the growth of children from 0–2 years in an urban West African community. *American Journal of Clinical Nutrition* **47:** 134–138.

Roy, S. K., Chowdhury, A. K. M. A., Rahaman, M. M. (1983). Excess mortality among children discharged from hospital after treatment of diarrhoea in rural Bangladesh. *British Medical Journal* **287:** 1097–1099.

Roy, S. K., Haider, R. *et al.* (1990). Persistent diarrhoea: clinical efficacy and nutrient absorption with a rice-based diet. *Archives of Disease in Childhood* **65:** 294–297.

Sarker, S. A., Wahed, M. A. *et al.* (1986). Persistent protein-losing enteropathy in post measles diarrhoea. *Archives of Disease in Childhood* **61:** 739–743.

Schorling, J. B., Guerrant, R. L. (1990). Diarrhoea and catch-up growth. *Lancet* **335:** 599–600.

Scrimshaw, N. S., Taylor, C. E., Gordon, J. E. (1968). *Interactions of nutrition and infection*. WHO Monograph Series No. 57. World Health Organization, Geneva.

Selvaraj, R. J., Bhat, K. S. (1972). Metabolic and bactericidal activities of leucocytes in protein-calorie malnutrition. *American Journal of Clinical Nutrition* **25:** 166–174.

Smith, I. F., Taiwo, O., Golden, M. H. N. (1989). Plant protein rehabilitation and iron supplementation of the protein-energy malnourished child. *European Journal of Clinical Nutrition* **43:** 763–768.

Smythe, P. M., Schorland, M. *et al.* (1971). Thymolymphatic deficiency and depression of cell-mediated immunity in protein-calorie malnutrition. *Lancet* **2:** 939–944.

Sommer, A., Katz, J., Tarwotjo, I. (1984). Increased risk of respiratory disease and diarrhea in children with pre-existing mild vitamin A deficiency. *American Journal of Clinical Nutrition* **40:** 1090–1095.

Sommer, A., Tarwotjo, I., Katz, J. (1987). Increased risk of xerophthalmia following diarrhea and respiratory disease. *American Journal of Clinical Nutrition* **45:** 977–980.

Srinivas, U., Braconier, J. H. *et al.* (1988). Trace element alterations in infectious diseases. *Scandinavian Journal of Clinical Laboratory Investigation* **48:** 495–500.

Stephenson, L. S. (1987). *The impact of helminth infections on human nutrition*. Taylor and Francis, London.

Stephenson, L. S., Crompton, D. W. T. *et al.* (1980). Relationships between *Ascaris* infection and growth of malnourished preschool children in Kenya. *American Journal of Clinical Nutrition* **33:** 1165–1172.

Suskind, R. M. (ed) (1977). *Malnutrition and the immune response*. Kroc Foundation Series, vol. 7. Raven Press, New York.

Thurnham, D. I. (1989). Vitamin A deficiency and its role in infection. *Transactions of the Royal Society of Tropical Medicine and Hygiene* **83:** 721–723.

Tomkins, A. M. (1981). Tropical malabsorption: recent concepts in pathogenesis and nutritional significance. *Clinical Science* **60:** 131–137.

Tomkins, A. M. (1983). Nutritional cost of protracted diarrhoea in young Gambian children. *Gut* **24:** 495A.

Tomkins, A. M. (1986). Protein-energy malnutrition and risk of infection. *Proceedings of the Nutrition Society* **45:** 289–304.

Tomkins, A. M. (1991). Recent developments in the nutritional management of diarrhoea. 1. Nutritional strategies to prevent diarrhoea among children in developing countries. *Transactions of the Royal Society of Tropical Medicine and Hygiene* **85:** 4–7.

Tomkins, A. M., Hussey, G. (1989). Vitamin A, immunity and infection. *Nutrition Research Reviews* **2:** 17–28.

Tomkins, A. M., Watson, F. (1989). *Malnutrition and infection. A review*. Advisory

Committee on Co-ordination/Subcommittee on Nutrition. World Health Organization, Geneva.

Tomkins, A. M., Dunn, D. T., Hayes, R. J. (1989). Nutritional status and risk of morbidity among young Gambian children allowing for social and environmental factors. *Transactions of the Royal Society of Tropical Medicine and Hygiene* **83**: 282–287.

Tomkins, A. M., Garlick, P. J. *et al.* (1983). The combined effects of infection and malnutrition on protein metabolism in children. *Clinical Science* **65**: 313–324.

Torun, B., Chew, F. (1991). Practical approaches towards dietary management of acute diarrhoea in developing communities. *Transactions of the Royal Society of Tropical Medicine and Hygiene* **85**: 12–17.

Ulijaszek, S. J. (1990). Nutritional status and susceptibility to infectious disease. In Harrison, G. A., Waterlow, J. C. (eds) *Diet and disease in traditional and developing societies*. Cambridge University Press, Cambridge, UK, pp. 137–154.

Usha, N., Sankaranarayanan, A. *et al.* (1990). Early detection of vitamin A deficiency in children with persistent diarrhoea. *Lancet* **335**: 422 (letter).

Van Lerberghe, W. (1990). Growth, infection and mortality: is growth monitoring an efficient screening instrument? In Tanner, J. M. (ed) *Auxology 88. Perspectives in the science of growth and development*. Smith-Gordon, Nishimura/London, pp. 101–110.

Wade, S., Parent, G. *et al.* (1988). Thymulin (Zn-FTS) activity in protein-energy malnutrition: new evidence for interaction between malnutrition and infection on thymic function. *American Journal of Clinical Nutrition* **47**: 305–311.

Waterlow, J. C. (1984). Protein turnover with special reference to man. *Quarterly Journal of Experimental Physiology* **69**: 409–438.

Weinberg, R. M. (1984). Iron withholding: a defense against infection and neoplasia. *Physiological Reviews* **64**: 65–102.

World Health Organization (1976). *Treatment and prevention of dehydration in diarrhoeal diseases*. WHO, Geneva.

World Health Organization (1986). *Oral rehydration therapy for treatment of diarrhoea in the home*. Report WHO/CDD/SER/86.9. WHO, Geneva.

World Health Organization (1988). Persistent diarrhoea in children in developing countries: memorandum from a WHO meeting. *Bulletin of the World Health Organization* **66**: 709–717.

World Health Organization (1990). *The rational use of drugs in the management of acute diarrhoea in children*. WHO, Geneva.

Zumrawi, F. Y., Dimond, H., Waterlow, J. C. (1987). Effects of infection on growth in Sudanese children. *Human Nutrition: Clinical Nutrition* **41C**: 453–462.

18
Malnutrition and mortality

Introduction

In developing countries, with some exceptions, official statistics of age-specific death rates are of limited accuracy and coverage, and often relate only to large towns. WHO, UNICEF and the UN statistical services have from time to time put together the available information, and often it is ten years or more out of date by the time that it reaches the reader. Conclusions in this chapter have to be seen in the light of these limitations.

Another kind of information is provided by prospective studies continuing over many years on defined population groups, usually rural. Examples are the demographic survey in Senegal by Cantrelle and Leridon (1971) and the numerous studies of the Matlab population in Bangladesh carried out by the International Centre for Diarrhoeal Disease Research in Dhaka. Long-continued investigations of mortality, morbidity, nutrition, etc. have been made on more limited groups, as in Kasongo, Zaïre (Van Lerberghe, 1990); the village of Santa Maria Cauqué and surrounding villages in the highlands of Guatemala (Mata, 1978); and the village of Keneba and its neighbourhood in The Gambia (McGregor, 1976). Such studies provide more accurate information on the mortality rates of children and on immediate and more remote causes of death. One limitation, however, is that it may be dangerous to generalize from small and localized samples. In The Gambia, for example, there were quite large differences in mortality rates between two adjacent villages (Billewicz and McGregor, 1981). A second problem is that the mere presence of health workers over many years can influence the situation, so that it is no longer typical.

Ten years ago it was estimated that of 120 million children born each year, between 10 and 18 million, or 8–15 per cent, would die by the age of five years (Gwatkin, 1980). This is an appalling figure, but it is well to remember also that 250 years ago the comparable figure in England was 75 per cent (Edmonds, 1835). Infant and child mortality rates worldwide and their changes over the past decades have been reviewed by Dyson (1977) and by Ashworth (1982a, b).

In most parts of the world these rates have been falling, although the debt crisis of the late 1980s is thought to have caused a setback. Because of increases in population the reductions in absolute numbers of deaths have been rather modest, with an actual increase in Sub-Saharan Africa (Figs. 18.1, 18.2).

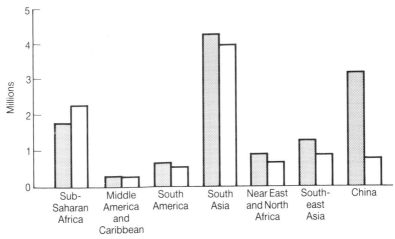

Fig. 18.1 Estimated numbers of infant deaths per year, by country group. ▨, 1960/65; ▯, 1980/85. From Carson and Wardlaw (1989).

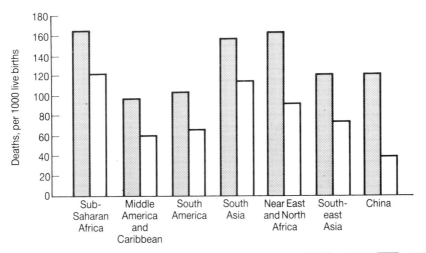

Fig. 18.2 Estimated infant mortality rates by country group. ▨, 1960/65; ▯, 1980/85. From Carson and Wardlaw (1989).

In Table 18.1 Feachem (1988) shows the relation between infant mortality rate (IMR), life expectancy and national wealth. However, as Feachem points out, there are some countries that are much healthier than their economic status predicts, and he lists as the five best performers Myanmar, China, Jamaica, Kerala State and Sri Lanka, with a median IMR of 36 in spite of a median GNP of only 310 US$ per head.

Table 18.1   Infant and child mortality rates and life expectancy in relation to GNP. Countries grouped according to mortality under 5 years

Mortality rate 0–5 years	Number of countries	Infant mortality rate[a]	Life expectancy[a] at birth	GNP per head[a] (US$, 1984)
> 175	32	136	46	260
95–174	31	83	57	740
30–94	29	44	67	1500
< 30	35	11	74	7300

[a] Median values for the group
From Feachem (1988)

We have to consider in this chapter the contribution of PEM to the high rates of death in early childhood. The IMR has long been regarded as an important index of public health in general. Some years ago it was suggested that the child mortality rate (CMR) from one year to the end of the fifth year of life (1–4+)* or, alternatively, mortality in the second year might give specific information about the nutritional state of children in a community (Wills and Waterlow, 1958; Gordon *et al.*, 1967). We reasoned, first, that in most reports the average age at which children presented at hospitals with severe PEM was between 12 and 24 months. Certainly there were exceptions, for example in Chile, where marasmus has for many years been the predominant form of PEM, presenting often in the first six months of life (Mönckeberg *et al.*, 1988). At the other extreme, the older literature shows that in Central Africa and India full-blown kwashiorkor was quite often seen in school-age children. In general, however, the highest prevalence was in the second year; this has been confirmed more recently by global UN figures showing that the peak prevalence of wasting also occurs at this time (Carlson and Wardlaw, 1990).

The second reason was that, by comparison with rates in well-to-do countries, the CMR in the Third World was relatively much higher than the IMR. In the 1950s–60s the death rate in the second year of life in a number of countries was 50–100 per 1000 (Gordon *et al.*, 1967). Dyson (1977) estimated the average CMR in the countries of tropical Africa to be 40 per 1000, which is some 50 times the CMR in Western Europe, whereas the ratio of IMRs was only about 15. Some examples are shown in Table 18.2. Although many of the figures are rather old, they suffice to reinforce the general point made by Dyson. The high relative CMRs stimulated many nutritional programmes specifically directed to this age-group, to a large extent neglecting infants. This was logical: the majority of child deaths should be preventable, since in Western countries they are prevented. However, in absolute terms more deaths occur in the first year than in any subsequent year, so if the aim is to reduce the number of deaths, infants should have priority.

---

* 4+ means to the end of the year beginning at age 4.0. The usual term 1–5 can be misleading. Hence CMR = average deaths per year between 1 and 4+ years per 1000 children alive at 1 year.

Table 18.2   Comparison of infant (IMR) and child (CMR) mortality rates in various countries at different epochs

Country	IMR[a]	CMR[b]	In relation to UK rates IMR	In relation to UK rates CMR	Reference
UK, 1978	13	0.55	–	–	1
France, 1901	148	17	×11	×31	1
Berlin, 1870	262	46	×20	×89	2
Brazil, 1970	109	11.5	×8	×21	1
Guatemala, 1958–64	100	30	×8	×55	3
India, Punjab, 1957–59	187	27	×14	×49	3
India, Tamil Nadu, 1973	119	19.5	×9	×35	4
Bangladesh, 1980	143	34	×11	×62	5
Senegal, 1971	205	89	×16	×162	6
The Gambia, 1951–75	239	85	×18	×154	7
Ghana, 1969	133	16	×10	×29	8

[a] IMR: per 1000 live births; [b] CMR: per 1000 alive at 1 year *per year* 1–4[+]

References:
1. Ashworth (1982a,b)
2. Prausnitz (1906)
3. Gordon *et al.* (1967)
4. Vellore (1973)
5. Chen *et al.* (1980b)
6. Cantrelle and Leridon (1971)
7. Billewicz and McGregor (1981)
8. Gaisie (1975)

Patterns of infant mortality

In Britain, France and Germany at the beginning of this century the IMR (deaths per 1000 live births) was more than 100 (Medical Research Council, 1917), comparable to that in many developing countries at the present time. There was, however, this difference, that in Britain the rate was much higher in the towns (150–160) than in the country (50–60), whereas the opposite is usually the case in the Third World, presumably due to better availability of medical services in the cities.

The temporal distribution of deaths in the first year has important implications for prevention. Cross (1979) introduced the concept of 'lethal day 50' (LD50), which is the number of days after birth by which 50 per cent of first year deaths have occurred. Table 18.3 shows how in Britain the LD50 has moved progressively to an earlier age as the IMR falls. In both advanced and less developed countries perinatal and neonatal deaths dominate the picture. Many of these deaths have special causes, such as prematurity, obstetric

Table 18.3   Infant mortality in the UK and lethal day 50 in four selected years

Year	Infant mortality /1000 live births	Lethal day 50	Causes of change	
1901	151	91 ⎫	Public health, water,	⎫
1935	57	28 ⎬	sewage, milk	⎬ Immunization,
1957	23	3 ⎱	Applied	⎰ medicine
1975	15.7	3 ⎰	physiology	

From Cross, 1979

complications, congenital defects and neonatal tetanus. For example, in the Matlab area of Bangladesh in 1975–77 tetanus neonatorum accounted for 26 per cent of infant deaths (Chen *et al.*, 1980*b*). Therefore in examining the effects of nutrition on mortality it is best to concentrate on post-neonatal deaths, which should be the most readily preventable.

Information on post-neonatal deaths month by month is difficult to obtain, but UN statistics do divide the post-neonatal period into two parts, one to six and six to 12 months. Figure 18.3 shows two contrasting examples. The data in Table 18.4 suggest, as in Fig. 18.3, that there are two patterns of distribution of deaths. In the first, seen in Latin America and Asia, there are more deaths between one and five months than between six and 12 months. The high mortality in the early post-neonatal period has little to do with nutrition. In developing countries most children are still breast-fed for at least the first few months of life (Chapter 16), and although growth failure may have begun it is not yet far advanced. Lower respiratory tract infections are a major cause of death in this period. It has been estimated that pneumonia accounts for 25 per cent of deaths between birth and five years, two-thirds occurring in infancy (Leoswki, 1986). It is only in the last decade that serious attention has been given to this subject (WHO, 1984; Shann, 1985; Lancet, 1985).

Diarrhoeal disease also plays a part in the early mortality, and is dominant

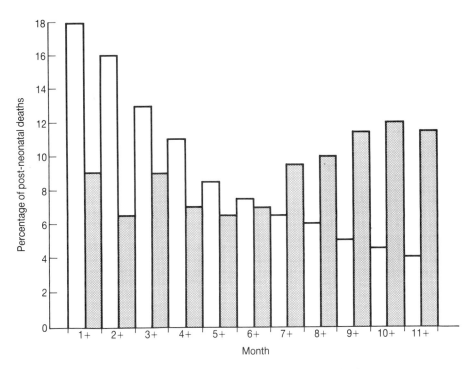

Fig. 18.3 Distribution of post-neonatal deaths: deaths in each month of age as percentage of all post-neonatal deaths. ☐, Latin America and the Caribbean; drawn from data of Puffer and Serano (1973); ▨, Senegal; drawn from data of Cantrelle and Leridon (1971).

Table 18.4   Distribution of infant deaths within the first year in various countries

Country	IMR	Neonatal	1–5+ months (A)	6–11 months (B)	A/B	Reference
		% of infant mortality rate[a]				
UK, 1984	9.5	32	32	10	3.2	1
Brazil, 1984	61	27	39	21	1.9	1
Guatemala, 1981	64	32	35	33	1.05	1
Costa Rica, 1983	18.5	60	30	12	2.5	1
Egypt, 1979	76.1	15.5	43.5	41	1.06	1
Sri Lanka, 1980	34.4	64.5	22	12.5	1.74	1
Thailand, 1984	11.3	39	35	15	2.35	1
Pakistan, 1979	94.5	52	35	13	2.70	1
Senegal, 1971	205	24	29	47[b]	0.62	2
The Gambia, 1951–75	239	31	20	35.5	0.56	3
Ghana, 1975	–	51	22.5	26.5[b]	0.85	4

[a] Except where otherwise indicated, perinatal deaths not included, so that the total of percentages is less than 100
[b] Neonatal includes perinatal deaths
References:
1. UN Demographic Yearbook, 1985, Table 22.
2. Cantrelle and Leridon (1971)
3. Billewicz and McGregor (1981)
4. Gaisie (1975)

in the later months of the first year. In Costa Rica Mata (1981) showed a close correlation between diarrhoeal deaths and total infant mortality rate. In the PAHO study in Latin America (Fig. 18.3), diarrhoeal disease was cited as a causal factor in 40–45 per cent of deaths over the whole post-neonatal period. In many countries the prevalence of diarrhoea peaks at around the end of the first year, in the weaning period. Thus it appears that children below six months are less likely to contract gastrointestinal infections, but when they do they are more likely to die.

In the other pattern, which seems from the limited data to be characteristic of tropical Africa two decades ago, mortality is higher in the second six months. If comparisons are made with India, Bangladesh or Guatemala, it is difficult to attribute these late infant deaths to the usual causes—low birth-weight, malnutrition or diarrhoeal disease. In the Kasongo study in Zaïre, although infant mortality figures were not considered to be reliable, four times as many deaths were recorded between six and 12 months as between one and six months, attributed mainly to measles (Van Lerberghe, 1990). In The Gambia malaria and meningitis are important factors (Greenwood *et al.*, 1987). The high IMR and CMR persisted unchanged in the Gambian village of Keneba for 25 years, from 1951 to 1975 (Billewicz and McGregor, 1981), and have only been reduced by the presence of a permanent medical team in the area (Lamb *et al.*, 1984). Even in a well-vaccinated rural Gambian population a recent report gave the IMR as 142 and the CMR as 43 per 1000 per year (Greenwood *et al.*, 1987).

The point being emphasized here is that the temporal pattern of deaths may give important clues to causes, particularly in regions where there are seasonal variations in the prevalence of diseases such as gastroenteritis and malaria (Billewicz and McGregor, 1981). Wherever infant mortality figures are collected, it would be possible to report them by month of age and by season, but this unfortunately is seldom done.

Patterns of child mortality

Disaggregated figures for deaths between one and five years are not available for many countries, but some examples are shown in Table 18.5. The mortality is highest in the second year of life (year 1+), and in most cases falls off rather gradually over the next two years. From Cross's rule (p. 328) one would expect the fall-off to be steeper when the absolute levels of CMR (Column 1) are lower, but there is no indication of this. All one can say is that, as in the first year of life, the younger the child the greater the risk. When resources are limited it would be sensible for programmes aimed at reducing child deaths to concentrate on the first two years of life.

Table 18.5 Pattern of child deaths at ages 1–4+ years in various countries

Country	Deaths 1–4+ years per 1000 alive at 1 year	% of child deaths by year				Reference
		1+	2+	3+	4+	
Berlin, 1870	46	47	24	17	12	1
Guatemala, 1958–64	30	46	27	17	10	2
Bangladesh, 1980	34	36	31	21	12	3
India, Tamil Nadu, 1973	19.5	30	29	23	18	4
India, Punjab, 1957–59	27	70	19	7	3	2
Zaïre, Kasongo, 1990	62	52	26	13	9	5
Senegal, 1971	89	54	31	11	4	6
The Gambia, 1951–75	85.5	43	30	16	11	7

References:
1. Prausnitz (1906)
2. Gordon *et al.* (1967)
3. Chen *et al.* (1980*b*)
4. Vellore (1973)
5. Van Lerberghe (1990)
6. Cantrelle and Leridon (1971)
7. Billewicz and McGregor (1981)

Effect of low birth weight on mortality

One of the most important contributors to infant and perhaps to child mortality is low birth weight. In 1980 it was estimated that of some 120 million babies born annually, 21 million were of low birth weight (LBW), according to the WHO definition of equal to or less than 2500 g (WHO, 1980; Hofvander, 1982). Ninety per cent of these LBW babies are born in developing countries and more than half of them in South-East Asia. Table 18.6 gives some examples of the distribution of birth weights. Table 18.7 shows the increased risk of neonatal and post-neonatal deaths associated with LBW. In terms of numbers, the most important group is that with birth weights between 2001 and 2500 grams. It is interesting that for both neonatal

Table 18.6   Percentage distribution of birth weights in various countries

Country	≤ 2000 g	2001–2500 g	2501–3000 g	Average birth weight (g)
England and Wales (1970)	2.3	4.6	18.9	3310
Mexico City (1970)	2.9	8.8	33.9	3025
Brazil (Ribeirao Preto, 1968)	2.7	6.0	23.5	3140
Guatemala (rural, 1964–71)	7.0	31.9	45.0	2551
Nigeria (Lagos, 1960)	4.1	9.0	10.7	3230
Senegal (Dakar, 1959)	3.0	6.9	26.4	3115
India (Bombay, 1970)	7.0	31.2	42.3	2636
Thailand (Bangkok, 1979)	1.7	8.9	37.0	2940
Indonesia (Jakarta, 1968)	8.7	14.4	54.7	2760

From WHO (1980)
Note that all the Third World figures, except for those from Guatemala, relate to big cities and are therefore not nationally representative, nor are they up-to-date.
   For further details on birth weights in Latin America, see Puffer and Serrano, 1987.

Table 18.7   Relative risk of death for low birth-weight children compared with risk for birth weight 2501–3000 g

Country	Neonatal deaths			Post-neonatal deaths			Reference
	Mortality rate[a]	Relative risk		Mortality rate[b]	Relative risk		
		1501 –2000	2001 –2500		1501 –2000	2001 –2500	
UK	5.2	13.4	3.4	4.2	4.3	1.8	1
Brazil (Ribeirao Preto)	28.2	23.3	4.0	–	–	–	2
India (Delhi)	21.2	30.8	4.5	25.3	5.3	2.2	2
India (rural)	45.6	16.1	3.3	–	–	–	3
Guatemala (rural)	39.0	27.3	3.4	60.0	7.0	0.8	2

[a] per 1000 live births
[b] per 1000 survivors
References:
1. Office of Population Censuses and Surveys (1988)
2. Ashworth and Feachem (1985)
3. Pratinidhi *et al.* (1986)

and post-neonatal deaths the relative risk at this range of birth weight is much the same in four very different environments. For neonatal deaths it is about four-fold, for post-neonatal about two-fold.

   Low birth weight should be divided into two categories, pre-term and small for gestational age (SGA), although this is seldom possible in national statistics. It is the latter group that is probably the most important from the nutritional point of view. The proportion of LBW infants who are SGA tends to be somewhat higher in developing than in affluent countries, although the difference is not very clear-cut. The mortality rate of SGA babies tends to be lower than that of preterm, particularly in the neonatal period (Pratinidhi *et al.*, 1986).

The risk that results from LBW is evidently not confined to the first year. In a cohort of children studied in The Gambia in the 1970s, the average age of post-neonatal deaths was 19 months and 78 per cent of these were children born in the hungry season, when mothers' body weights were depressed and birth weights were low (A. M. Prentice, personal communication).

Kramer (1987) has examined in detail the determinants of LBW. It is generally accepted that birth weight is related to the mother's weight (e.g. Thomson *et al.*, 1968) and to her gain in weight during pregnancy. In a study in Senegal there was also a significant correlation between birth weight and mother's height (Briend, 1985), and in Guatemala a close relationship was found between maternal height and infant mortality (Martorell, 1989).

Several attempts have been made to increase birth weight by supplementary feeding of the mother during pregnancy. In The Gambia a supplement of 400 kcal/day improved birth weight by a mean of 230 g and reduced the incidence of LBW from 28 per cent to 5 per cent, but this happened only in the wet season; in the dry season the supplement had no effect (Prentice *et al.*, 1983). In Colombia a supplement of 800 kcal/day in the third trimester of pregnancy produced an increase of nearly 200 g in the birth weight of babies whose mothers were thin (weight/height < 360 g/cm) (Herrera *et al.*, 1980). In Guatemala an energy supplement of 20 000 kcal, amounting to 25 per cent of the total extra requirement for pregnancy (FAO/WHO/UNU, 1985), produced an increase of only 110 g in birth weight (Lechtig *et al.*, 1975). A later analysis of this study showed that when a mother continued to lactate well into the next pregnancy—a situation that would produce particular stress—there was some decrease in her fat stores, but no effect on the birth weight (Merchant *et al.*, 1990). These mothers did, however, take more of the supplement that was made available to them. Ramachandran (1990) concluded that the impact of such feeding programmes on birth weight was very limited. What we do not know is the effect on mortality of small differences in birth weight, e.g. between 2300 and 2500 g.

It may be that the problem starts earlier than the actual pregnancy. Teenage pregnancies are notorious in resulting in low birth weight. In a study in India girls were divided at the age of five into nutritional groups according to their height. By the time that they became pregnant the height differential between the groups had disappeared; nevertheless, the early nutritional state did have a small effect on birth weight and on infant mortality rate (Ramachandran, 1989). In the words of McCarrison 50 years ago, quoted by Lind (1984): 'The satisfaction of nutritional needs in pregnancy begins with the antenatal lives of the mothers of our race.'

Birth interval is also important, for both infant and neonatal mortality (see Chapter 20). The effect is most evident for birth intervals of less than two years, and it is here that the influence of prolonged breast feeding is crucial (Chapter 16).

Contribution of PEM to mortality

Mortality statistics do not give a clear picture of the contribution of PEM to infant and child mortality. There are obvious problems over the accuracy of the diagnoses, which are frequently retrospective. Malnutrition is often not mentioned. In an analysis of nearly 13 000 infant and child deaths in Bangladesh malnutrition was not included in a list of ten specific causes of death (Chen *et al.*, 1980*b*). In their very extensive survey in Latin America Puffer and Serrano (1973) found that malnutrition was not very often cited as a direct cause, but they considered that it was a contributory cause in nearly 50 per cent of infant and child deaths.

The contribution of malnutrition must vary with the prevailing pattern of disease, since diseases differ in the extent to which malnutrition is a predisposing factor. If there is a common and powerful cause of death that has only a weak relation to nutritional status, anthropometric indicators will have very little value for the purpose of prediction. An example here is malaria: Trape *et al.* (1987), on the basis of WHO statistics, estimated that malaria might account for 15 deaths per 1000 children between birth and four years in the world as a whole. In The Gambia chemoprophylaxis reduced the mortality rate in children between one and four years from 60 per 1000 to 27 (Greenwood *et al.*, 1988). In an area where malaria is endemic, the child mortality rate would bear little or no relation to the prevailing state of nutrition.

At the other end of the spectrum is diarrhoeal disease, which is inextricably interwoven with malnutrition (Chapter 17). To give two examples: in a study in Uganda the risk of death was increased ten-fold in children with diarrhoea if their weight for age was below −2 SD or their mid-arm circumference less than 12 cm (Vella *et al.*, 1991). These relationships were essentially unchanged when social and environmental factors were allowed for. In Bangladeshi children who weighed less than 55 per cent weight for age the death rate was 14 per cent within three months of discharge from a diarrhoeal disease treatment centre, compared with 1 per cent if the children's weight for age was 75 per cent or more at the time of discharge (Roy *et al.*, 1983). In Senegal the fatality rate for children admitted to hospital with diarrhoea was increased more than two-fold if weight for height was less than 80 per cent, and six-fold in those with oedema (Beau *et al.*, 1987).

Measles perhaps occupies an intermediate position. Morley (1969) drew attention to the remarkable severity of measles in Nigeria, and attributed it to malnutrition, whereas Chen *et al.* (1980*b*) in Bangladesh considered that malnutrition played little part in this infection. In one study in West Africa the severity was attributed to overcrowding, which allowed a child to receive a very large dose of virus over a short period of time (Aaby *et al.*, 1984, 1988). Case fatality rates in measles have been reviewed by Van Lerberghe (1990). There is certainly a remarkable and unexplained difference in the severity of measles in Africa and the Indian sub-continent. Some representative case fatality rates are: USA 0.1 per cent; The Gambia 14–15 per cent (Hull *et al.*, 1983); West Bengal 1.1 per cent (Sinha, 1977). One reason for the high fatality rates is that measles occurs at a younger age in the Third World, but this does not explain the difference between the two continents.

The importance of lower respiratory tract infections has already been mentioned. The commonest causative organisms of pneumonia are *Streptococcus pneumoniae* and *Haemophilus influenzae*. Bang *et al.* (1990) have reported a significant reduction in mortality from pneumonia by treatment with cotrimoxazole. This successful programme in India was carried out by paramedics, village health workers and traditional birth attendants, who were trained in the recognition and management of pneumonia according to the guidelines proposed by WHO (1982, 1988). The case-fatality rate was reduced to 0.8 per cent, compared with 13.5 per cent in control villages. After a year of intervention the pneumonia-specific mortality in children under five was more than halved, the effect being greatest in children under one year. There is little information about the extent to which malnutrition predisposes to these infections or influences the fatality rate.

Vitamin A deficiency and mortality

Mention has been made in the previous chapter (pp. 309, 310) of the effect of vitamin A deficiency on morbidity from respiratory infections and diarrhoeal disease. Here we are concerned with mortality, although admittedly the separation is artificial. McLaren *et al.* (1965) observed higher rates of mortality in severely malnourished children who were xerophthalmic compared with those who were not, as did Sommer *et al.* (1983) in children in the community who were only slightly xerophthalmic. Great interest has been aroused by a study of Sommer *et al.* (1986) in Indonesia which indicated that supplements of vitamin A (200 000 IU six-monthly) reduced mortality by 34 per cent compared with a control group. A more recent study in Indonesia using monosodium glutamate fortified with vitamin A showed a similar reduction in mortality (Muhilal *et al.*, 1988).

Replication of this work in India has given contradictory results. In one study in which vitamin A was given, as in Indonesia, in a massive dose, there was no difference between groups receiving vitamin A and placebo (Vijayaraghavan *et al.*, 1990). In both groups the mortality fell well below the national average and was inversely related to the number of capsules that the children received. It is argued that this is an indication of their contact with the health services, which, rather than the supplement, is the crucial factor (Gopalan, 1990). In a second trial in India weekly supplements of vitamin A were given in amounts that would potentially be available in foods (approximately 8000 IU per week). Mortality was reduced by 34 per cent in the treated group, particularly in children less than three years old and in those who were stunted (Rahmathullah *et al.*, 1990).

The interpretation of these four studies has been discussed by Forman (1989). A fifth trial recently reported from Nepal has shown a 30 per cent decrease in mortality, compared with controls, in children aged six months to six years who received 60 000 retinol equivalents of vitamin A every four months for a year (West *et al.*, 1991). Thus four out of five community trials have shown an effect.

In a study in Tanzania vitamin A supplements reduced the case-fatality rate from measles in malnourished children in hospital (Barclay *et al.*, 1987). It is currently recommended by WHO that vitamin A capsules should be given in all cases of measles where the case-fatality rate customarily exceeds 1 per cent.

Mortality is also influenced by social and cultural factors such as breast feeding (Chapter 16), sanitary facilities (Rahman *et al.*, 1985), the mother's education, the time available for looking after children etc. In a community study in The Gambia a significant risk factor for death was animals being kept in the compound (Pickering *et al.*, 1986). Another was the mother being self-employed; those who had regular paid work left their children with grandmothers—a pattern that is also found in the Caribbean, but in that culture does not appear to be disadvantageous (Sinha, 1988). Allowance has to be made for these confounding variables in assessing the specific contribution of PEM to mortality.

Anthropometric assessment of the risk of death

Prospective studies of mortality require large numbers of children to be followed over a substantial period of time. This is a major undertaking and therefore not many such studies have been done. The first was that of Sommer and Loewenstein (1975) in Bangladesh, who used arm circumference for height (QUAC stick) as the predictor. They found a clear relation between arm circumference and mortality rate, particularly in children of three years and below. Kielmann and McCord (1978) in the Punjab used weight for age, and showed that at all levels of weight for age the risk was greater in children initially below one year of age than in those aged one to three years. The threshold for a significant increase in risk was 80 per cent weight for age by the Harvard standard below one year, and 70 per cent in the older children.

Two years later Chen *et al.*, (1980*a*) published a study of key importance from Bangladesh. The initial ages of the children in their cohort ranged from 15 to 26 months, so no infants were included, and they were followed for two years. Four indices were used: weight for age, weight for height, height for age and arm circumference. The results in Fig. 18.4 show a clear threshold

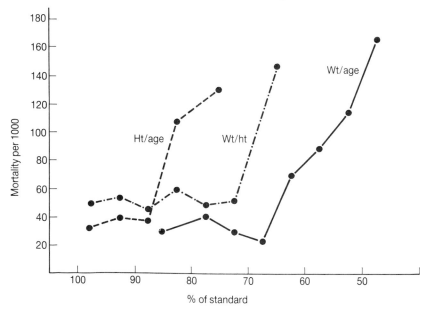

Fig. 18.4 Relation of deaths per 1000 children in Matlab, Bangladesh, to anthropometric estimates of nutritional status. Reproduced by permission of the American Society for Clinical Nutrition from Chen *et al.* (1980*a*).

effect. Very similar findings were reported by Heywood (1982) from Papua-New Guinea. It would seem from these figures that mild and moderate degrees of deficit had little predictive power. In the Bangladesh study, for all three indices the mortality rate in children classified as severe was greater in the second year of follow-up. This led Chen *et al.* to suggest that these severely malnourished children might represent a special sub-group particularly exposed to social and environmental handicaps.

Subsequent discussion centred round the relative value of the different indices in terms of their sensitivity and specificity (Chapter 14). Weight for height is a useful predictor over the short term; weight for age and height for age perform better over the longer term, i.e. one to two years. No advantage was found in correcting arm circumference for age or height.

A problem discussed in detail by Habicht *et al.* (1982) is to identify the cut-off points that give the best predictive power. If the cut-off is too low, many children who subsequently die will be missed (low sensitivity); if it is too high, the number of children expected to die will be over-estimated (low specificity), making the process of screening inefficient. Table 18.8, from a study in Uganda (Vella, 1990), illustrates the predictive performance of the various indicators at the conventional cut-off points. All have rather low specificity. The poor performance of the two measures of thinness may be because the interval between the initial measurements and follow-up was one year. It is likely that the predictive power of the different indicators depends on how far ahead they are predicting.

Table 18.8 Efficiency of various anthropometric indicators in predicting death over an interval of one year in rural Uganda. Total number of deaths, 96

Index	Deaths predicted	Deaths not predicted
Weight for age < −2 SD	37	59
Height for age < −2 SD	40	56
Weight for height < −2 SD	12	84
Mid-upper arm circumference < 12.5 cm	25	71

Data from Vella (1990)

Bairagi *et al.*, (1985) extended their studies in Bangladesh to take account of season and to include weight and height velocities as indicators. The velocities showed no advantage over the standard indicators for periods over a year, but weight velocity was found to be a good predictor of short-term mortality (two months). Briend *et al.* (1987), working in the same area, have taken the anthropometric identification of risk a stage further. They followed 5000 children initially aged six to 36 months at monthly intervals, using arm circumference as the only indicator. Common infectious diseases were also examined as risk factors (Table 18.9). In contrast to the results in Fig. 18.4, there was no threshold effect, but a suitable cut-off point could be chosen according to local conditions and resources. Two other points stand out in this study: the rather low relative risk imposed by diarrhoea and the high risk related to the presence of oedema. This is not really in contradiction with the clinical finding (Chapter 12) that in severe PEM the presence or absence of oedema has little prognostic significance, because in the clinical situation the risk is being

Table 18.9   Relative risk of death associated with various factors in Matlab, Bangladesh

Risk factor	Relative risk
Female gender	2.6
No breast-feeding	2.1
Any diarrhoea	4.8
Diarrhoea > 7 days	7.6
Bloody diarrhoea	11.3
Acute respiratory infection	11.6
Oedema	84.1
Mid-upper arm circumference ≤ 10 cm	48.0
Mid-upper arm circumference ≤ 11 cm	20.1
Mid-upper arm circumference ≤ 12 cm	11.1
Mid-upper arm circumference ≤ 13 cm	6.3

From Briend *et al.* (1987)

related not to that in normal children but to that in other children with severe PEM but without oedema.

Briend *et al.* (1989) reported that the absolute arm circumference (AC) was the best predictor of death, without any correction for age. They proposed that the risk of death depended on the extent to which the protein reserves of the body, as represented by muscle, are depleted. A given value of the AC, e.g. 11 cm, carries the same risk in a child at one year or three years: in the older child the deficit is greater compared with the expected AC; in the younger child the deficit is less, but this is counterbalanced by the increased risk that results from being young.

All these reports suggest strongly that PEM as assessed by the usual anthropometric criteria (Chapter 14) is indeed associated with a high mortality rate. Chen (1986) calculated that in the Matlab area of Bangladesh 45 per cent of deaths were nutrition-related. It is remarkable that this estimate from prospective studies agrees closely with that found in the retrospective PAHO child mortality survey (Puffer and Serrano, 1973).

Most of the studies described so far were made in South-East Asia. In Africa the most detailed investigation that has been reported to date is the Kasongo study in Zaïre (Kasongo Project Team, 1983; Van Lerberghe, 1990). Some 6000 children were followed, but the age-group below six months was under-represented, so that reliable figures were not obtained for infant mortality. The child mortality in the Kasongo group was 15.5 per year per 1000 children alive at one year, which is similar to that of Matlab children—13.1 per 1000 per year (Chen, 1986). In spite of this similarity, the relationships between anthropometric indices and risk of death were quite different from those found in Matlab. The specificities and sensitivities of all the indicators were lower in Kasongo. With weight for age as indicator, in Matlab the risk of death for the lowest 10 per cent was 4.5 times that for the highest 10 per cent, whereas the comparable risk ratio in Kasongo was 1.4. The weights and heights of the children who died were not significantly different from those of the whole cohort, but height velocities in the months before death were significantly lower, particularly in younger children.

Van Lerberghe (1990) suggests that the difference between the results in Zaïre and Bangladesh arises from the greater homogeneity of the Kasongo children. There does not seem to be the same high-risk sub-group related to low socioeconomic status that was postulated by Chen *et al.* (1980*a*). Another factor may be that the immediate causes of death were different in the two groups. As mentioned earlier, measles was a far more common cause in Kasongo, whereas diarrhoea was less important.

A certain amount of additional information has been provided by nutrition intervention studies, summarized by Ashworth (1982*b*) and Martorell and Ho (1984). The large-scale projects at Narangwal (Punjab) and INCAP (Guatemala) did not give very clear-cut answers, probably because of the confounding effect of providing medical care as well as food. However, a striking reduction in mortality was obtained in a programme in which supplementary food was given to all members of the family without medical intervention (Baertl *et al.*, 1970).

In conclusion, PEM, as judged by any of the anthropometric indicators, contributes to death. It is impossible to make a general estimate of the strength of the relationships, because other factors such as age and the prevailing pattern of disease have to be taken into account. Much has been written about the definition of indicators that are the best predictors of death, in terms of sensitivity and specificity. For operational purposes this quest does not seem to be particularly useful, since the best compromise will vary from one population to another, and for short-term screening will be determined mainly by the resources available, as discussed in Chapter 14.

References

Aaby, P., Bukh, J. *et al.* (1984). Determinants of measles mortality in a rural area of Guinea-Bissau: crowding, age and malnutrition. *Journal of Tropical Pediatrics* **30**: 164–167.

Aaby, P., Bukh, J. *et al.* (1988). Decline in measles mortality: nutrition, age at infection or exposure? *British Medical Journal* **296**: 1225–1228.

Ashworth, A. (1982*a*). International differences in infant mortality and the impact of malnutrition. *Human Nutrition: Clinical Nutrition* **36C**: 7–23.

Ashworth, A. (1982*b*). International differences in infant mortality and the impact of malnutrition. *Human Nutrition:Clinical Nutrition* **36C**: 279–288.

Ashworth, A., Feachem, R. G. (1985). Interventions for the control of diarrhoeal diseases among young children: prevention of low birth weight. *Bulletin of the World Health Organization* **63**: 165–184.

Ashworth, A., Waterlow, J. C. (1982). Infant mortality in developing countries. *Archives of Disease in Childhood* **57**: 882–884.

Baertl, J. M., Morales, E. *et al.* (1970). Diet supplementation for entire communities. *American Journal of Clinical Nutrition* **23**: 707–715.

Bairagi, R., Chowdhury, M. K. *et al.*, (1985). Alternative anthropometric indicators of mortality. *American Journal of Clinical Nutrition* **42**: 296–306.

Bang, A. T., Bang, R. A. *et al.* (1990). Reduction in pneumonia mortality and total child-based mortality by means of community-based intervention trial in Gadchiroli, India. *Lancet* **336**: 201–206.

Barclay, A. J. G., Foster, A., Sommer, A. (1987). Vitamin A supplements and mortality related to measles. *British Medical Journal* **294**: 294–296.

Beau J-P., Garenne, M. *et al.* (1987). Diarrhoea and nutritional status as risk factors of child mortality in a Dakar hospital (Senegal). *Journal of Tropical Pediatrics* **33**: 4–9.

Billewicz, W. Z., McGregor, I. A. (1981). The demography of two West African (Gambian) villages, 1951–1975. *Journal of Biosocial Science* **13**: 219–240.

Briend, A. (1985). Do maternal energy reserves limit fetal growth? *Lancet* **1**: 38–40.

Briend, A., Wojtyniak, B., Rowland, M. G. M. (1987). Arm circumference and other factors in children at high risk of death in rural Bangladesh. *Lancet* **2**: 725–728.

Briend, A., Garenne, M. *et al.* (1989). Nutritional status, age and survival: the muscle mass hypothesis. *European Journal of Clinical Nutrition* **43**: 715–726.

Cantrelle, P., Leridon, H. (1971). Breast feeding, mortality in childhood and fertility in a rural zone of Senegal. *Population Studies* **25**: 505–533.

Carlson, B. A., Wardlaw, T. M. (1989). Draft report on global, regional and country assessment of child malnutrition. UNICEF, New York.

Chen, L. C. (1986). Primary health care in developing countries: overcoming operational, technical and social barriers. *Lancet* **2**: 1260–1265.

Chen, L. C., Chowdhury, A. K. M. A., Huffman, S. L. (1980*a*). Anthropometric assessment of energy-protein malnutrition and subsequent risk of pre-school mortality among pre-school aged children. *American Journal of Clinical Nutrition* **33**: 1836–1845.

Chen, L. C., Rahman, M., Sarder, A. M. (1980*b*). Epidemiology and causes of death among children in a rural area of Bangladesh. *International Journal of Epidemiology* **9**: 25–33.

Cross, K. W. (1979). La chaleur animale and the infant brain. *Journal of Physiology* **294**: 1–21.

Dyson, T. (1977). Levels, trends, differentials and causes of child mortality—a survey. *World Health Statistics Report* **30**: 282–311. World Health Organization, Geneva.

Edmonds, T. R. (1835). On the mortality of infants in England. *Lancet* **1**: 690–695.

FAO/WHO/UNU (1985). Energy and protein requirements. Report of a Joint FAO/WHO/UNU Consultation. *Technical Report Series No. 724*. World Health Organization, Geneva.

Feachem, R. G. (1988). Epidemiology and tropical public health: current and future contributions with particular emphasis on the role of the London School of Hygiene and Tropical Medicine. *Transactions of the Royal Society of Tropical Medicine and Hygiene* **82**: 790–798.

Forman, M. R. (1989). Research priorities and strategies for investigating the influence of vitamin A supplementation on mortality. *Food and Nutrition Bulletin* **11**: 25–35.

Gaisie, S. K. (1975). Levels and patterns of infant and child mortality in Ghana. *Demography* **12**: 21–34.

Gopalan, C. (1990). Vitamin A and child mortality. *Bulletin of the Nutrition Foundation of India* **11**: no. 3.

Gordon, J. E., Wyon, J. B., Ascoli, W. (1967). The second year death rate in less developed countries. *American Journal of Medical Sciences* **254**: 357–380.

Greenwood, B. M., Greenwood, A. M. *et al.* (1987). Deaths in infancy and early childhood in a well-vaccinated, rural West African population. *Annals of Tropical Paediatrics* **7**: 91–99.

Greenwood, B. M., Greenwood, A. M. *et al.* (1988). Comparison of two strategies for the control of malaria within a primary health care programme in The Gambia. *Lancet* **1**: 1121–1127.

Gwatkin, D. R. (1980). How many die? A set of demographic estimates of the annual number of infant and child deaths in the world. *American Journal of Public Health* **70**: 1286–1289.

Habicht J-P., Meyers, L. D., Brownie, C. (1982). Indicators for identifying and counting the improperly nourished. *American Journal of Clinical Nutrition* **35**: 1241–1254.

Herrera, M. G., Mora, J. O. *et al.* (1980). Maternal weight/height and the effect of food supplementation during pregnancy and lactation. In Aeti, H., Whitehead, R. G. (eds) *Maternal nutrition during pregnancy and lactation*. Hans Huber, Bern, pp. 252–263.

Heywood, P. (1982). The functional significance of malnutrition—growth and prospective risk of death in the highlands of Papua-New Guinea. *Journal of Food and Nutrition* **39**: 13–19.

Hofvander, Y. (1982). International comparisons of potential growth of low birth weight infants with special reference to differences between developing and affluent countries. *Acta Paediatrica Scandinavica* **296**: (Suppl.) 14–18.

Hull, H. F., Williams, P. J., Oldfield, F. (1983). Measles mortality and vaccine efficacy in rural West Africa. *Lancet* **1**: 972–975.

Kasongo Project Team (1983). Anthropometric assessment of young children's nutritional status as an indicator of subsequent risk of dying. *Journal of Tropical Pediatrics* **29**: 69–75.

Kielmann, A. A., McCord, C. (1978). Weight for age as an index of risk of death. *Lancet* **1**: 1247–1250.

Kramer, M. S. (1987). Determinants of low birth weight: methodological assessment and meta-analysis. *Bulletin of the World Health Organization* **65**: 663–737.

Lamb, W. H., Foord, F. A. *et al.* (1984). Changes in maternal and child mortality rates in three isolated Gambian villages over ten years. *Lancet* **2**: 912–914.

Lancet (1985). (Leading article). Acute respiratory infections in under-fives: 15 million deaths a year. *Lancet* **2**: 699–701.

Lechtig, A., Habicht, J. P. *et al.* (1975). Effect of food supplementation during pregnancy on birth weight. *Pediatrics* **56**: 508–520.

Leoswki, J. (1986). Mortality from acute respiratory infections in children under 5 years of age: global estimates. *WHO Statistical Quarterly* **39**: 138–144.

Lind, T. (1984). Could more calories per day keep low birth weight at bay? *Lancet* **1**: 501–502.

McGregor, I. A. (1976). Health and communicable diseases in a rural African environment. *Oikos* **27**: 180–192.

McLaren, D. S., Shirajian, E. *et al.* (1965). Xerophthalmia in Jordan. *American Journal of Clinical Nutrition* **17**: 117–130.

Martorell, R. (1989). Body size, adaptation and function. *Human Organization* **48**: 15–20.

Martorell, R., Ho, T. J. (1984). Malnutrition, morbidity and mortality. In Mosley, W. H., Chen, L. C. (eds) *Malnutrition, morbidity and mortality*. Population and Development Review Suppl. **10**: 49–68.

Mata, L. J. (1978). *The children of Santa Maria Cauqué: a prospective field study of health and growth*. MIT Press, Cambridge, Mass.

Mata, L. J. (1981). Epidemiological perspective of diarrhoeal disease in Costa Rica and current efforts in control, prevention and research. *Revista Latinoamericana de Microbiología* **23**: 109–119.

Medical Research Council (1917). *Infant mortality*. Special Report Series No. 10. HM Stationery Office, London.

Merchant, K., Martorell, R., Haas, J. D. (1990). Consequences for maternal nutrition of reproductive stress across consecutive pregnancies. *American Journal of Clinical Nutrition* **52**: 616–620.

Mönckeberg, F. (ed) (1988). *Desnutricion infantil: Fisiopathología, clínica, tratamiento y prevenciòn: Neustra experiencia y contribución*. Instituto de Nutrición y Tecnologia de los Alimentos. Santiago, Chile.

Morley, D. (1969). Severe measles in the tropics—I and II. *British Medical Journal* **1**: 297–300 and 363–365.

Muhilal, Permeisih, D. *et al.* (1988). Vitamin A-fortified monosodium glutamate and health, growth and survival of children: a controlled field trial. *American Journal of Clinical Nutrition* **48**: 1271–1276.

Office of Population Censuses and Surveys (1988). *Mortality statistics, 1986. Perinatal and infant deaths. Social and biological factors, Table 7d*. HM Stationery Office, London.

Pickering, H., Hayes, R. J. *et al.* (1986). Social and environmental factors associated with the risk of child mortality in a peri-urban community in The Gambia. *Transactions of the Royal Society of Tropical Medicine and Hygiene* **80**: 311–316.

Pratinidhi, A., Shah, U. *et al.* (1986). Risk-approach strategy in neonatal care. *Bulletin of the World Health Organization* **64**: 291–297.

Prausnitz, W. (1906). Mortalität und Morbidität im Säuglingsalter. In Pfaundler, M., Schlossmann, A. (eds) *Handbuch der Kinderheilkunde*, 1st edn. Vogel, Leipzig, p. 279.

Prentice, A. M., Whitehead, R. G. *et al.* (1983). Prenatal dietary supplementation of African women and birth weight. *Lancet* **1**: 489–492.

Puffer, R. R., Serrano, C. V. (1973). *Patterns of mortality in childhood.* Scientific Publication no. 262. Pan American Health Organization, Washington, DC.

Puffer, R. R., Serrano, C. V. (1987). *Patterns of birthweights.* Scientific Publication no. 504. Pan American Health Organization, Washington DC.

Rahman, M., Rahaman, M. M. *et al.* (1985). Impact of environmental sanitation and crowding on infant mortality in rural Bangladesh. *Lancet* **2**: 28–31.

Rahmathullah, L., Underwood, B. A. *et al.* (1990). Reduced mortality among children in Southern India receiving a small weekly dose of vitamin A. *New England Journal of Medicine* **323**: 929–935.

Ramachandran, P. (1989). Nutrition in pregnancy. In Gopalan, C., Suminder Kaur (eds) *Women and nutrition in India.* Special Publication Series no. 5. Nutrition Foundation of India, New Delhi, pp. 153–193.

Roy, S. K., Chowdhury, A. K. M. A., Rahaman, M. M. (1983). Excess mortality among children discharged after treatment of diarrhoea in rural Bangladesh. *British Medical Journal* **287**: 1097–1099.

Shann, F. (1985). Pneumonia in children: a neglected cause of death. *World Health Forum* **6**: 143–145.

Sinha, D. P. (1977). Measles and malnutrition in a West Bengal village. *Tropical Geographical Medicine* **29**: 125–134.

Sinha, D. P. (1988). *Children of the Caribbean 1945–1984: progress in child survival, its determinants and implications.* Caribbean Food and Nutrition Institute, Kingston, Jamaica.

Sommer, A., Loewenstein, M. S. (1975). Nutritional status and mortality: a prospective validation of the QUAC stick. *American Journal of Clinical Nutrition* **28**: 287–292.

Sommer, A., Tarwotjo, I. *et al.* (1983). Increased mortality in children with mild vitamin A deficiency. *Lancet* **2**: 585–588.

Sommer, A., Tarwotjo, I. *et al.* (1986). Impact of vitamin A supplementation on child mortality. *Lancet* **1**: 1169–1173.

Thomson, A. M., Billewicz, W. Z., Hytten, F. E. (1968). The assessment of fetal growth. *Journal of Obstetrics and Gynaecology of the British Commonwealth* **75**: 903–916.

Trape, J. F., Quinet, M. C. *et al.* (1987). Malaria and urbanization in Central Africa: the example of Brazzaville. Part V: Pernicious attacks and mortality. *Transactions of the Royal Society of Tropical Medicine and Hygiene* **81**: (Suppl. 2). 34–42.

United Nations (1985). Demographic Yearbook, table 22.

Van Lerberghe, W. (1990). *Kasongo: child mortality and growth in a small African town.* Smith-Gordon, Nishimura/London.

Vella, V. (1990). Nutrition and mortality among Ugandan children. Ph.D. thesis, University of London.

Vellore (1973). *Longitudinal studies in human reproduction.* Monograph no. 6. Department of Biostatistics, Christian Medical College, Vellore, India.

Vijayaraghavan, K., Radhaiah, G. *et al.* (1990). Effect of massive dose vitamin A on morbidity and mortality in Indian children. *Lancet* **336**: 1342–1345.

West, K. P., Pokhrel, R. P. *et al.* (1991). Efficacy of vitamin A in reducing pre-school child mortality in Nepal. *Lancet* **338**: 67–71.

Wills, V. G., Waterlow, J. C. (1958). The death rate in the age-group 1–4 years as an index of malnutrition. *Journal of Tropical Pediatrics* **3:** 167–170.

World Health Organization (1980). Division of Family Health. Incidence of low birth weight—a critical review of available information. *World Health Statistics Quarterly* **33:** 197–224.

World Health Organization (1982). Guidelines for research on acute respiratory infections. Memorandum from a WHO meeting. *Bulletin of the World Health Organization* **60:** 521–533.

World Health Organization (1984). A programme for controlling acute respiratory infections in children. Memorandum from a WHO meeting. *Bulletin of the World Health Organization* **62:** 47–58.

World Health Organization (1988). *Respiratory infections in children: management in small hospitals. A manual for doctors.* WHO, Geneva.

19

The effect of malnutrition on mental development

S. M. Grantham-McGregor

Introduction

In 1956 Geber and Dean reported that severely malnourished children had low developmental levels in the acute stage. In 1959, Robles *et al.* also showed that the children's development improved with nutritional rehabilitation. At that time Stoch and Smythe began the first longitudinal study of survivors of severe malnutrition (Stoch and Smythe, 1963). A further impetus was given to research in the field when Dobbing and Winick showed that severe malnutrition resulted in permanent changes to rat brains (Davison and Dobbing, 1966; Winick and Noble, 1966). Dobbing found that the rat brain was especially vulnerable during the brain growth spurt. He suggested that this coincided with the last trimester of pregnancy and the first two years of life in humans.

A large number of studies followed in the 1960s and 70s. However it soon became clear that unravelling the role of malnutrition was enormously complicated. The heterogeneous nature of undernutrition may explain some of the complications. In addition to protein and energy, many other nutrients may be deficient, such as trace elements and vitamins. Deficiencies vary in severity and duration, ranging from a relatively short severe episode to less severe undernutrition *in utero* and throughout childhood. Further, children may be affected at different stages of development. They are also exposed to very different types of sociocultural and economic backgrounds. All these factors probably modify the effects of undernutrition on children's development.

Effect of undernutrition on behaviour

When assessing the effects of undernutrition on behaviour it may be useful to divide them into transient and long-term effects.

Transient effects

Transient effects would include behaviours which are readily induced and reversed and are almost certainly mediated through altered metabolic pathways. There are many examples. Torun and Viteri (1981) showed that children rapidly reduced their activity levels when their energy intake was reduced. In another study (Grantham-McGregor *et al.*, 1991*a*), 18 severely malnourished children in hospital were compared with 14 other children who were adequately nourished but ill with other diseases. Every week time-scheduled observations were made of the children while they were alone in their cribs. On admission to hospital the malnourished children were significantly less active and more apathetic than the comparison children and when presented with a standard set of toys they explored them less. After a short period of nutritional rehabilitation, their activity levels (Fig. 19.1), mood and amount of exploration (Fig. 19.2) became similar to the comparison group. It is not known precisely which nutrients were responsible for these changes.

In adequately nourished subjects, eating lunch has transient effects on mood and performance in certain cognitive tasks (Craig, 1986). It has recently been shown that missing breakfast adversely affected the cognitive functions of school children who were stunted or wasted, and those who had survived an episode of severe malnutrition in early childhood. In contrast, adequately nourished children were either not affected or actually improved (Simeon and Grantham-McGregor, 1989). These findings suggest that short-term metabolic changes interact with underlying differences between the groups causing transient behaviour changes. It could be that undernourished or previously severely malnourished children are more vulnerable to stressors, and other stressors may produce similar effects.

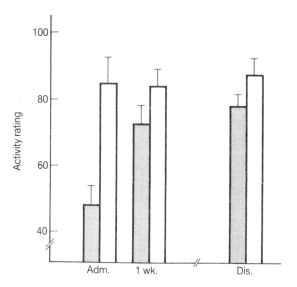

Fig. 19.1   Activity ratings, means with standard errors, observed during three periods of 10 minutes on each day, on admission to hospital, one week later, and when ready for discharge from hospital. ▨, 18 severely malnourished children; ▯, 14 adequately nourished children.

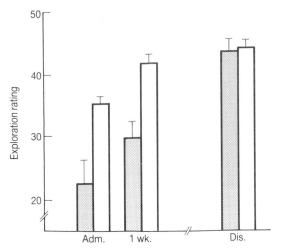

Fig. 19.2 Exploration ratings, means with standard errors, observed during 15 minutes after the child was presented with a standard set of toys; on admission to hospital, one week later, and when ready for discharge from hospital.☐, 17 severely malnourished children;☐, 14 adequately nourished children.

There is an increasing number of reports which suggest that iron deficiency has a transient effect on behaviour. Iron supplementation has been given to iron-deficient, anaemic children in several clinical trials (Pollitt *et al.*, 1989). In children over two years of age improvements have usually been found in the performance of tests of specific cognitive functions and in school achievement after three months of treatment. Pollitt has suggested that these improvements are mediated through changes in children's level of arousal and attention (Pollitt *et al.*, 1986). It is possible that other specific nutrient deficiencies may also affect behaviour.

Long-term effects

There are several possible mechanisms which could explain the link between nutritional deficiencies and more permanent behavioural changes. Firstly, if the deficiencies which cause transient changes persist for long periods of time, children may acquire skills more slowly than normal. They may consequently develop substantial lags in mental development and school achievement which are difficult to reverse, especially in deprived environments. Mild to moderately undernourished children have been shown in several studies to be less active and explore less than better nourished children (Graves, 1976, 1978; Chavez and Martinez, 1982). These behaviours may well lead to poor development; however, a time sequence linking behavioural change to poor development has not been established.

Further, the children's apathetic behaviour may induce changes in their caretakers which reinforce their poor development. Chavez and Martinez (1982) showed that when undernourished children were given nutritional supplementation their parents became more responsive and stimulating towards them than parents of non-supplemented children. A similar type of interaction may occur with older children in school. Once teachers have low expectations of children's ability, they tend to reinforce the situation.

Lastly, malnutrition may be linked to poor development through permanent anatomical and biochemical changes in the central nervous system. Fetal iodine deficiency is a classic example of drastic CNS damage causing mental retardation.

Children with severe malnutrition have small heads (Brown, 1965) and EEG changes for at least one year following the episode (Barnet *et al.*, 1978). However, most evidence for CNS changes comes from animal research. It is well established that following an episode of severe undernutrition brains of rats have permanent neuroanatomical changes; these include decreased brain weight, especially the cerebellum, decreased number of glial cells and cerebellar granule cells, deficits in granular to Purkinje cell ratio, and deficits and alterations to dendritic spines, network size and branching patterns (Bedi, 1987). Although rats also show impaired problem-solving ability (Smart, 1986), there is no evidence directly linking CNS changes to function.

The precise role of the quality of environmental stimulation in the link between malnutrition and mental development has not been elucidated. Bedi and Bhide (1988) reviewed studies on environmental enrichment in rats. They found that brains of malnourished rats showed changes with increased stimulation but the changes were similar to those shown by well-nourished animals. There were no signs of an interaction. However, the behavioural abnormalities observed in malnourished rats are reduced when they are exposed to sensory stimulation (Levitsky, 1979).

Problems in malnutrition and mental development research

Investigators have encountered several problems in this field. Firstly, there are problems with measuring mental development. Most investigators have used tests from developed countries. Infant developmental assessment tests such as the Griffiths or Bayley scales have been used with young children. These contain different subscales of motor and mental function which are averaged to give a developmental quotient. Intelligence quotient tests such as the Stanford Binet and the Wechsler Intelligence Scale for children (WISC) are suitable with older children; they do not usually include motor function. Tests of specific cognitive functions such as short-term memory and visual perception have been used in a few studies. Tests from another culture have doubtful validity (Pollitt and Thomson, 1977). At best, these tests are useful in comparing groups, and then measures of stability over time are needed. Also they need to be validated against other measures of how the child functions in his society.

School achievement tests are measures of what the children learn in school; they usually comprise reading, spelling and arithmetic, but sometimes other subjects are included. Scores on these tests reflect school attendance and sociocultural characteristics of the family as well as the ability of the child.

A further problem is that malnutrition is invariably associated with a host of sociocultural deprivations (Grantham-McGregor, 1984). Many of these conditions independently affect mental development. Investigators have been unable to separate these effects entirely satisfactorily from those of malnutrition.

Studies of severely malnourished children

Many observational studies have been carried out in which survivors of severe malnutrition have been compared with other children. In early studies no attempt was made to control for social factors. More recently investigators have compared malnourished children with carefully matched controls or siblings. In addition they have attempted to measure social background factors and control for them in statistical analyses. In this review I will only discuss studies which used carefully matched controls or siblings, and reported sufficient detail to allow evaluation.

Studies with siblings

Studies comparing school-age children who have survived severe PEM with their siblings are listed in Table 19.1. Some of them also had a group of matched controls. In four of the eight studies the previously malnourished children performed significantly worse than their siblings. These studies were from Mexico (Birch *et al.*, 1971), Jamaica (Hertzig *et al.*, 1972), Nigeria (Nwuga, 1977), and India (Pereira *et al.*, 1979).

In one South African study there were no differences between the groups on an IQ test, but the previously malnourished group performed worse on a drawing test (Evans *et al.*, 1971). In the three remaining studies no significant differences were found. In one from Peru (Graham and Adrianzen, 1979) only school achievement measures were looked at. The other two were both from South Africa. The outcome measures were motor speed, coordination and grip strength in one study (Bartel *et al.*, 1978) and school achievement, employment status and social adjustment in the other (Moodie *et al.*, 1980).

Studies with matched controls

Four studies in which carefully matched controls were used are listed in Table 19.2. In addition three of the sibling studies in Table 19.1 had a group of matched controls. In six of the total of seven, the index child performed worse than the controls. These studies were from Uganda (Hoorweg and Stanfield, 1976), Barbados (Galler, 1984), Jamaica (Hertzig *et al.*, 1972; Grantham-McGregor *et al.*, 1987), India (Champakam *et al.*, 1968) and Nigeria (Nwuga, 1977).

The only study with matched controls in which no differences were found between the groups was the South African one (Bartel *et al.*, 1978) (Table 19.1) in which the outcome measures were grip strength, motor speed and coordination.

Behaviours affected

There was no consistent evidence across studies of any specific cognitive

Table 19.1 Studies of survivors of severe malnutrition compared with siblings and matched controls

Reference	Subjects	Type of PEM	Siblings or comparisons	Results of index group
Birch et al. (1971) Cravioto, DeLicardie (1975) (Mexico)	37, aged 5–13 years	Kwashiorkor	37 siblings nearest in age	Lower scores on verbal, performance and fullscale of WISC[a] Poorer on intersensory integration
Hertzig et al. (1972) Richardson et al. (1973) (Jamaica)	74 boys, aged 5–10 years	Mixed severe PEM	38 male siblings 6–12 years 74 classmates or yardmates	Lower scores on verbal and fullscale of WISC, no difference in school achievement
Nwuga (1977) (Nigeria)	52, aged 9–10 years	Kwashiorkor	34 siblings	Lower scores on verbal, performance and fullscale of WISC. Lower school grades Lower scores in WISC: visual memory, picture arrangement, block design and Ravens Scale
			32 classmates	Lower in all of the above and shape discrimination
			38 upper class children	Upper class group had higher scores in all subtests
Pereira et al. (1979) (India)	130, 6–12 years	Kwashiorkor or marasmic-kwashiorkor	88 siblings	Significantly worse school grades
Evans et al. (1971) (South Africa)	31, aged 9–15 years	Kwashiorkor	31 siblings	No difference on New South African Scales. Lower on Goodenough Drawing Test
Graham and Adrianzen (1979) (Peru)	110, 6–12 years	Marasmus or marasmic-kwashiorkor	188, 6–12 years siblings	No difference in school grade child enrolled
Bartel et al. (1978) (South Africa)	31, aged 6–12 years	Kwashiorkor or marasmic-kwashiorkor	31 siblings 31 yardmates	No difference in grip strength, motor development, finger tapping and motor speed No difference in above (except 2 of 93 items) No effect of age of hospital admission
Moodie et al. (1980) (South Africa)	116, 15 years after acute episode	Kwashiorkor	116 siblings	No difference in school grades, or employment and social adjustment

[a] WISC, Wechsler Intelligence Scale for Children

Table 19.2 Studies of survivors of severe malnutrition compared with matched controls

Reference	Subjects	Type of PEM	Comparisons	Results of index group
Hoorweg and Stanfield (1976) (Uganda)	60, 11–12 years	Mixed severe malnutrition	20 classmates, matched for age, sex, SES[a]	Lower scores in tests of motor functions, block design, memory for design, Ravens matrices, and incidental learning. No difference in arithmetic, vocabulary, Proteus mazes, Knox cubes
Galler (1984) (Barbados)	129, 5–11 years	Underweight or marasmus	Classmates, yardmates, matched for age	Lower scores in verbal performance and full scale of WISC,[b] poorer school grades, more neurological soft signs
Champakam et al. (1968) (India)	19, 8–11 years	Kwashiorkor	53 classmates matched for age, religion, caste, SES, family size, birth order, parental education	Lower scores on tests of neurosensory integration and intelligence. Lowest in tests of perceptual and abstract abilities
Grantham-McGregor et al. (1987)	17, 7–8 years	Mixed, severe malnutrition	18 children in hospital matched for age and SES	Lower scores on Griffiths and Stanford Binet

[a] SES, socioeconomic status
[b] WISC, Wechsler Intelligence Scale for Children

deficit. In three cases (Richardson *et al.*, 1972, 1975; Hoorweg and Stanfield, 1976; Galler, 1984) the children's behaviour at school or home was investigated.

Compared with the control groups, the index children were found to be easily distracted, shy, withdrawn, emotionally immature, restless and unable to stay still. They also made poor relationships with peers, had difficulties in maintaining attention, and rested more.

Critique of observational studies

In no study were the index children better than the comparisons. In general, differences were more often found between previously malnourished children and matched controls than with siblings. Siblings are probably the best control for social background in spite of differences in age and birth order. However, the main problem with siblings is that they are very likely to have been mildly to moderately undernourished themselves; in which case the only difference in nutritional status between the groups may have been the occurrence of an acute episode of oedema or wasting.

There is some evidence that the acute episode *per se* does not have a marked effect on children's development (Hoorweg and Stanfield, 1976). In a Jamaican intervention study of severely malnourished children who were admitted to hospital, we examined the relationship between initial anthropometry and the children's level of development one month after recovery. After controlling for age and intervention, the children's initial height for age was associated with their mental development but the presence of oedema or their degree of wasting was not (Table 19.3) (Grantham-McGregor, 1982).

Table 19.3 Relative effect of independent variables on the developmental quotient in 39 malnourished children

Variable	Standardized regression coefficient	*P*-value
Intervention	.3723	< 0.01
Age	.17077	NS
Height for age, % expected	.4857	< 0.005
Weight for height, % expected	.1558	NS
Oedema	.0460	NS

In another Jamaican study (Grantham-McGregor *et al.*, 1989) 29 children who had recently recovered from severe malnutrition were matched with 29 stunted children of the same height, age and social background but who had not had an episode of severe malnutrition. All the children had development assessments on the Griffiths Mental Development Scales. In addition, 15 non-stunted children of the same age and from similar but not identical social backgrounds were tested. There was only a small non-significant difference between the previously malnourished group and the stunted group. Both groups had markedly lower scores than the non-stunted group (Table 19.4). It would appear that in these children, an episode of severe malnutrition had only a small effect on development over and above that associated with stunting. Comparisons with siblings are therefore likely to minimize differences between the groups.

Table 19.4 Mean scores adjusted for age, on the Griffiths Mental Development Scales in three groups of children

Scale	Acutely malnourished (n = 29)		Stunted, not acutely malnourished (n = 29)		Non-stunted controls (n = 15)	
	Mean	s.d.	Mean	s.d.	Mean	s.d.
Developmental quotient**	97.9	10.3	100.4	13.4	107.9	14.6
Hearing and speech	104.5	16.3	103.5	22.0	110.1	20.3
Hand and eye*	98.2	12.9	102.1	10.4	109.2	19.3
Performance**	90.8	11.6	95.4	15.7	104.6	14.3

Analysis of covariance with age as covariate: $*P < 0.05$, $**P < 0.01$, covariate $P < 0.01$ for each analysis

On the other hand when matching controls, it is not possible to match for all factors which affect mental development (Richardson, 1974). Even when 'macroenvironmental' factors are similar, differences may still exist in the microenvironment (Cravioto and DeLicardie, 1972). Controlling for social background factors statistically is also fraught with difficulties. Accurate measurement of all relevant social factors is probably not possible.

Another confounding variable affecting both types of studies was that the index children were in hospital, which may have contributed to their poor development. Only one study had controls who were also in hospital (Grantham-McGregor *et al.*, 1987).

The malnourished children in most of the studies would have returned to poor environments and probably poor nutrition. It is not possible to determine to what extent their continuing poor development was due to these conditions rather than a result of the original acute episode. A further difficulty associated with retrospective case-control studies is that we cannot be sure whether the children's level of development preceding the onset of malnutrition was the same. There has only been one prospective study (Cravioto and DeLicardie, 1972). In this, a cohort of children from a Mexican village were followed from birth. The children who became severely malnourished had normal levels of development preceding the onset of malnutrition.

Conclusions from observation studies

None of the studies has provided conclusive evidence that severe malnutrition leads to poor mental development. However, in view of the consistency of the findings from different countries, it is reasonable to attribute cause to the relationship in certain conditions: that is, when severe PEM occurs in the first two years of life in the presence of sociocultural deprivation it appears to have a detrimental effect on mental development which lasts at least through childhood.

Studies from developed countries

Studies from developed countries of children with malnutrition secondary to other diseases potentially separate the effects of malnutrition from those of poverty. Several studies have been reviewed by Rush (1984). Children who suffered from pyloric stenosis or cystic fibrosis in early childhood have been compared with siblings or matched controls, or between groups of different severity. Small differences or differences in younger children only or no differences have been reported.

It appears that the findings are inconsistent with those from less developed countries. However, there are many problems in interpreting these data. In some studies the groups were small, in others the outcome measures were inadequate. Perhaps the most important problems are that the duration of malnutrition was often not reported or short, and the difference in severity between groups was sometimes small. Few of the children would have suffered a severe episode followed by long-term undernutrition as is usually the case in developing countries.

The role of stimulation may be critical. It possibly affords some protection against the detrimental effects of malnutrition on behaviour, as has certainly been shown in animals (Levitsky, 1979). Unfortunately, the studies from industrialized countries did not include measures of development just after the illness, but it is likely that a stimulating environment would facilitate catch-up in development after the insult. The data of Lloyd-Still *et al.* (1974) suggest that this may occur.

Rehabilitation studies with severely malnourished children

Adoption

There are no well-designed studies in which children recovering from severe PEM have been exposed to both adequate nutrition and stimulation. However, Winick and colleagues (Winick *et al.*, 1975) reported on the development of malnourished Korean children, who were adopted by North American families before two years of age. At school age they reached normal North American standards in school achievement and IQ levels, but differences, related to their early nutritional status, remained.

We have reported one case in which a marasmic child was adopted and showed remarkable improvement in developmental levels (Grantham-McGregor and Buchanan, 1982).

Stimulation

In a Jamaican study (Grantham-McGregor *et al.*, 1987), the effect of increased stimulation on the development of severely malnourished children was evaluated. The children were provided with a simple play programme in hospital. They were then visited at home for an hour a week for two years, then every two weeks for a third year. Community health aides conducted the visits and left homemade toys with the mothers which were changed every week. The children were compared with two other groups, who were also in hospital: an adequately nourished group with diseases other than malnutrition and another severely malnourished group. These groups received standard medical care only. Both malnourished groups had similar low levels of development on admission to hospital, and were seriously behind the adequately nourished group. The stimulated malnourished group showed marked improvements in development. Three years after intervention stopped, benefits were still apparent in their IQs (Fig. 19.3). They were significantly

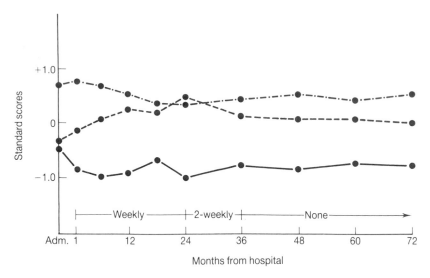

Fig. 19.3 Developmental quotient and IQ scores transformed to standard scores for each test session from admission to hospital to 72 months following discharge. ·—·●—·· , 20 adequately nourished; ——●—— , 16 non-intervened malnourished; ——●—— , 18 intervened malnourished children. Reproduced by permission from Grantham-McGregor *et al.*(1987).

ahead of the non-intervened malnourished group, and only slightly below the adequately nourished children. Six years after intervention, the intervened group showed benefits in school achievement compared with the non-intervened malnourished group (unpublished data).

The results of this study and of the adoption studies illustrate the importance of the quality of the environment for children's development. However, there is no evidence that malnourished children respond more to stimulation than adequately nourished ones. It does indicate that stimulation should be included in the treatment and rehabilitation of malnourished children.

Studies of mild to moderate malnutrition

Observation studies

Many studies of moderately undernourished children have shown a relationship between undernutrition and developmental levels in young children (e.g. Lasky *et al.*, 1981; Powell and Grantham-McGregor, 1985), and with school achievement (e.g. Johnson *et al.*, 1987) and neurosensory integration in older children (Cravioto *et al.*, 1966). In general children's development is more often related to height for age than weight for height (Grantham-McGregor *et al.*, 1990). However, because of the inevitable association between undernutrition and poor social backgrounds it is not possible to attribute cause to the relationship.

Supplementation studies

Several experimental studies have been conducted in which nutritional supplementation was given to prevent undernutrition or to treat it. These studies allow us to come closer to inferring a causal link between mild to moderate malnutrition and poor mental development. They have been extensively reviewed (Rush, 1984; Grantham-McGregor, 1987). Only the well documented studies from developing countries with reasonably adequate designs will be discussed here. Most of them have involved giving supplements from pregnancy through early childhood in communities where malnutrition is common (Table 19.5).

Table 19.5 Studies of nutritional supplementation in children or mothers exposed to malnutrition in developing countries

Reference	Treatment group	Results
Joos *et al.* (1983) (Taiwan)	a. Supplement in pregnancy and lactation b. Placebo	Benefits to children's motor development at 8 months
Waber *et al.* (1981) (Bogota, Colombia)	a. Supplement in pregnancy and first 3 years b. Supplement combined with stimulation for 3 years c. Stimulation for 3 years, no supplementation d. Nothing	Supplement gave increase in activity at 4 months; benefit to motor skills mainly at 18 months and to all areas of development at 36 months. Stimulation benefit to language. Interaction at 18 months, not at 36 months.
Freeman *et al.* (1980) (Guatemala)	a. Supplement in pregnancy and first 7 years in different amounts	Small association between cognitive functions and amount of supplementation
Chavez and Martinez (1982) (Mexico)	a. Supplement in pregnancy and lactation and first 7 years b. Nothing	Benefit to all subscales of Gesel Test and increase in activity

Supplementation from pregnancy

In Taiwan (Joos *et al.*, 1983) mothers were supplemented throughout pregnancy and lactation. At eight months of age the treated group had slightly higher scores on the motor scale but not the mental scale of the Bayley Infant Scales than a control group.

In the Bogota study (Waber *et al.*, 1981) there were several groups of which four will be considered; one was supplemented from pregnancy throughout the first three years of life, in another the children had stimulation for three years, another group had both treatments, and a fourth served as a control. Supplementation gave a small benefit to all areas of the children's development at 36 months of age, with a tendency to favour motor skills at 18 months. Stimulation benefitted only language and personal-social behaviour. There was a significant interaction between the treatments at 18 but not at 36 months of age.

Freeman *et al.* (1980) in Guatemala gave supplements to pregnant mothers and young children at centres in four villages. Benefits were found in several tests of specific cognitive function in those who received large amounts of supplement compared with those who received little. A major problem with this study is that supplement was given on a self-selection basis, which must have introduced bias.

In Mexico (Chavez and Martinez, 1982) pregnant mothers and children up to seven years of age were supplemented. They were compared with a group of children born in the same village one year previously but the extra attention they received was not controlled for. The supplemented children showed substantial benefits in all areas of development on infants' tests, and in first grade at school. They also showed a marked increase in activity in the first two years of life.

Supplementation of children already undernourished

In three studies supplement was given to children already malnourished. In Cali, Colombia (McKay *et al.*, 1978), supplementation had no benefit on the performance of three-year olds in tests of cognitive function, whereas supplementation with stimulation produced marked benefits which were proportional to the duration of the programme. This study highlights the importance of stimulation. No anthropometric or dietary intake data were reported and it is difficult to interpret the lack of response in the supplemented group.

Both undernourished and adequately nourished children in Bogota were supplemented (Mora *et al.*, 1974). After one year the supplemented undernourished children showed small improvements on the Griffiths Test compared with the other groups; no details of this study have been published.

In a recent Jamaican study (Grantham-McGregor *et al.*, 1991*b*), stunted children between nine and 24 months of age were randomly assigned to four treatment groups for two years. One group was a control, one received psychosocial stimulation, one received nutritional supplementation, while one had both treatments. Supplementation had a significant benefit on the children's developmental quotients on the Griffiths Test. The locomotor and performance subscales also showed significant improvements and the improvement in the hearing and speech subscales approached significant levels ($P < 0.01$). There was no significant interaction between treatments and the effects were additive. The group which received both treatments showed the most benefit (Fig. 19.4). The scores for a group of non-stunted children are shown in the figure for comparison.

Critique of supplementation studies

There are many problems with the interpretation of these findings (Grantham-McGregor, 1987). First, only a limited increase in dietary intake was generally achieved. This was due to substitution, sharing, morbidity and failure to collect supplement. Random assignment was often not used and in only two studies was there an attempt to control for the extra attention the children received (Joos *et al.*, 1983; Grantham-McGregor *et al.*, 1991*b*).

There are also insufficient findings on the long-term effects of supplementation. A preliminary report of the Bogota study of supplementation from pregnancy showed that some benefits were still apparent three years later (Herrera and Super, 1983). However, their loss of subjects was extremely

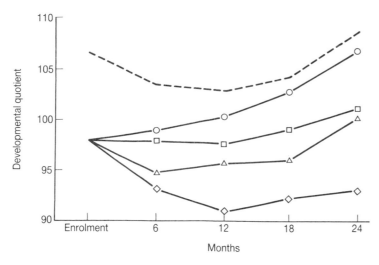

Fig. 19.4 Mean developmental quotients of stunted children adjusted for initial age and score, compared with non-stunted children adjusted for age only. Results of intervention over two years. ▬ ▬ ▬ ▬ , non-stunted; stunted: □▬▬▬□ , stimulated; △▬▬▬△ , supplemented; ○▬▬▬○, stimulated and supplemented; ◇▬▬▬◇ , non-stimulated and unsupplemented controls. Reproduced by permission from Grantham-McGregor *et al.* (1991*b*).

large. The children who received both stimulation and supplementation in the Cali study (McKay *et al.*, 1978) showed small benefits throughout the first three school grades (McKay and McKay, 1983).

Conclusions from supplementation studies

In spite of the difficulties in conducting supplementation studies, the findings are reasonably consistent. Supplementation appears to have concurrent benefits under certain circumstances, i.e. if supplement is given from the last trimester of pregnancy and through early childhood in poor communities where undernutrition is prevalent. There is less evidence of an effect of supplementation on children who are already malnourished. However, findings from the recent Jamaican study of stunted children (Grantham-McGregor *et al.*, 1991*b*) suggest that their development also benefits from supplementation. This provides reasonably strong evidence that the poor levels of development commonly found in stunted children are at least partly mediated through poor nutrition. There is insufficient evidence to determine whether there are long-term benefits from supplementation, and whether there is an interaction with stimulation.

References

Barnet, A. B., Weiss, A. P. *et al.* (1978). Abnormal auditory evoked potentials in early infancy malnutrition. *Science* **201**: 450–452.

Bartel, P. P., Griesel, R. D. *et al.* (1978). Long term effects of kwashiorkor on psychomotor development. *South African Medical Journal* **53**: 360–362.

Bedi, K. S. (1987). Lasting neuro-anatomical changes following undernutrition. In

Dobbing, J. (ed) *Early nutrition and later achievement*. Academic Press, London, pp. 1–49.

Bedi, K. S., Bhide, P. G. (1988). Effects of environmental diversity on brain morphology. In Jones, D. G. (ed) *Current topics in research on synapses*. A. R. Liss, New York.

Birch, H. G., Pineiro, C. *et al.* (1971). Relation of kwaskiorkor in early childhood and intelligence at school age. *Pediatric Research* **5:** 579–585.

Brown, R. E. (1965). Decreased brain weight in malnutrition and its implications. *East African Medical Journal* **42:** 584–595.

Champakam, S., Srikantia, S. G., Gopalan, C. (1968). Kwashiorkor and mental development. *American Journal of Clinical Nutrition* **21:** 844–852.

Chavez, A., Martinez, C. (1982). *Neurological maturation and performance on mental tests. Growing up in a developing community*. INCAP, Guatemala City.

Craig, A. (1986). Acute effects of meals on perceptual and cognitive efficiency. *Nutrition Reviews* **44:** 163–171.

Cravioto, J., DeLicardie, E. (1972). Environmental correlates of severe clinical malnutrition and language development in survivors from kwashiorkor and marasmus. In *Nutrition, the nervous system and behaviour*. PAHO Scientific Publication no. 251, Washington, pp. 73–94.

Cravioto, J., DeLicardie, E. R. (1975). Neurointegrative development and intelligence in children rehabilitated from severe malnutrition. In Prescott, J. W., Read, M., Coursin, D. (eds) *Brain function and malnutrition. Neuropsychological methods of assessment*. John Wiley, New York, pp. 53–71.

Cravioto, J., DeLicardie, E., Birch, H. (1966). Nutrition, growth and neurointegrative development: an experimental and ecological study. *Pediatrics* **38:** (Suppl.) 319–372.

Davison, A. N., Dobbing, J. (1966). Myelination as a vulnerable period in brain development. *British Medical Bulletin* **22:** 40–44.

Evans, D. E., Moodie, A. D., Hansen, J. D. L. (1971). Kwashiorkor and intellectual development. *South African Medical Journal* **25:** 1413–1426.

Freeman, H. E., Klein, R. E. *et al.* (1980). Nutrition and cognitive development among rural Guatemalan children. *American Journal of Public Health* **70:** 1277–1285.

Galler, J. (1984). The behavioral consequences of malnutrition in early life. In Galler, J. (ed) *Nutrition and behavior*. Plenum Press, New York, pp. 63–118.

Geber, M., Dean, R. F. A. (1956). The psychological changes accompanying kwashiorkor. *Courrier* **6:** 6–15.

Graham, G. G., Adrianzen, B. T. (1979). Status in school of Peruvian children severely malnourished in infancy. In Brozek, J. (ed) *Behavioral effects of energy and protein deficits*. DHEW (NIH) Publication no. 79–1906, pp. 185–194.

Grantham-McGregor, S. M. (1982). The relationship between developmental levels and different types of malnutrition in children. *Human Nutrition: Clinical Nutrition* **36C:** 319–320.

Grantham-McGregor, S. M. (1984). A social background of childhood malnutrition. In Brozek, J., Schürch, B. (eds) *Malnutrition and behavior: critical assessment of key issues*. Nestlé Foundation, Switzerland, pp. 358–374.

Grantham-McGregor, S. M. (1987). Field studies in early nutrition and later achievement. In Dobbing, J. (ed) *Early nutrition and later achievement*. Academic Press, London, pp. 128–174.

Grantham-McGregor, S. M. (1989). The effects of undernutrition on mental development. In Shepherd, R. (ed) *Psychobiology of human eating and nutritional behavior*. Wiley Psychophysiology Series. J. Wiley and Sons Inc., Chichester, England, pp. 321–339.

Grantham-McGregor, S. M., Buchanan, E. (1982). The development of an adopted child recovering from severe malnutrition. Case report. *Human Nutrition: Clinical Nutrition* **36C:** 251–256.

Grantham-McGregor, S. M., Meeks-Gardner, J. *et al.* (1990). The relationship between undernutrition, activity levels and development in young children. In Schürch, B., Scrimshaw, N. (eds) *Activity, energy expenditure and energy requirements in young children.* Nestlé Foundation, Switzerland, pp. 361–383.

Grantham-McGregor, S., Powell, C., Fletcher, P. (1989). Stunting, severe malnutrition and mental development in young children. *European Journal of Clinical Nutrition* **43:** 403–409.

Grantham-McGregor, S. M., Schofield, W., Powell, C. (1987). Development of severely malnourished children who received psychosocial stimulation: six year follow up. *Pediatrics* **79:** 247–254.

Grantham-McGregor, S., Stewart, M., Powell, C. (1991a). Behaviour observations of severely malnourished children in a Jamaican hospital. *Developmental Medicine and Child Neurology* **33:** 706–714.

Grantham-McGregor, S. M., Powell, C. *et al.* (1991b). Nutritional supplementation, psychosocial stimulation and development of stunted children: the Jamaican study. *Lancet* **338:** 1–5.

Graves, P. L. (1976). Nutrition, infant behavior and maternal characteristics: a pilot study in West Bengal, India. *American Journal of Clinical Nutrition* **29:** 305–319.

Graves, P. L. (1978). Nutrition and infant behaviour: a replication study in the Katmandu valley, Nepal. *American Journal of Clinical Nutrition* **31:** 541–551.

Herrera, M., Super, C. (1983). *Social performance and physical growth of underprivileged children: results of the Bogota project at seven years.* Report to World Bank. Harvard School of Public Health, Cambridge, Mass.

Hertzig, M. E., Birch, H. G. *et al.* (1972). Intellectual levels of school children severely malnourished during the first two years of life. *Pediatrics* **49:** 814–824.

Hoorweg, J., Stanfield, J. P. (1976). The effects of protein energy malnutrition in early childhood on intellectual and motor abilities in later childhood and adolescence. *Developmental Medicine and Child Neurology* **18:** 130–150.

Johnson, F. E., Low, S. M. *et al.* (1987). Interaction of nutritional and socioeconomic status as determinants of cognitive development in disadvantaged urban Guatemalan children. *American Journal of Physical Anthropology* **73:** 501–506.

Joos, S. K., Pollitt, E. *et al.* (1983). The Bacon Chow Study: maternal nutritional supplementation and infant behavioral development. *Child Development* **54:** 669–676.

Lasky, R. E. M., Klein, R. E. *et al.* (1981). The relationship between physical growth and infant behavioural development in rural Guatemala. *Child Development* **52:** 219–226.

Levitsky, D. A. (1979). Malnutrition and hunger to learn. In Levitsky, D. A. (ed) *Malnutrition, environment and behavior.* Cornell University Press, Ithaca and London, pp. 161–179.

Lloyd-Still, J. D., Wolff, P. H., Schwachman, H. (1974). Intellectual development after severe malnutrition in infancy. *Pediatrics* **54:** 306–311.

McKay, A., McKay, H. (1983). Primary school progress after preschool experience: troublesome issues in the conduct of follow-up research and findings from Cali, Colombia study. In King, K., Meyers, R. (eds) *Preventing school failure: the relationship between preschool and primary education.* International Development Research Center, Ottawa, pp. 32–42.

McKay, H., Sinesterra, L. *et al.* (1978). Improving cognitive ability in chronically deprived children. *Science* **200:** 270–278.

Moodie, A. D., Bowie, M. D. *et al.* (1980). A prospective 15-year follow-up study of kwashiorkor patients. *South African Medical Journal* **58:** 677–681.

Mora, J. O., Amezquita, A. *et al.* (1974). Nutrition, health and social factors related to intellectual performance. *World Review of Nutrition and Dietetics* **19:** 205–236.

Nwuga, U. C. B. (1977). Effect of severe kwashiorkor on intellectual development among Nigerian children. *American Journal of Clinical Nutrition* **30:** 1423–1430.

Pereira, S. M., Sundararaj, R., Begum, A. (1979). Physical growth and neurointegrative performance of survivors of protein-energy malnutrition. *British Journal of Nutrition* **42**: 165–171.

Pollitt, E., Thomson, C. (1977). Protein-calorie malnutrition and behavior: a view from psychology. In Wurtmann, R., Wurtmann, J. (eds) *Nutrition and the brain*, vol. 2. Raven Press, New York, pp. 261–306.

Pollitt, E., Haas, J., Levitsky, D. (1989). International conference on iron deficiency and behavioral development. *American Journal of Clinical Nutrition* **50**: (Suppl.): 566–705.

Pollitt, E., Saco-Pollitt, C. *et al.*, (1986). Iron deficiency and behavioral development in infants and preschool children. *American Journal of Clinical Nutrition* **43**: 555–565.

Powell, C. A., Grantham-McGregor, S. (1985). The ecology of nutritional status and development in young children in Kingston, Jamaica. *American Journal of Clinical Nutrition* **41**: 1322–1331.

Richardson, S. A. (1974). The background history of school children severely malnourished in infancy. In Schulman, I. (ed) *Advances in pediatrics*, vol. 21. Yearbook Medical Publishers Inc., Chicago, pp. 167–195.

Richardson, S. A., Birch, H. G., Hertzig, M. (1973). School performance of children who were severely malnourished in infancy. *American Journal of Mental Deficiency* **5**: 623–632.

Richardson, S. A., Birch, H. G., Ragbeer, C. (1975). The behavior of children at home who were severely malnourished in the first two years of life. *Journal of Biosocial Science* **7**: 255–256.

Richardson, S. A., Birch, H. G. *et al.* (1972). The behavior of children in school who were severely malnourished in the first two years of life. *Journal of Health and Social Behaviour* **13**: 276–283.

Robles, B. R., Ramos-Galván, R., Cravioto, J. (1959). Valoracion del conducta del nino con desnutricion avanzada y de sus modificaciones durante la recuperacion. *Boletin Medical del Hospital Infantil de Mexico* **16**: 317–324.

Rush, D. (1984). The behavioral consequences of protein-energy deprivation and supplementation in early life: an epidemiological perspective. In Galler, J. (ed) *Human nutrition. A comprehensive treatise.* Plenum Press, New York and London, pp. 119–154.

Simeon, D., Grantham-McGregor, S. M. (1989). Effects of missing breakfast on the cognitive functions of school children of differing nutritional status. *American Journal of Clinical Nutrition* **49**: 646–653.

Smart, J. L. (1986). Undernutrition, learning and memory: review of experimental studies. In Taylor, T. G., Jenkins, N. K. (eds) *XIII International Congress of Nutrition*. John Libbey, London, pp. 74–78.

Stoch, M. B., Smythe, P. M. (1963). Does undernutrition during infancy inhibit brain growth and subsequent intellectual development? *Archives of Disease in Childhood* **38**: 546–552.

Torun, B., Viteri, F. E. (1981). Energy requirements of preschool children and effects of varying energy intakes on protein metabolism. In Torun, B., Young, V. R., Rand, W. M. (eds) *Protein energy requirements of developing countries: evaluation of new data*. Food and Nutrition Bulletin Suppl. 5. UNU, Tokyo, pp. 229–241.

Waber, D. P., Vuori-Christiansen, L. *et al.* (1981). Nutritional supplementation, maternal education, and cognitive development of infants at risk of malnutrition. *American Journal of Clinical Nutrition* **34**: 807–813.

Winick, M., Noble, A. (1966). Cellular response in rats during malnutrition at various ages. *Journal of Nutrition* **89**: 300–306.

Winick, M., Meyer, K. K., Harris, R. (1975). Malnutrition and environmental enrichment by early adoption. *Science* **190**: 1173–1175.

20
Prevention of protein-energy malnutrition

Introduction

It would not be appropriate to end a book on PEM without some attempt to wrestle with the subject of prevention, on which a great deal has been written by economists and social scientists as well as by nutritionists and health scientists. Mosley (1984) has made a plea, which has not gone unheeded, for bringing more closely together the biological and social sides of the debate. The literature is consequently enormous. All that can be attempted here is some brief notes on the background, the strategies and the inputs needed for the prevention of PEM.

The scene is dominated by the Declaration of Alma Ata in 1978, which has been accepted by the great majority of the world's governments. The basic philosophy of the Declaration is that health is a fundamental human right: people have the right and the duty to participate individually and collectively in the planning and implementation of their health care. The objective laid down in the Declaration is 'Health for All by the Year 2000'. The policies that are called for to achieve this objective are:

political commitment of the state;
more equitable distribution of resources;
involvement of the community in social control of the health infrastructure and technology and in shaping its health and economic future;
technical and economic co-operation among countries;
integration of the activities of the health sector with those of other sectors: agriculture, animal husbandry, food, industry, education, housing, public works and transport.

This last policy element will apply particularly to the improvement of nutrition. It has been well said that, because of its multiple causation, malnutrition is often considered as everybody's concern but no-one's responsibility (WHO, 1981).

The basic strategy for achieving Health for All is primary health care (PHC), which is conceived as an integral part not only of the health system but of overall social and economic development of the community (Mahler, 1988). PHC is defined in the Declaration of Alma Ata as:

> . . . essential health care based on practical, scientifically sound and socially acceptable methods and technology made universally accessible to individuals and families in the community through their full participation and at a cost that the community and country can afford to maintain at every stage of their development in the spirit of self-reliance and self-determination.

Operationally, PHC is said to include eight essential elements, which are listed in Table 20.1.

Table 20.1   Essential elements of primary health care

Education on health problems
Promotion of adequate food supplies and proper nutrition
Adequate supply of safe water and basic sanitation
Maternal and child health care, including family planning
Prevention and control of locally endemic diseases
Immunization against major infantile diseases
Appropriate treatment of common diseases and injuries
Provision of essential drugs

In the sections that follow we attempt to examine some of the political, strategic and tactical questions that link the prevention of PEM to primary health care as conceived by Mahler (1988).

The political and economic background

Since PEM is the product of poverty and deprivation, in the long run it can only be eliminated by political action to reduce the inequalities between and within countries. It is surely an unacceptable state of affairs that, according to the Executive Director of UNICEF, adequate investments in human development, including health services, nutrition, education and housing would amount to 30–50 billion dollars a year, which is only 5 per cent of world military spending. According to the World Bank, the re-allocation of only 2–3 per cent of world income per year would eradicate poverty by the year 2000 (Streeter, 1981). It would be Utopian to suppose that such adjustments will happen quickly. As the reports of UNICEF on the State of the World's Children remind us every year, it requires political will, although they prudently stop short of saying exactly what that phrase means. It means a will by the people, as well as the governments, of the rich countries to accept more responsibility and perhaps some sacrifices; and a will by the governments and people of the poorer countries to move towards a reduction of inequality.

The three decades up to 1980 were a period of rapid economic growth in the world as a whole. There were impressive increases in food production which, except in Africa, managed to keep up with rising populations (Mellor,

1986). In Asia the increased production resulted mainly from scientific advances leading to increased yields; in Africa such increase as has occurred has been largely through bringing in more land (Chandler, 1989). It seems unlikely that either of these two processes can continue at the same rate. Blaxter (1986) has discussed the discernible limits to world food production on the basis of the cultivable area available and the thermodynamics of energy transduction in the green leaf, and estimates that the carrying capacity of the world is 7–8 billion people, not quite double our present population. Further rises in crop yields, through the application of genetics and biotechnology, will require a parallel increase in water supplies and expensive fertilizers.

At the same time during this period there were substantial falls in infant mortality rate (Chapter 18) and increases in life expectancy, but because of the expanding population the absolute number of child deaths has not fallen.

Many felt that progress was too slow, and that such benefits as did arise were unequally distributed and did not trickle down to the poor. Against this it was argued that there are three components to development: economic and industrial growth, infrastructure and social development, and they must be allowed to grow in that order. Money devoted to social development, which is essentially recurrent expenditure, drains away capital resources that are needed for decreasing poverty and raising income levels. Gopalan (1988) has emphasized the importance of the time-scale of development. In Europe and North America the process of industrialization and the creation of wealth took 150 years. It was only during the latter part of this period that serious attention was given to social development and by that time the infrastructure had been laid and the resources were available. In fact, from the evidence of changes in stature it seems that both in Europe and North America deteriorations in health were occurring precisely at the time when national wealth was increasing (Chapter 13). The advances in health technology came towards the end of this period of rapid economic growth.

There may be questions about how far improvements in public health have been achieved by progress in medical science or by general social development. The fact remains that we now know that it is possible to reduce mortality and prolong life—surely important components of well-being. Naturally a duty is felt to apply these advances world-wide. This represents in effect an attempt to short-circuit the historical development process and the result has simply been to produce a vast increase in the world's population without the resources to support it. Moreover, there have also been harmful effects of unbalanced economic and industrial development (Gopalan, 1986). It is true that some countries—Sri Lanka and Jamaica are often quoted as examples —have done much to fulfil social needs without significant economic growth, but it has been questioned whether this policy is sustainable.

The World Bank, rejecting these arguments, developed the Basic Needs Approach, which Streeter (1981) described as 'thrice blessed: it is good in its own right; it raises productivity and it lowers reproductivity'. Underlying this approach are two concepts: the first is the ideal of equity and the right of all human beings to education, work, food and health, as laid down in the UN Declaration of Human Rights. The right to health is enshrined in the Declaration of Alma Ata, but it is a nebulous right, since it cannot be enforced. Secondly, there is the concept of human capital which is just as essential for development as material capital, and should not be squandered.

Galbraith (1986) has said: 'No error in the advice given to the new countries in recent decades has rivalled that which places investment in industrial apparatus ahead of investment in human capital.' It is interesting that there was intense opposition in the Third World to the Basic Needs Approach being adopted by the donor countries on the grounds that the rich countries were trying to deprive the poor ones of the means of economic and industrial growth by which they had themselves become rich; and that the approach represented an unwarranted intrusion into their decisions about priorities.

In the 1980s the situation changed. Now we see Third World countries overburdened with debt, the servicing of which eats up the export earnings that are needed for developing a sound infrastructure and has caused governments to cut back on health budgets (Musgrove, 1986; Stewart, 1989). In the words of Grant (1990).

> The blame [for the debt crisis] lies with irresponsible borrowers and irresponsible lenders, and with international economic arrangements, including trade regulations and commodity prices over which the developing world has little control but within which it must earn a living. Meanwhile the consequences are falling in highly disproportionate measure on those who have least responsibility for the debt and least capacity to repay.

As the British Chancellor of the Exchequer pointed out, in an address to Commonwealth finance ministers in 1990: 'the cost to developing countries of protectionism by the industrialized countries greatly exceeds the total value of aid flows'.

However, to be fair, money is not the only determinant. In an earlier analysis of mortality trends in 43 countries between 1938 and 1963 it was concluded that income growth accounted for only 16 per cent of the increase in life expectancy (Evans *et al.*, 1981). Moreover, an economic crisis does not simply put the machine into reverse. Many of the earlier achievements, such as the extension of education and water supplies and the strengthening of infrastructures, remain, at least for a time, although of course it will be necessary to struggle to maintain them.

The contribution of developed countries

Both peoples and governments of the richer countries express feelings of responsibility for health and nutrition in the Third World. According to a joint resolution of the United States Congress in 1975: 'Every person in this country and *throughout the world* (my italics) has the right to food—the right to a nutritionally adequate diet . . . this right is henceforth to be recognized as a cornerstone of US policy' (quoted by Byron, 1988). The problem is to convert words and good intentions into deeds. In spite of this resolution, between 1977 and 1986, a period of transition from expansion to depression, US military aid increased by a factor of three, from $2 to $6 billion a year, whereas food aid increased hardly at all, from $1.17 to $1.30 billion (Byron, 1988). This is surely not an isolated example.

The setback of the 1980s suggests that it is unrealistic to rely on continuing growth of the world economy. It follows, then, that a decent standard of life for the peoples of the Third World cannot be achieved in a reasonable time without some transfer of resources from the rich to the poor. The radical approach to resource transfer is by restructuring the world economy to produce the New International Economic Order, an important part of which is 'fairer' terms of trade for developing countries. According to the Brandt report, published in 1980, serious discussions of this approach began in the early 1970s. To a non-economist it is not apparent that very much progress has been made in this direction, particularly in the face of the debt crisis of the late 1980s.

The more familiar method of transferring resources is by aid from the richer to the poorer countries, direct or through the UN Agencies and their special programmes. A substantial part of overseas aid is indeed devoted to helping the poorer countries to fulfil their basic needs and to building up the necessary infrastructure—schools, housing, roads, water supplies and health. Nevertheless, it is a drop in the bucket. Few of the rich countries have reached the UN target of 0.7 per cent of GNP being spent on overseas aid (Table 20.2).

Table 20.2 Aid contributions as a percentage of the gross national product

Country	1960	1983
Belgium	0.88	0.59
Canada	0.20	0.45
Denmark	0.09	0.73
France	1.38	0.74
Germany	0.33	0.49
Netherlands	0.31	0.91
Norway	0.11	1.06
Sweden	0.05	0.85
UK	0.56	0.35
USA	0.54	0.24
Total	0.55	0.36

From Hopkins (1987)

Quite apart from the quantity of aid, there is a widespread view that aid often does more harm than good. It distorts the economy of the receiving countries and creates an undesirable state of dependence. The controversy has been particularly intense over food aid. A large part of the food given as aid is sold on the open market and represents import substitution (Singer and Longhurst, 1986). The money so raised is meant to be spent by the local government on social and other kinds of development. However, it is argued that food aid is inconsistent with self-reliance (Stewart, 1986) and that it tends to depress local food production and reduce the incomes of farmers. Some hold that it would be better to give money, to enable the receiving governments to buy food, either locally or from outside, but this would not meet the needs of donor countries to dispose of surplus stocks. Only a lesser part of food aid is used for the direct benefit of the poor, in food for work programmes, for school-feeding and for supplements to vulnerable groups.

Another criticism is that aid is usually given on a relatively short-term basis whereas it is useless to initiate programmes that cannot be sustained. Health and education, for example, are labour-intensive, and governments crippled by debt or trade imbalance cannot sustain the recurrent costs. Aid, therefore, as organized at present, is criticized as not going to the root of the problem.

This brings us back to the political question. In the Western democracies, as Seaman and Poore (1990) have pointed out, 'the size of aid budgets and the way in which they are spent are ultimately in the power of the public'. In the rich countries public interest is mainly aroused by disasters, and to communicate a more basic understanding of the problems seems to be very difficult. King (1990) has injected a new element by linking the subject of child health and survival in the Third World to that of ecological disaster. The failure to transfer resources is forcing less developed countries into methods of land and fuel use and of industrial development that must add to the destruction of the world's environment. Although King's article aroused much controversy and disagreement, this linking of child survival to an issue over which there is much public concern could in the long run be very helpful.

Most donor countries, implicitly or explicitly, have a policy of 'aid to the poorest'. In the UK this was the policy established in the 1970s by Dame Judith Hart, when disillusionment with the 'trickle-down' theory was setting in, and officially it remains in force. However, experience shows that it is difficult to reach the poor. The former Prime Minister of India, Mr Gandhi, has said that, out of every six rupees allocated for development, only one reached the poor, quite apart from 'hidden leaks'. One reason for the difficulty is that, almost by definition, the poorest countries have the weakest infrastructure, both material and human, for operating programmes effectively. Another reason is that the community participation, so essential for success at the grass-roots level, may in some cases be politically unacceptable. The non-governmental agencies are better able than governments to get round this particular problem.

The difficulty of reaching the poor, and the consequent disillusion with donors, are reflected in this plaint by an anonymous Indian:

I was hungry and you formed a committee to investigate my hunger;
I was homeless and you filed a report on my plight;
I was sick and you held a seminar on the situation of the underprivileged;
You investigated all aspects of my plight—and yet I am still hungry,
homeless and sick. (quoted by Ulbricht, 1976).

There is one form of aid about which there should be no controversy—the strengthening of human resources, not only by training programmes and technical co-operation but by support of universities and other institutions in the Third World. Economic and social growth depends not only on money, but on people who know what to do, in all sectors and at all levels. It could be argued that the relative success of India since independence is because she has built up so many institutions for training and research, whereas in Africa, which has been described as a bottomless pit for aid (House of Commons, 1985) such institutions are much less well advanced (Odhiambo, 1988). Therefore it would be reasonable, as a slogan for policy, to link 'Aid to the Poorest' with 'The Development of Self-reliance'.

Technical co-operation and training programmes are important also for the young of industrial countries, who are eager to make a contribution and to share their technical skills. Unfortunately, training of Third World people in the richer countries is not always geared to what they have to do when they return home. Moreover, research programmes, large or small, usually have to be related to the criteria of outside aid agencies, and there is often an element of paternalism, of 'we know what is best for you', in decisions about what should be supported. Aid agencies are unwilling to provide money, even on a small scale, for institutions in developing countries to spend as they think best. The development of self-reliance requires some change in this attitude.

Strategies for prevention

Everyone agrees that the prevention of PEM cannot be an isolated objective, separated from more general measures to meet the basic needs of the poor. The prevention of malnutrition can only be achieved and sustained within a framework of more general advance in other sectors. However, just as disillusionment with economic development and attempts at income generation led to the 'Basic Needs Approach' and 'Development with a Human Face', so these concepts in turn have led to the strategy of concentrating efforts on those at greatest risk, as the most likely way of achieving some results within a reasonable time. The slogan of WHO's Risk Approach (Backett *et al.*, 1984) is: 'something for all but more for those in need *in proportion to that need*' (my italics). The risk strategy is seen as a guide to resource allocation which necessarily involves positive discrimination.

As a consequence, there have been many programmes that concentrated specifically on disadvantaged individuals or groups, and some success stories. Gwatkin *et al.* (1981) posed the question: can health and nutrition interventions make a difference? and concluded that the answer was 'Yes'. They analysed the outcome of ten projects in terms of the effect on mortality. The most impressive was that of Arole (1988) in Jamkhed, India, where the infant mortality fell between 1971 and 1976 from 97 to 39, while in control areas it remained at 90. Berg (1987; summarized in The Lancet, 1988) examined four World Bank projects in Brazil, Colombia, India and Indonesia. The elements of the programmes were targeted food distributions and subsidies; integration of nutrition intervention with primary health care and family planning; nutrition education; and involvement of the community in health and nutrition programmes. Berg concluded that 'a well-managed and targeted programme is able to reduce serious and severe malnutrition more than a less focussed programme and at a significantly lower cost'.

Others, however, are less optimistic and in the nutrition community at the present time there is very active debate about policies and strategies. The principle of 'targeting' on those specially at risk would appear, particularly to medical people, to be obviously sensible and sound; in reality things are not so simple. Pacey and Payne (1985) have discussed the problems, both theoretical and practical, that are involved in the targeted approach, and their book is an important contribution to the debate. Their position could be summarized in the words of Seckler (1982, quoted by Payne, 1987), in relation to stunting: '. . . except where people are in clear and present danger of functional impairment due to malnutrition, interventions should be targeted to poor environments and not to poor individuals'.

In an ideal world it should not be necessary to make the choice implied by Seckler. In reality a Third World government, faced with constraints on its resources, has to make a choice on how far they should be narrowly focussed and how far more widely spread. It is not within the scope of this book to make judgements or recommendations about such choices. The fact is that as far as concerns the health sector and the prevention of PEM, targeted policies are to some extent inevitable and the question to be considered here is not so much whether they are the right policies but how they should best be executed.

The activities concerned in the prevention of PEM are of two kinds: those that operate at the regional or country level and those that impinge directly on the individual family or child. The distinction is of course not clear-cut, because activities at the level of the individual have to be backed up by some organizational structure at a higher level. Furthermore, there are some general principles which have a bearing on all activities, and whose importance has been increasingly recognized in recent years: the special role of women and the necessity of community participation in decision-making as well as in actual activities (see below).

It is useful to distinguish between aims, scope and methods. The *aim* of the lead agencies in this field, WHO and UNICEF, is to promote child survival and, more specifically, to eliminate severe PEM and halve the prevalence of moderate PEM by the year 2000. In response to criticisms (see below) that child survival is too narrow an objective, the latest version of UNICEF strategy (UNICEF, 1990) is described as the 'Principle of First Call'—'that the lives and the *normal development* (my italics) of children should have first call on society's concern and capacities and that children should be able to depend on that commitment in good times and in bad . . .'. The words 'normal development' represent a very important extension of the commitment.

The focus on child survival has an obvious appeal, as shown, for example, by a statement by Mr Christopher Patten, when he was Minister of Overseas Development in the British Government: 'If development and aid programmes have one easily measurable and fundamental purpose, it is to stop so many babies dying' (Patten, 1989). It has a particular appeal, perhaps, for those trained in medicine, since death of children from malnutrition is technically preventable and it is not tolerable that efforts should not be made to prevent it.

The philosopher of science, Sir Karl Popper, has said: '. . . we should demand the elimination of suffering rather than the promotion of happiness' (quoted by Payne, 1987). Thus one argument for regarding the promotion of child survival as a priority aim is the moral imperative.

The second argument, supported by the World Bank (Lancet, 1988), relies on the concept that malnutrition is a cause as well as an effect of poverty and that successful adjustments and growth cannot occur if a population is prevented by ill-health and undernutrition from achieving its physical, intellectual and social potential. In the words of Jolly (1987):

> It is almost a reflex of the economic mind to think of adjustment with a human face as a welfare programme. In contrast, I would stress that it is primarily one of enhancing production and investment . . .

To this may be added the effect, or alleged effect, on the birth rate of reducing infant and child deaths (see below).

Strong criticisms have been expressed of both foundations of the child survival strategy. The moral imperative is not conclusive. Thus Gopalan (1982) has called the strategy 'a policy of brinkmanship', which simply reduces the size of the tip of the iceberg without going to the root of the problem. The argument based on the preservation of human capital and future productivity has been criticized by Payne (1987). His view follows logically from the concept discussed in Chapter 13, that if Third World children are for the most part adapted to the stresses of their environment, then by definition their human potential is preserved.

What is the appropriate target?

Newell and Nabarro (1989) suggest that the infant mortality rate and hence the question of infant and child survival no longer has the general public health significance that it used to, now that there are specific techniques for preventing death which have no effect on the health of the survivors. They express concern that concentration on child survival is opting for an easy solution that relies on technical measures and is more concerned with the means than the real ends. Such an approach, in their view, cannot lead to a sustainable solution.

Perhaps the concentration should be on the family rather than the child. Much lip-service is paid to community participation, but has anyone consulted the community about priorities? Newell and Nabarro (1989) put a point of view which deserves to be quoted in full:

> We know of no society where the death of an infant is not thought of as a personal or a family tragedy. However, there are many societies where these tragedies have a ranking different from that in ours. There are groups which consider that the illness, death or disability of a breadwinner, or even the death of a buffalo, may threaten the structure or survival of the family. There are others which may consider the pressure of an extra mouth to feed a mixed blessing. These realities cannot be viewed as right or wrong. What is wrong is to assume that all societies think alike and that their actions should be conditioned by our views. Infant deaths . . . may not be the first priority in all societies.

Pacey and Payne (1985) have raised a similar point: a poor family may be in a very delicate balance between productive members and those who have to be looked after and fed—the very young and very old. The balance alters with time (Fig. 20.1), and a new mouth to feed at the wrong time may affect it disastrously.

Nabarro (1984) has provided an excellent description of the stresses faced by such families in a 'typical' village in Nepal, if, as he says, any village can be regarded as typical. This general description could be applied equally well to the urban poor, if for seasonal changes are substituted fluctuations in opportunities for earning money, in the price of food, etc.

The lynch-pin of the family is the mother. Rural women make a very important contribution to food production. For example, Edmundson and

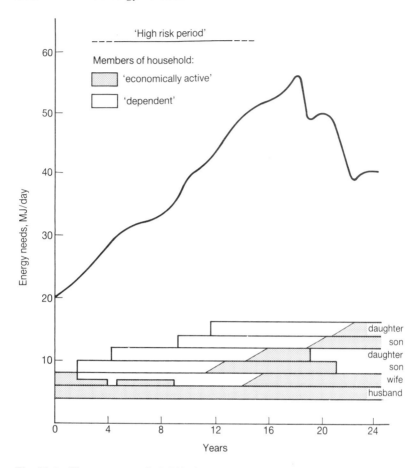

Fig. 20.1   The energy needs (MJ/day) of a household with four children for 25 years after its formation. The peak value, before the eldest daughter leaves home at the age of about 17 years, is about 56 MJ (13 500 kcal) per day. Reproduced by permission from Pacey and Payne (1985).

Edmundson (1988) found that in an Indian village women spent 27 per cent more time in the fields than men although their energy intake was 27 per cent less. It is the women who have to fetch water and fuel, often from long distances. They have to keep the house, prepare food, look after children; if the older children share these tasks, as they often do, they cannot go regularly to school. In the cities it is probable that women can find work more easily than men, as domestics, street vendors or in factories, work that takes them away from home for very long hours. In the Third World maternal deaths amount to 100 – 300 per 100 000 live births, compared to 7 – 15 in developed countries (Hammam and Youssef, 1986). The death of the mother in childbirth must be a disaster for these marginal families that rely so heavily on the mother.

We have also become more aware in recent years of the enormous pressures under which poor women operate and their difficulties of choice. (See Nabarro, 1984; also Food and Nutrition Bulletin (4), 1989, for a series of highly informative papers on this subject.) In the words of McGuire and Popkin (1989):

> Crucial conflicts face poor women in low-income countries as they try to fulfil their economic, biological and social roles at each stage in the life-cycle, particularly during the child-bearing years. Changes in behaviour that enhance their contribution to one role can have crucial negative effects on their other roles and activities.

Joseph (1985) points out a global trend towards increased social and economic mobility of women and discusses how this may reflect on child care.

How, then, can women, with these pressures on their energy and time, be expected to do all the things that experts think they ought to do—breast-feed more often, prepare more nutritious weaning foods in a cleaner way, spend more time playing with their children, take them to health centres, etc.?

Inputs and tools

Rifkind and Walt (1988) have said: 'The basis of *sustained* good health will depend on community decisions to act on low-cost techniques, not just on the provision of such technologies'. Habicht and Berman (1987) make a useful distinction between the technologies, where the criterion is efficiency, and the organization for delivering the technologies, where the criteria are equity, cost and participation. Perhaps the conflict of opinion on strategies is more apparent than real. Governments or other agencies have to make services available, but a working primary health care system is necessary for the services to be properly used. These are two sides of the same coin. It is against this background that we have to look at the various inputs, tools and methods that are proposed or used for the prevention of PEM.

'Inputs' refers to resources to which poor people must have access if there is to be a decrease in the prevalence of malnutrition; 'tools' are what Newell and Nabarro (1989) call the technologies. They are conveniently covered by the UNICEF acronym GOBI-FFF: growth-monitoring, oral rehydration, promotion of breast-feeding, immunization, female education, family planning and food, although not necessarily in that order.

All that is said here has been said many times before. An excellent short account is given by Tomkins (1987).

Education

At the top of the list comes the education of women. Thirty years ago Cravioto *et al.* (1967) in Mexico showed that in a homogeneous community the mother's level of education was a dominant factor in whether or not a child became malnourished. This observation has been confirmed many times. In a report prepared for the World Bank, Hicks (quoted by Streeter, 1981) attempted to rank the factors that determined whether a child survived or died. The education of women came out on top, above food, water and sanitation.

This correlation between female literacy and child survival has been found worldwide and is independent of differences in wealth or general standards of living (Lovel, 1989). Rohde has aptly said: 'teach a man and you teach an individual; teach a woman and you teach a nation'.

How this relationship works is unknown. One might suppose that more educated women are better at organizing their time and resources, however meagre; make more use of health services; start child-bearing later and have longer birth intervals. Perhaps the mechanism does not matter; the fact is enough, so long as more girls have access to the schooling which is their right. One favourable aspect of urbanization may be that it makes this access easier. Sinha (1988) has pointed out that in the Caribbean not only are more girls being educated but 70 per cent of women are gainfully employed, earning money outside the home. This has not, as might have been anticipated, prevented massive declines in infant and child mortality over the last 25 years, which may be an indication of the key role of the grandmother in Caribbean society.

Better access to the educational system is one thing; conventional health and nutrition education provided by an outsider, based on the idea that mothers are 'ignorant', is quite a different matter and many believe that it does not work (Praun, 1982). The family is part of a community, which has conventions and customs based on long experience and perhaps religious beliefs. As several authors have noted, a common belief of many mothers that needs to be changed is that sick children should not be fed. However, it is not so easy to break away from customs ingrained for generations and to do so there must be a perceived advantage as well as a real advantage (Nabarro, 1984). Moreover, the poorest in any community are the weakest. In the words of Praun (1982): '. . . within deprived and oppressed groups there is the feeling of insecurity and of despair at ever being able to do something by themselves. This translates into conformism and dependency . . .'. She describes a programme of nutrition education in Central America which surmounted these difficulties by developing real participation. In this process the community health worker must play a key role. In a more sophisticated situation (South Africa) it was found that even though a programme of nutrition counselling increased the mothers' knowledge, there was no effect on the nutritional status of the children (Glatthaar *et al.*, 1986).

Water supplies and sanitation

The International Water Decade (1981–90) has seen significant increases in the proportion of people with access to clean water and sanitary facilities, but Table 20.3 shows that there is still a long way to go.

Table 20.3   Water supplies and sanitation in the developing world (excluding China)

| | Percentage of people served | | | |
| | Water | | Sanitation | |
Year	Urban	Rural	Urban	Rural
1970	65	13	34	11
1980	74	32	56	14
1985	86	44	62	15

From UNICEF (1987)

Although technical improvements in pumps, pipes and latrines have increased the reliability and reduced the cost, the investments needed are still large, and the question of effectiveness compared with other interventions has to be considered. Esrey *et al.* (1985) reviewed 67 studies of the effect on diarrhoeal disease of improving water supplies and disposal of excreta. The impact on diarrhoea morbidity was inversely related to the level of hygiene before the intervention, for which, interestingly, the authors took literacy as a proxy. This is a clear indication for targeting at the community or population level. It is to be expected that the impact of improvements in water supply and sanitation will vary for different infections, according to the dose needed to produce symptoms. For enterotoxigenic *E.coli* the dose is high and the impact should be great, whereas the reverse holds for rotavirus.

Only a minority of the studies reviewed by Esrey *et al.* (1985) were considered to be well-designed and technically satisfactory, but they were consistent in reporting a positive impact: a median reduction of 27 per cent in diarrhoea morbidity and 30 per cent in mortality. Improvements in water quality had a lesser impact than improvements in the availability of water and the disposal of excreta.

An important point emerged in a recent report from Bangladesh (Aziz *et al.*, 1990). Tube-wells, pit latrines and health education were provided in one area, but not in a neighbouring control area. After three years the number of episodes of diarrhoea was 25 per cent lower in the intervention area, but the incidence of prolonged diarrhoea (> 14 days) was 40 per cent lower. This is important, because it is the prolonged diarrhoea syndrome (PDS, Chapter 17) which carries the greatest risk of producing PEM and death.

Diarrhoeal pathogens are transmitted not only by water but also by food and by direct contact of the child with people's hands, utensils, etc. Rowland *et al.* (1978) showed how porridges and gruels that were allowed to stand about for several hours after being cooked operated as culture media. No doubt this source of transmission could be reduced by education of the mother, but to have to cook children's food freshly before every meal makes yet more demands on her time and resources. Another possibility that needs further investigation is how far traditional processes used in some parts of the world in the preparation of weaning foods, such as fermentation, may have bacteriostatic effects (Mensah *et al.*, 1990) (Chapter 16).

A United Nations report (1985), quoted by Sinha (1988), suggested that attitudes and behaviour related to health practices and personal hygiene may be more important than physical facilities. It has indeed been found in some cases that hand-washing is effective in reducing direct transmission of infectious agents (Feachem, 1984). Torun (1982) in Guatemala found a reduction of 30 per cent in the incidence rate of diarrhoea in the peak season and 50 per cent in the number of days ill as a result of an education programme. A study in Bangladesh (Khan, 1982) showed how hand-washing could reduce the transmission of shigellosis within a family, once one member had become infected.

It may be concluded that improvements in water supply, sanitation and hygiene do reduce the incidence of diarrhoea, but Briend *et al.* (1989) in particular have questioned whether they have any impact on nutritional state. For example, in a group of villages in Bangladesh the provision of tube wells, latrines and education in hygiene reduced the incidence of diarrhoea by 30 per cent compared with a control area, but there was no effect on nutritional state (Hasan *et al.*, 1989). As discussed in Chapter 17, it is far from clear whether over the longer term diarrhoeal and other infections have the major effects on nutrition and growth that have sometimes been claimed.

The impact of these programmes should in any case not be thought of only in terms of morbidity and mortality; it has been said that 'an economic analysis has shown that the saving of women's time from the chore of water collection is itself a sufficient economic justification for investments in water supply' (Anonymous, 1987). If human rights have any reality, access to plentiful and clean water is surely one of them.

Oral rehydration therapy

It could be argued that if priority is being given in health and nutrition policy to reduction of infant and child deaths, oral rehydration therapy (ORT) is one of the cheapest and most effective ways of achieving that aim. Dehydration is probably responsible for a substantial proportion of deaths, but it only occurs in a minority of episodes of diarrhoea, perhaps about 10 per cent (Lovell, 1989), and diarrhoea has its main prevalence in a rather restricted age-range, six to 24 months. A programme for promoting ORT must therefore be one that is highly targeted, and it can surely only succeed through community health workers and community participation (see below). When treatment is needed, it is needed urgently, and even in a well organized system local health centres or posts are not within easy range of everyone and are unlikely to be open 24 hours a day and seven days a week. Therefore the community health worker must be the first line of defence.

ORT is undoubtedly effective in the treatment of individual children. The problem is that not enough mothers know about it, have access to it, or recognize the need for it. ORT may conflict with strongly held cultural beliefs, which vary greatly in different parts of the world, about how sick children should be treated. Here anthropologists can make a particularly important contribution (Kendall *et al.*, 1984). Coreil and Mull (1988) draw a parallel with the obvious need for sociocultural research to make family planning programmes acceptable.

However, it has to be recognized that ORT is a palliative; it is argued by Henry *et al.* (1990*b*) that programmes focussing on ORT are unlikely to reduce mortality due to diarrhoea substantially unless in the context of a broader policy to tackle the diarrhoea-malnutrition syndrome. In their surveys in Bangladesh 63 per cent of all diarrhoeal deaths occurred in children with persistent diarrhoea associated with malnutrition. Clearly there is an urgent need for research on the causes of the persistent diarrhoea. (See also Chapter 17.)

Immunization

Although at the time of writing vaccines (except against pertussis) are not available for the respiratory and diarrhoeal diseases that make the largest contribution to infant and child mortality, immunization against other infections, particularly measles, is very important, especially in populations where a large number of children are to some extent malnourished. With many types of infection even a moderately malnourished child is likely to have a more severe and prolonged illness (Chapter 17) and to need more food on recovery to make good the losses incurred when ill.

WHO's Expanded Programme of Immunization (EPI) covers six diseases: diphtheria, pertussis, tetanus (DPT), tuberculosis, poliomyelitis and measles. There has been an encouraging increase in coverage over the last decade. As of 1989 it is estimated that two-thirds of children in developing countries have received three doses of DPT and polio vaccine, more that 70 per cent have been vaccinated with BCG and nearly 60 per cent with measles vaccine (Henderson *et al.*, 1988; Henderson, 1989; Hall *et al.*, 1990). So successful has been the programme that polio is on the verge of being eradicated from the WHO Western Hemisphere region (G. A. O. Alleyne, personal communication). Prevention of neonatal tetanus by the administration of tetanus toxoid to pregnant women has lagged behind. According to Warren (1990) full coverage with existing vaccines could reduce mortality under five years of age by 20 per cent.

Four problems remain. Of the diseases covered by EPI, the most lethal is measles. It has been estimated that 51 million cases and 1.6 million deaths occur annually from this cause in the Third World. Overcrowding increases the intensity of transmission and hence the case fatality. This is likely to be an important factor in urban slums. The main causes of death associated with measles are bronchopneumonia and diarrhoea. According to Feachem and Koblinsky (1983) *Shigella* may play a major role as the cause of post-measles diarrhoea. These authors calculated that measles immunization, with a coverage of 45–90 per cent, could prevent between 6 and 26 per cent of diarrhoeal deaths. In current practice measles vaccination at 9–11 months produces sero-conversion rates of 80–90 per cent, provided that the vaccine is in good condition. Earlier vaccination has not been recommended because of interference by maternal antibodies. Although the peak prevalence of measles seems generally to be in the second year (e.g. Van Lerberghe, 1990) cases do occur earlier and the development of a vaccine that could be given to younger infants would be an important advance.

In one region of The Gambia, where vaccine-preventable deaths have been largely eliminated, the main causes of death under five are now respiratory infections, diarrhoea and malaria (Hall *et al.*, 1990). It is probable that the pattern is the same elsewhere. Respiratory deaths are due largely to *Pneumococcus sp.* and *H.influenzae*. Current vaccines are not protective under 15 months of age, when most of the deaths occur, so there is a need for new vaccines. The causes of severe diarrhoea in young children are so numerous (Chapter 17) that the prospects of effective vaccines being developed at an affordable cost seem rather remote.

Malaria has been somewhat neglected in the recent literature as a cause of death in infants and young children, but in regions where the disease is, holo-endemic such as The Gambia it is surely very important (McGregor, 1982). It may be overlooked as a cause of death, particularly in children who are malnourished, for two reasons. First, such a child may be unable to produce a typical pyrexia (Chapter 12), and in my experience the presenting feature is often diarrhoea; secondly, malaria has a general immunosuppressive effect and its action in promoting the severity of other infections may not be recognized (Chapter 17). Much research is being done on malaria vaccines, but there is a long way to go.

Breast feeding

As discussed in Chapter 16, breast feeding during infancy and partial breast feeding prolonged into the second year are important for the baby's nutrition, for protection from infection, for prolonging the birth interval and no doubt for psychological reasons also. In view of the different traditional patterns of infant feeding in different parts of the world, it may be unwise to insist on exclusive breast feeding for a certain number of months. There is something illogical about involving community participation on the one hand, on the other trying to alter traditional practices unless there is a very good reason for it.

It is another matter to try to discourage mothers from abandoning their traditional practices as they come into contact with what we are pleased to call civilization. This problem is not new; feeding bottles were used in ancient Greece and Rome. There are two elements in it: one is social class and the other is urbanization. Surveys in countries such as Mexico, Malaysia and Kenya (Dimond and Ashworth, 1987) have shown that better-off urban women are least likely to start breast feeding, and if they do start, most likely to continue for only a short time. One of the pressures to prefer formula feeding has been reduced, if not entirely removed, by the WHO/UNICEF code of practice for the promotion of infant formulae. However, these women may regard breast feeding as old-fashioned, uncivilized or even disgusting (Harfouche, 1980). Here education is important and can be effective, as has been shown by experience in industrialized countries such as Britain.

Only recently has attention begun to be paid to the urban poor, who will soon constitute 50 per cent of the world's population. It is they who present the really difficult problem, particularly unmarried teenage mothers. Anyanyu and Ewonwu (1987), in a study on poor urban women in Lagos, Nigeria, found that virtually all women expressed strong positive feelings about breast feeding, but there was a large discrepancy between their expressed intentions and what they actually did. These authors conclude that it is superficial to attribute the decline in breast feeding under these conditions simply to attitudes imported from the developed world. 'It is clear that such explanations are over-simplified . . . and ignore the hard realities of urban existence that may make prolonged breast-feeding difficult.' Obviously everything should be done to promote the provision of crèches at the place of work for those who work in offices and factories, but it is probable that most poor urban women are earning what they can in the so-called informal sector. It may be worthwhile to advise that the baby should continue to be breast-fed at least at night, but, as the Nigerian authors point out, nutrition education is useless when it simply extols virtues already accepted. They would prefer emphasis to be given on how to prepare better and more hygienic supplementary foods.

Supplementary feeding

It has already been mentioned (Chapter 16) that supplementary feeding of pregnant women has in some instances resulted in increases in birth weight and reductions in the proportion of low birth weight infants. There are numerous well controlled research studies in which food supplements for infants and young children have produced increases in growth, e.g. those of Hanumantha Rao and Naidu (1977) in India and Mora *et al.* (1981) in Colombia. However, when it comes to large-scale routine feeding programmes the results are much less encouraging. Beaton and Ghassemi (1982) reviewed a large number of programmes in which food had been distributed to pre-school children either under the auspices of the World Food Programme or through various charities. They concluded that there was very little evidence of benefit in terms of improvement of growth. In a later paper Beaton (1982) suggested that this may be an inappropriate criterion. There may be unmeasured benefits such as an increase in physical activity. In these large-scale programmes no-one really knows what the effect is on children's actual food intakes. There is undoubtedly leakage; if the food is given to be taken home it is shared with the family; if it is consumed by the child on the spot, perhaps it eats less at home. This leakage surely does not particularly matter; the families receiving the supplement are presumably poor, so it may be regarded as a form of income transfer, though probably not a very efficient one. Other non-nutritional benefits often claimed are that a feeding programme attracts mothers to clinics, that it is a vehicle for nutrition and health education and that it encourages community participation.

Opponents of supplementary feeding programmes argue that they are expensive, they divert staff from more useful activities, they discourage breast feeding and promote diarrhoea and they create a dependence on imported foods (Maxwell, 1978). In one study in Khartoum, specifically designed to test some of these objections, dried skim milk regularly distributed in the health centres was replaced in some centres by a ration of local beans, which would be consumed by the whole family. The weight gain of infants was similar in both groups and there was no evidence that the dried milk decreased breast feeding or promoted diarrhoea (Zumrawi *et al.*, 1981).

The effectiveness of feeding programmes could theoretically be increased by targeting the supplements more closely to children most in need, identified by anthropometric screening. Many such programmes are 'vertical' operations, in which food is regularly distributed at a central point by special staff. It is difficult to imagine that under these conditions it is really possible to separate those children or mothers who will receive food from those who will not, without causing bad feeling. Surely the solution is for food, like drugs, to be available to community health workers, who know the families and can distribute it according to their perception of needs.

Before leaving this subject, it may be of interest to recall something of its early history. In the depression of the 1930s British farmers were unable to sell their milk because people could not afford to buy it. The Government consulted Sir John Boyd Orr, later the first Director-General of FAO, who suggested that it should be distributed free in schools. An attempt was made to monitor the effects, and although there were only small, barely significant, increases in growth the teachers reported that the children became more active and difficult to control. Free or subsidized milk for pregnant women, infants and pre-school children was provided in Britain throughout the last war and for many years after, and is still available in the UK for those in need. My view, perhaps simplistic, is that what is considered necessary for British children is necessary for the children of poor countries, particularly as there is a surplus of milk in the industrialized world. The Nobel Laureate Hans Singer considers it by no means inevitable that this should have a bad effect on local agriculture (Singer and Longhurst, 1986).

Growth monitoring

Growth monitoring (GM) is an even more contentious subject than sup-plementary feeding. The basic objective of GM is to detect faltering in growth at an early stage in order to prevent a child from becoming malnourished. This has to be distinguished from anthropometric screening to select for special attention those children who are already undernourished (Gopalan, 1987; Hendrata and Rohde, 1988). GM is pointless unless it is followed by some kind of action. However, as Jelliffe and Jelliffe (1987) have observed, there is no consensus either on what constitutes inadequate growth, or on what action is appropriate when faltering occurs. More research is undoubtedly needed on the risks associated with different patterns of growth and on the costs of GM in terms of field-workers' and mothers' time (Nabarro and Chinnock, 1988).

GM depends on measurements of velocity and the idea is that it will provide a sensitive indicator of what is happening and a predictor of what is likely to happen. It has already been pointed out (Chapter 13) that growth velocities over short periods such as a month are so variable that it is extremely difficult to organize the information in a way that is useful. Henry *et al.* (1990*a*) have claimed that weight at six months is a better predictor of weight at subsequent periods than weight gain or growth velocity. If that is so, it would be possible to decide at this critical age on a particular weight, e.g. the 5th NCHS centile, which should be regarded as a trigger for action. This would include a number of false positives—5 per cent of the normal population, plus infants who, perhaps because of a low birth weight, are growing along a low centile track —but that is not very important. Healy *et al.* (1988) have suggested that in addition to an 'action limit' at the 5th centile, a 'warning limit' might be specified, say at the 25th centile. If the next measurement was below the 25th centile, it would indicate a need for intervention.

A number of authors have stressed the practical difficulties of GM: that it is unrealistic to expect relatively untrained health workers to make accurate measurements, record them accurately on charts and understand how to inter-pret them. Jelliffe and Jelliffe (1987) say: 'All procedures are more difficult to carry out than was previously realized . . . these difficulties are magnified enormously by the rapid spread of primary health care'. Others have found it difficult to persuade women to bring their children long distances to a clinic for an operation whose purpose they do not understand. In the experience of Nabarro and Chinnock (1988) village-based weighing sometimes deterred women from participating in other health activities, because they felt that their time was being wasted. Figure 20.2 gives a graphic account of the effect of an attempt to monitor growth in a Himalayan village, which illustrates the results of failure to involve the community.

There is general agreement than GM must not be seen as an isolated activity. In the words of Arole (1988), one of the pioneers of primary health care, 'When placed clearly in the hands of villagers, GM becomes the tool of development and an integral part of the community participatory process'. Introduction of GM into his community was facilitated by the establishment of a small rural hospital. This point of view has been stressed also by Hendrata and Rohde (1988) in an article with the provocative title 'Ten pitfalls of growth monitoring and promotion'. The ideal is to have duplicate records of the growth chart, one of which is kept by the mother as part of the child's

FROM A VILLAGE IN THE HIMALAYAS

Why irate mothers put the outsider to flight

Within hours of her arrival in the village, the young woman knew she was on probation. One false move and she could be sent packing, as other strangers had been. The villagers had, astutely, let her have the hut next to the drummer who was also the community's watchman. He closely observed her comings and goings for several days.

He concluded that she was not an interfering busybody. Unlike most town people, Anjana – officially designated as a "health worker" – didn't turn up her nose at the dirt in which they all wallowed. Everybody relaxed. The women, distrustful at first, soon warmed to her, asked her what to do if their babies had colic or conjunctivitis, or just cried too much. Gradually, they came to trust her enough to do as she said – sometimes.

All seemed well until one cold winter day, when taking advantage of the new road linking the village to the district town, Anjana's superior arrived in a Jeep. He had come, the doctor told Anjana – caught unawares – to launch a new project designed to induce village women to take better care of their children. The idea was simple: one, two and three-year-olds would be weighed on the scales – the latest that modern technology could provide – which he had brought with him. The three children who weighed the most, and were the cleanest, would receive cash prizes.

The women, puzzled at first, were soon splitting their sides with laughter. What? Weigh children in kilos? Rice, wheat, potatoes – those you weigh. But children? Perhaps the doctor had been a shopkeeper once? Or did he want to set up a trade in children? "How much" they finally asked Anjana, earnestly, "is he going to pay us per kilogramme of child?" "Seventy-five rupees for the first prize, 50 for the second, 30 for the third," Anjana tried to clarify.

Each woman, convinced that her child was the healthiest in the village, and would win the money, good-humouredly picked up her offspring and hurried towards the tin-roofed shelter under which the doctor had set up his equipment. He was appalled. The children, always barefoot, had feet encrusted with layers of dirt; many had dripping noses; several had dirty bottoms; most wore torn, filthy clothes. "Send them back," he told Anjana, "and explain to them again the importance of cleanliness. The prizes will go to children who are both healthy and clean."

The women left, peeved, and some didn't return, but the poorest did, with the children all scrubbed and neat: they were thinking of the money. Three hours passed before the last child had been weighed and inspected. The sun began to dip behind the high mountains in the West. Many women were now restive. When

the doctor, beaming, announced the prizewinners, there was a moment of tense silence. The winners stepped forward proudly with their children and accepted the cash. Then all hell broke loose.

"What about my baby? Who says he's not healthy?" "And mine!" "What about mine?" another woman snarled, closing in on the doctor. Confronted with a barrage of questions, he soon disappeared from Anjana's sight as a crowd of women pushed and jostled and shrieked abuse. "We know what happened," one of them yelled. "There was money for each of us, but you and Anjana have split it between yourselves. You can't fool us. Take that, and that . . ."

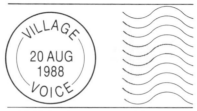

Afraid that her presence might stoke the inflamed tempers, Anjana quietly withdrew. The doctor, retrieving his weighing machine and papers, fled down the hill pursued by a horde of furious women, many with wailing babies in their arms.

We too joined the chase, trying to catch up with him: he had promised to talk to us about his projects. "Wait, doctor, wait," we called out. But he jumped into the Jeep and raced off, churning up a cloud of dust.

We climbed back to our own hut and were preparing supper when we heard an altercation. All over the village squabbles were breaking out like little fires flaring up. Men were shouting at their wives; the women were answering back. The husbands, their day's work over, had come back hungry, but their food was not ready. What had the women been up to?

One by one the little fires went out. Now the men were laughing: "Just like women, to stand in line for three hours, for nothing . . ."

We walked to the temple square to hear the villagers talk about the day's events, but they fell silent just as we approached. Everybody was watching the lone figure of a woman trudging wearily up the path.

Anjana stopped, then climbed slowly towards her hut, a picture of dejection even in the grey light of dusk.

Six months' work gone to waste. She would have to start building bridges all over again.

© *Victor Zorza & Veenu Sandal, 1988*

Fig. 20.2 Difficulties faced by community health workers over growth monitoring in a Himalayan village. Reproduced by permission of *The Times*, London.

'health passport', containing records of immunization, illnesses, etc. In this way Morley's advocacy of growth charts as the 'road to health' can be fulfilled (Morley, 1973).

There is little objective evidence of the effectiveness of GM in preventing PEM. That reviewed by Ashworth and Feachem (1986) is not particularly convincing. Time will no doubt show. GM is likely to be most effective when combined with health education.

Family planning and the control of fertility

As everyone now realizes, reduction in the accelerating growth of the world's population is a matter of profound concern, not only in relation to probable limits on food supply, but in the wider context of the environment: the conflict between natural resources and man's need for water, food and clothing. It has been said by many authorities on the environment that in the last analysis the only effective way of counteracting the increase of carbon dioxide will be to reduce the growth of the world's population.

Here the prevention of PEM and of the deaths associated with it can, paradoxically, make a major contribution. Therefore this section ends, as it began, with one of the most important indirect factors related to infant and child mortality—family planning and the control of fertility.

This relationship is in two directions. Numerous reports, of which Fig. 20.3 is an example, illustrate the influence of child spacing on mortality. In Williams' original description (Chapter 1) kwashiorkor was described as the disease of the displaced child. Better birth spacing is promoted by prolonged breast feeding and the consequent lactational amenorrhoea (Chapter 16). The other side of the coin is that falls in child mortality are accompanied or followed by falls in birth rate. Demographers have questioned any causal

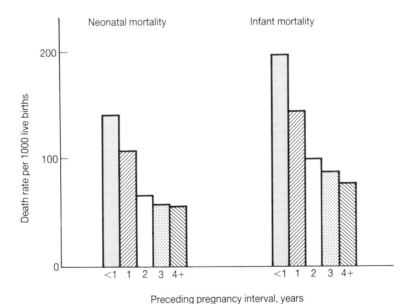

Fig. 20.3 Effect of birth spacing on neonatal and infant mortality rates. Reproduced by permission from Omran and Standley (1976).

relationship, but according to Rohde (1991) 'modern demographic analysis invariably identifies mortality decline as a precondition to fertility decline, the only uncertainty being the timing'. It seems that when social and economic conditions improve fertility rises at first and then falls (Lipton, 1988). Fig. 20.4 is a good example of this inverted U-shaped response.

In South-East Asia the under-five mortality rate has fallen from 260 per 1000 live births in 1950 to 110 in 1986, and the crude birth rate has fallen in the same period from 45 to 30 per 1000 population (UNICEF, 1987). At first sight it may seem that the 30 per cent decrease in birth rate does not compensate for the 60 per cent reduction in deaths, but this is not so. In 1950, per 1000 population, 33 children were born and survived to five years of age, whereas the comparable figure in 1986 is 27. This represents a significant decrease in the rate of population growth.

The growth of populations can be described in three stages.

(i)　High birth rate and high death rate. This has been the characteristic condition world-wide until modern times. From the classical period until the 18th century the average expectation of life at birth was only

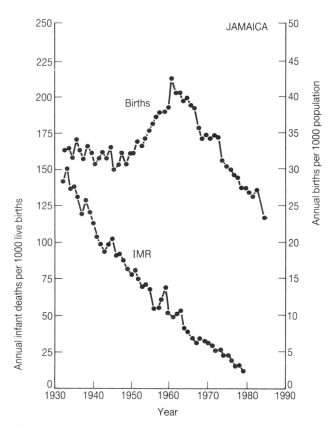

Fig. 20.4　Relationship between birth rate and infant mortality rate in Jamaica between 1930 and 1980. Reproduced by permission from Sinha (1988).

about 30 years for men and 25 for women and changed very little (for references see Waterlow, 1989).

(ii)   High birth rate and low death rate. This is the situation in which Third World countries are beginning to find themselves today. Births still exceed deaths, but the rate of population increase is beginning to slow down.

(iii) Low birth rate and low death rate, the current condition of industrialized countries leading to relatively stable populations.

The fear is that Third World countries will be caught in a 'demographic trap' and instead of moving on to stage (iii) will revert to stage (i), with consequences far worse, in terms of famine and social conflict, than in the old days because the absolute populations are so much larger. Reducing child mortality should make some contribution to averting this catastrophe.

Primary health care and community participation

In the preceding sections a number of inputs and tools have been briefly described which, working together, can contribute to prevention of PEM, reduction in child mortality and enhancement of the quality of life. Some of the inputs can only be made at the level of the government or regional administration, such as improvement in the education and literacy of women, and the provision of water supplies. Some services may best be provided by 'vertical' programmes with special staff, for example immunization, malaria control, possibly supplementary feeding, possibly family planning, although vertical programmes are nowadays very much frowned on. At the end of the line, however, the inputs and the services have to be provided to *people*, whether in a village or an urban slum. There is general agreement that people can only be reached effectively through the primary health care system (PHC), the fundamentals of which were outlined at the beginning of this chapter. The GOBI-FFF programme, whose elements have been discussed, seems at first sight to fit well with the PHC concept. Recently, however, it has come in for much criticism (e.g. Newell, 1988; Wiesner, 1988), which could also be aimed at many other governmental and multilateral programmes.

Criticisms of the GOBI-FFF programme

There are three main lines of attack.

(i)   The programme takes poverty and inequality for granted and seeks only to alleviate their effects, not to eradicate them. It proposes technologies as a substitute for social transformation.

(ii)   It represents a selection of elements of health care, rather than a comprehensive approach. In the words of Newell (1988): 'Selective PHC has a list; when you start with any list, it becomes the objective'.

(iii) It represents messages imposed from outside and increases depen-

dency on the central state, i.e. the ideas of the élite and the bureau-
cracy. Lip service may be paid to community participation, but that
participation is viewed simply as a means of getting messages across,
not as a source of actual decisions and of popular control.

The case for the defence is that polarizations between selective and comprehensive health care, between horizontal and vertical programmes, etc. are
artificial—'men of straw' in the words of Taylor and Jolly (1988). It was never
envisaged at Alma Ata that everything could be done at once. In order to
get something done it is necessary to select those activities most likely to be
feasible and productive. Selective activities are not regarded as a substitute
for comprehensive PHC, but as a leading edge which, by achieving something,
will promote confidence and facilitate further achievements.

It seems to me that there is a real philosophical difference between the two
points of view, which could perhaps be summed up as the difference between
idealist and empiricist, a difference that cannot be resolved by logical argument and that is repeated over and over again in the history of human development. As Taylor and Jolly admit, there is a major difficulty in relating the
objective priorities set by experts to the felt needs of the community. This is
a difficulty that we constantly see in any system that attempts to operate
democratically and that must at the same time lead and follow the wishes of
the people.

It is agreed that no inputs or programmes can succeed and be sustained
unless they are accepted by the community, but there are different kinds of
acceptance: there is active and enthusiastic acceptance which reflects self-
reliance, and there is passive acceptance of authority which is considered to
be contrary to human dignity. Clearly some programmes, such as family
planning and the promotion of breast feeding, depend totally on real acceptance of the first kind, but others, such as immunization, may have to make
do with passive acceptance. It is surely difficult to persuade people that a
procedure such as an injection, with which they may be totally unfamiliar,
can cause something *not* to happen. Convincing demonstration of cause and
effect, which is necessary for real acceptance, is much more difficult for
prevention than for cure. According to Walt *et al.* (1989), few communities
see the advantage of preventive care whether or not they have to pay for
it.

As Chen (1986) has pointed out, for the success of programmes demand
may be as important as supply, citing as an example the extremely low uptake
of a well-planned programme for the prevention of neonatal tetanus in
Bangladesh. Similarly, Malison *et al.* (1987) have described the disappoint-
ingly low utilization of health services in Uganda. The solution to this problem
is seen to lie through the community health worker, who will stimulate
demand by engaging the understanding and participation of the community.

The community health worker

It seems from the experience of the ten years since Alma Ata that the programme of PHC based on the community health workers (CHWs) has run
into many more difficulties than had been expected (WHO, 1989). These
difficulties are of two kinds. First, there are the problems of how the CHWs

function within the community, graphically described by Walt *et al.* (1989) with examples from many countries. The community as a whole is supposed to select the CHWs, but in reality it may be dominated by an élite with its own interests and power structure. In India caste is very important. Governments originally assumed that communities would be willing to support their CHWs in kind or in cash, but many have been reluctant to do so, at least on a sustained basis. High levels of dedication and leadership are needed (Flahault and Roemer, 1986). The CHW may not be well enough trained to have self-confidence or to inspire the confidence of the community, who may be willing to accept curative hand-outs, such as drugs or food, but suspicious of preventive activities, such as health education. For all these reasons in many countries the CHWs have been weak and inactive and there has been a very high rate of attrition. However, this gloomy picture is not universal. As Walt *et al.* (1989) point out: 'Religion plays an important part. In Buddhism voluntarism is a positive value. It is possibly no accident that some of the largest health volunteer programmes are in Buddhist countries: Thailand, Myanmar and Sri Lanka'.

From the more limited perspective of the prevention of PEM, weakness of the CHW programmes is very serious. Only the CHW can know which families are most at risk, or which are most in need of extra food or education in health and nutrition. It is the CHW who can operate a system of informal and informed targeting provided that she or he has the confidence of the community.

It seems likely that outside agencies and the training programmes inspired by them are unrealistic in their expectations of what the CHW should do. Table 20.4, from UNICEF (1990), is a list of what a 'typical health worker

Table 20.4   What a typical health worker with 3 months' training should be able to do

I.   Advise parents on:
       importance of immunization
       birth spacing
       breast feeding
       hand washing
       treatment of diarrhoea
       feeding during weaning
       feeding during illness
       giving up harmful traditional practices
II. Stimulate the community to:
       protect water supplies
       construct latrines
       keep environment clean
     Treat common illnesses
     Recognize and refer serious illnesses
     Give first aid for injuries
     Give vaccinations
     Give nutritional supplements
     Organize growth monitoring
     Identify children at special risk
III. Help teachers to teach about health
     Assist health teams e.g. in malaria control
     Work with community and religious leaders

Summarized from UNICEF (1990)

with 3 months' training should be able to do'. Such a worker is supposed to be responsible for 200–250 families. It seems doubtful if anyone could do all these things effectively, month in and month out. In India, which has extensive experience of various systems of PHC, the list of the responsibilities of an Anganwardi worker (i.e. village health worker) is not so long, but still formidable (Table 20.5).

Table 20.5 Function of Anganwardi workers (India)

Survey community and enlist beneficiaries
Non-formal education of children 3–6 years
Supplementary feeding of children 0–6 years
Supplementary feeding of pregnant and nursing mothers
Primary health care and first aid
Assist in immunization
Organize referral for the sick
Health and nutrition education of mothers

Summarized from Nutrition Foundation of India (1988)

The basic health system

This leads on to the second area of difficulty. To fulfil their responsibilities the CHWs need support, not only from the community but from the basic health care system, with its chain of command from Ministry to health post. The health system has to provide the supplies without which the CHW cannot operate credibly—basic drugs, food for the needy, materials for oral rehydration and family planning; it has to provide in-service training and technical back-up. On the other side, as mentioned above, technical inputs and vertical programmes, as of immunization or malaria control, need the co-operation of CHWs if they are to work well. Clearly the two systems should operate in a complementary way, but this does not always happen. Chabot and Bremners (1988), based on their experience in Mali, describe the mutual relation of the two systems as one of almost continuous conflict. 'They need each other for their daily functioning but they are seldom partners in a development process.' These words could equally well have been written about the situation often found in industry! As in most human affairs, the development of partnership, confidence and trust depends as much on personal characteristics as on management systems. Perhaps this is achieved more easily when part of the health service input comes from non-governmental sources, as described by Costello (1989) in Nepal.

The health post itself needs back-up at the secondary level. It has been common in recent years to castigate governments for spending too large a proportion of the health budget on hospitals. It is certainly bad if the hospitals are unnecessarily elaborate and if only the better-off have access to them, but the pendulum should not swing too far. No health service can command confidence and support if it cannot deal with problems such as tuberculosis, fractures and injuries, difficult deliveries and the resuscitation of severely ill children. Death or disability of the mother or father may spell ruin for the family and the children. Dr Arole, the pioneer of PHC in Jamkhet, Maharashtra, insists on the need for an operating theatre to back up the CHWs whom he has organized. WHO (1981) has stated that 'As a matter of principle, preventive services without curative ones are as unbalanced as curative services without prevention'. Gopalan (1989) goes further and says: 'The cause of rural health will not be served by our preventing the growth and development of advanced centres of learning and sophisticated diagnostic and treatment centres in cities'.

Lastly, there is the question of cost. Ashworth and Feachem (1986) estimated that in Indonesia an 'ideal' GOBI-FFF package, under the best conditions, would cost $31 per child per year, four times the annual expenditure per head on health. By contrast, Walsh and Warren (1979) calculated that a disease-oriented approach that concentrated on the top three priorities, diarrhoeal disease, measles and malaria, would cost $2 per head per year. Such an approach is clearly inadequate. The idea of a low-cost solution to the health problems of the Third World is a myth. It seems to follow that the costs of a PHC service, if estimated realistically, are inevitably more than can be afforded by very poor countries, so that there is probably no alternative to an injection of funds from outside. However, the hope is that if the service is successful in maintaining health and increasing productivity, it will generate at least some local support.

This description of some of the problems of putting PHC into practice has strayed from the topic of prevention of PEM, precisely because that aim cannot be achieved or even tackled in isolation from other activities inside and outside the health sector. One basic question remains, relating to ends rather than means, which was raised earlier in this chapter: does the community, which is supposed to be the source of decisions, give the same priority as we do to the promotion of child survival, or is this an ideal imposed from outside?

It is sad that this discussion of the role of PHC in the prevention of PEM should have to end with the admission of UNICEF, in their 'State of the World's Children' (1990): 'The PHC strategy, although fully inflated with rhetoric in all nations, has failed to lift off in all but a few'.

Conclusion

Those of us who work in the fields of nutrition and health will probably be asking ourselves: What part can we play in the prevention of PEM? WHO (1981), in an analysis of the role of the health sector in food and nutrition, listed the sector's responsibilities at the national level as: definition and analysis of nutrition problems; promotion of and participation in multisectoral food and nutrition strategies and programmes; and participation in setting up a food and nutrition surveillance scheme. To these should be added research —basic, epidemiological and operational—to fill gaps in the knowledge on which the analysis of nutritional problems must be founded. Sinisterra (1987) has said: 'It is not the function of scientists to change the economic and political structure of a society, but it is our responsibility to understand its inequalities and limitations because it is within this context that we must exercise our knowledge'. Newell (1988) put it succinctly: 'It is the responsibility of the health sciences to describe possible interventions and their implications and costs, but not to choose'.

The sting is in the tail of Newell's remark—'not to choose'. If the only real solution to PEM lies through political and social action; if, as is often the case, the health sector is relatively weak, and politicians and administrators choose not to apply the knowledge put at their disposal, then the training, experience and activities of professionals in health and nutrition may seem to be rather irrelevant. Professionals are also citizens, and perhaps a more productive way ahead for us would lie through promotion of political will. Some even hold that technical progress is counter-productive because it weakens the drive for more radical reorganization. The dilemma may be overstated, but I believe it to be a real one, particularly for those at the beginning of their careers, as I have discussed in a paper called 'Crisis for Nutrition' (Waterlow, 1981).

Nevertheless, when I look back over the time, ever since the last war, that I have been working on PEM, I feel some grounds for optimism about what has been achieved in improving nutrition and child health. There is greater awareness of nutritional problems by governments and international agencies, including awareness of their great complexity. In spite of limited resources there has been in many countries a reduction in infant and child mortality and an increase in the expectation of life. Table 20. 6, from India, is just one example, although there is indeed far to go. There has been an upsurge of interest in nutrition by social scientists and anthropologists, which will make an increasingly important contribution in the decades to come. Admittedly the rate of progress, whether fast or slow, depends on political and economic factors, but it is difficult to conceive that the momentum can be entirely lost.

Nutritionists have a special role, since they are the lynch pin of the co-operation between different sectors, on which the possibility of preventing PEM depends. It is therefore essential that nutrition should continue to develop as a discipline in its own right, if there is to be any hope of achieving the WHO/ UNICEF target of eliminating severe PEM and halving the prevalence of moderate PEM by the end of the decade.

Table 20.6   Changes in health indicators in India over 30 years

	1955	1985
Infant mortality rate	146	95
Child mortality rate	30	11
Life expectancy at birth, years	41	56

Data from Gopalan (1989)

References

Anyanyu, R. C., Enwonwu, C. O. (1985). The impact of urbanization and socio-economic status on infant feeding practices in Lagos, Nigeria. *Food and Nutrition Bulletin (UNU)* **7**: 33–37.

Anonymous (1987). The International Water Decade. *Lancet* **2**: 890–891.

Arole, M. (1988). A comprehensive approach to community welfare: growth monitoring and the role of women in Jamkhed (Maharashtra). *Indian Journal of Pediatrics* **55**: Suppl. S100–105.

Ashworth, A., Feachem, R. G. (1986). *Interventions for the control of diarrhoeal diseases among young children: growth monitoring programmes*. WHO paper CDD.86.1. World Health Organization, Geneva.

Aziz, K. M. A., Hoque, B. A. *et al*. (1990). Reduction in diarrhoeal diseases in children in rural Bangladesh by environmental and behavioural modifications. *Transactions of the Royal Society of Tropical Medicine and Hygiene* **84**: 433–438.

Backett, E. M., Davies, A. M., Petros-Barvazian, A. (1984). *The risk approach in health care*. World Health Organization, Geneva.

Beaton, G. H. (1982). Evaluation of nutrition interventions: methodologic considerations. *American Journal of Clinical Nutrition* **35**: 1280–1289.

Beaton, G. H., Ghassemi, H. (1982). Supplementary feeding programmes for young children in developing countries. *American Journal of Clinical Nutrition* **35**: 863–916.

Berg, A. (1987). *Malnutrition: what can be done? Lessons from World Bank experience*. Johns Hopkins University Press, Baltimore.

Blaxter, K. L. (1986). Food and people. Presidential address to the XIIIth International Congress of Nutrition. *Human Nutrition: Clinical Nutrition* **40C**: 95–102.

Brandt, W. (1980). *North-South: a programme for survival*. Pan Books, London and Sydney.

Briend, A., Hasan, K. Z. *et al*. (1989). Are diarrhoea control programmes likely to reduce childhood nutrition? Observations from rural Bangladesh. *Lancet* **2**: 319–322.

Byron, W. J. (1988). On the protection and promotion of the right to food: an ethical reflection. In LeMay, B. W. J. (ed) *Science, ethics and food*. Smithsonian Institution Press, Washington and London, pp. 14–30.

Chabot, H. T. J., Bremners, J. (1988). Government health services versus community: conflict or harmony? *Social Science and Medicine* **27**: 957–962.

Chandler, R. F. (1989). Toward a sustained agricultural economy. In Hirschoff, P. M., Kotter, N. G. (eds) *Completing the food chain: strategies for combating hunger and malnutrition*. Smithsonian Institution Press, Washington and London, pp. 134–139.

Chen, L. C. (1986). Primary health care in developing countries: overcoming operational, technical and social barriers. *Lancet* **2**: 1260–1265.

Coreil, J., Mull, J. D. (1988). Anthropological studies of·diarrhoeal illness. *Social Science and Medicine* **27**: 1–3.

Costello, A. M. de, L. (1989). Strengthening health care systems to improve infant health in rural Nepal. *Transactions of the Royal Society of Tropical Medicine and Hygiene* **83**: 19–22.

Cravioto, J., Birch, H. G. *et al*. (1967). The ecology of infant weight-gain in a pre-industrial society. *Acta Paediatrica Scandinavica* **56**: 71–84.

Dimond, H. J., Ashworth, A. (1987). Infant feeding practices in Kenya, Mexico and Malaysia. The rarity of the exclusively breast-fed infant. *Human Nutrition: Applied Nutrition* **41A**: 51–64.

Edmundson, W. C., Edmundson, S. A. (1988). Food intake and work allocation of male and female farmers in an impoverished Indian village. *British Journal of Nutrition* **60**: 433–439.

Esrey, S. A., Feachem, R. G., Hughes, J. M. (1985). Interventions for the control of diarrhoeal diseases among young children: improving water supplies and excreta disposal facilities. *Bulletin of the World Health Organization* **63**: 757–772.

Evans, J. R., Hall, K. L., Warford, J. (1981). Health care in the developing world: problems of scarcity and choice. *New England Journal of Medicine* **305**: 1117–1127.

Feachem, R. G. (1984). Interventions for the control of diarrhoeal diseases among young children: promotions of personal and domestic hygiene. *Bulletin of the World Health Organization* **62**: 467–476.

Feachem, R. G., Koblinsky, M. A. (1983). Interventions for the control of diarrhoeal diseases: measles immunization. *Bulletin of the World Health Organization* **61:** 641–652.

Flahault, D., Roemer, M. I. (1986). *Leadership for primary health care*. Public Health Paper no. 82. World Health Organization, Geneva.

Galbraith, J. K. (1986). Economic policy as a historical process: the meaning for agriculture and nutrition. In *Nutrition issues in developing countries for the 1980s and 1990s*. National Academy Press, Washington, DC, pp. 15–24.

Glatthaar, I. I., Fehrsen, G. S. *et al.* (1986). Protein-energy malnutrition: the role of nutrition education in rehabilitation. *Human Nutrition: Clinical Nutrition* **40C:** 271–285.

Gopalan, C. (1982). The nutrition policy of brinkmanship. *Bulletin of the Nutrition Foundation of India*, October 1982.

Gopalan, C. (1986). The effect of development programmes on the nutrition of populations. In Taylor, T. G., Jenkins, N. K. (eds) *Proceedings of the XIIIth International Congress of Nutrition*. John Libbey, London, pp. 9–18.

Gopalan, C. (1987). Growth monitoring—some basic issues. *Bulletin of the Nutrition Foundation of India* 8, no. 2.

Gopalan, C. (1988). In *Profiles of undernutrition and underdevelopment*. Scientific Report no. 8, p. vi. Nutrition Foundation of India, New Delhi.

Gopalan, C. (1989). Delivery of health care: challenges and strategies. In Gopalan, C. *Nutrition, health and national development*. Special Report Series no. 4, pp. 101–114. Nutrition Foundation of India, New Delhi.

Grant, J. (1990). In *The state of the world's children*. UNICEF and Oxford University Press.

Gwatkin, D. R., Wilcox, J. R., Wray, J. D. (1981). Can health and nutrition intervention make a difference? *World Health Forum* **2:** 119–128.

Habicht J-P., Berman, P. A. (1987). Strategies in primary health care. *American Journal of Public Health* **77:** 1396–1397.

Hall, A. J., Greenwood, B. M., Whittle, H. (1990). Modern vaccines: practice in developing countries. *Lancet* **335:** 774–777.

Hamman, M., Youssef, N. H. (1986). The continuum in women's productive and reproductive roles: implications for food aid and children's well-being. In *Food aid and the well-being of children in the developing world*. UNICEF, New York, pp. 85–104.

Hanumantha Rao, D., Nadamuni Naidu, A. (1977). Nutritional supplementation: whom does it benefit most? *American Journal of Clinical Nutrition* **30:** 1612–1616.

Harfouche, J. K. (1980). Psycho-social aspects of breast-feeding, including bonding. *Food and Nutrition Bulletin* **2:** 2–6.

Hasan Kh. Z., Briend, A. *et al.* (1989). Lack of impact of a water and sanitation intervention on the nutritional status of children in rural Bangladesh. *European Journal of Clinical Nutrition* **43:** 837–844.

Healy, M. J. R., Min Yang *et al.* (1988). The use of short-term increments in length to monitor growth in infancy. In Waterlow, J. C. (ed) *Linear growth retardation in less developed countries*. Nestlé Nutrition, Vevey/Raven Press, New York, pp. 41–52.

Henderson, R. H. (1989). Child survival—world survival: an epidemiologist's story. *Journal of the Royal College of Physicians (London)* **23:** 271–276.

Henderson, R. H., Keja, J. *et al.* (1988). Immunizing the children of the world: progress and prospects. *Bulletin of the World Health Organization* **66:** 535–543.

Hendrata, L., Rohde, J. E. (1988). Ten pitfalls of growth monitoring and promotion (GM/P). *Indian Journal of Pediatrics* **55:** Suppl. S9–S15.

Henry, F. J., Briend, A., Cooper, E. S. (1990*a*). Targeting nutritional interventions: is there a role for growth monitoring? *Health Policy and Planning* **4:** 295–300.

Henry, F. J., Briend, A., Fauveau, V. (1990*b*). Child survival: should the strategy be redesigned? Experience from Bangladesh. *Health Policy and Planning* **5:** 226–234.

Hopkins, A. F. (1987). Aid for development: what motivates the donors? In Clay, E., Shaw, J. (eds) *Poverty, development and food*. Macmillan Press, Basingstoke, UK, pp. 153–172.

House of Commons (1985). *Famine in Africa; Second Report from the Foreign Affairs Committee*. HM Stationery Office, London.

Jelliffe, E. F. P., Jelliffe, D. B. (1987). Algorithms, growth monitoring and nutritional interventions. *Journal of Tropical Pediatrics* **33**: 290–295.

Jolly, R. (1987). Adjustment with a human face: a broader approach to adjustment policy. In Clay, E., Shaw, J. (eds) *Poverty, development and food*. Macmillan Press, Basingstoke, UK, pp. 61–77.

Joseph, S. C. (1985). Realistic approaches to world hunger: public health measures. *Food and Nutrition Bulletin* **7**: 5–9.

Kendall, C., Foote, D., Martorell, R. (1984). Ethnomedicine and oral rehydration therapy: a case study of ethnomedical investigation and program planning. *Social Science and Medicine* **19**: 253–260.

Khan, M. U. (1982). Interruption of shigellosis by hand-washing. *Transactions of the Royal Society of Tropical Medicine and Hygiene* **76**: 164–168.

King, M. (1990). Health is a sustainable state. *Lancet* **336**: 664–667.

Lipton, M. (1988). *Attacking undernutrition and poverty: some issues of adaptation and sustainability*. Reprint no. 13. International Food Policy Research Institute, Washington, DC.

Lovel, H. (1989). Targeted interventions and infant mortality. *Transactions of the Royal Society of Tropical Medicine and Hygiene* **83**: 10–18.

McGregor, I. A. (1982). Malaria: nutritional implications. *Review of Infectious Diseases* **4**: 798–804.

McGuire, J., Popkin, B. M. (1989). Beating the zero-sum game: women and nutrition in the third world. *Food and Nutrition Bulletin* **11**: 38–63.

Mahler, H. (1988). Present status of WHO's initiative, 'Health for all by the year 2000'. *Annual Review of Public Health* **9**: 71–97.

Malison, M. D., Scheito, P. *et al.* (1987). Estimating health service utilization, immunization coverage and childhood mortality: a new approach in Uganda. *Bulletin of the World Health Organization* **65**: 325–330.

Maxwell, S. (1978). Food aid for supplementary feeding programmes. *Food Policy* **3**: 289–298.

Mellor, J. W. (1986). Food production, food supply and nutritional status. In *Nutrition issues in developing countries for the 1980s and 1990s*. National Academy Press, Washington DC, pp. 25–42.

Mensah, P. P. A., Tomkins, A. M. *et al.* (1990). Fermentation of cereals for reduction of bacterial contamination of weaning foods in Ghana. *Lancet* **336**: 140–143.

Mora, J. O., Sellers, S. G. *et al.* (1981). The impact of supplementary feeding and home education on physical growth of disadvantaged children. *Nutrition Research* **1**: 213–225.

Morley, D. (1973). *Pediatric priorities in the developing world*. Butterworth, London.

Mosley, W. H. (1984). Child survival: research and policy. In Mosley, W. H., Chen, L. C. (eds) *Malnutrition, morbidity and mortality*. Population and development review, Suppl. 10.

Musgrove, P. (1986). The impact of the economic crisis on health and health care in Latin America and the Caribbean. *WHO Chronicle* **40**: 152–157.

Nabarro, D. (1984). Social, economic, health and environmental determinants of nutritional status. *Food and Nutrition Bulletin* **6**: 18–32.

Nabarro, D., Chinnock, P. (1988). Growth monitoring: inappropriate promotion of an appropriate technology. *Social Science and Medicine* **27**: 941–948.

Newell, K. W. (1988). Selective primary health care: the counter-revolution. *Social Science and Medicine* **27**: 903–906.

Newell, K. W., Nabarro, D. (1989). Reduced infant mortality: a societal indicator, an emotional imperative or a health objective? *Transactions of the Royal Society of Tropical Medicine and Hygiene* **83**: 33–35.

Nutrition Foundation of India (1988). Integrated child development services (ICDS). A study of some aspects of the system. Scientific Report No. 7. Nutrition Foundation of India, New Delhi.

Odhiambo, T. R. (1988). The innovative environment for increased food production in Africa. In LeMay, B. W. J. (ed) *Science, ethics and food*. Smithsonian Institution Press, Washington and London, pp. 38–51.

Omran, A. R., Standley, C. C. (eds) (1976). *Family formation patterns and health*. World Health Organization, Geneva.

Pacey, A., Payne, P. R. (eds) (1985). *Agricultural development and nutrition*. Hutchinson, London.

Patten, C. (1989). *Times (London)*, 1 March.

Payne, P. R. (1987). Malnutrition and human capital: problems of theory and practice. In Clay, E., Shaw, J. (eds) *Poverty, development and food*. Macmillan Press, Basingstoke, UK, pp. 22–41.

Praun, A. (1982). Nutrition education: development or alienation? *Human Nutrition: Applied Nutrition* **36A**:28–34.

Rifkind, S. B., Walt, G. (1988). Health priorities and the developing world. *Lancet* **2**: 744.

Rohde, J. E. (1991). The demographic trap. *Lancet* (letter) **337**: 51.

Rowland, M. G. M., Barrell, R. A. E., Whitehead, R. G. (1978). Bacterial contamination in traditional Gambian weaning foods. *Lancet* **1**: 136–138.

Seaman, J., Poore, P. (1990). Overpopulation and death in childhood. *Lancet* (letter) **336**: 936–937.

Seckler, D. (1982). Small but healthy: a basic hypothesis in the theory, measurement and policy of malnutrition. In Sukhatme, P. V. (ed) *Newer concepts in nutrition and their implications for policy*. Maharashtra Association for the Cultivation of Science Research Institute, Pune, India, pp. 127–137.

Singer, H. W., Longhurst, R. (1986). The role of food aid in promoting the welfare of children in developing countries. In *Food aid and the well-being of children in the developing world*. UNICEF/World Food Programme. UNICEF, New York, pp. 27–66.

Sinha, D. P. (1988). *Children of the Caribbean 1945–1984. Progress in child survival, its determinants and implications*. Caribbean Food and Nutrition Institute, Kingston, Jamaica.

Sinisterra, L. (1987). Studies on poverty, human growth and development: the Cali experience. In Dobbing, J. (ed) *Early nutrition and later development*. Academic Press, London, pp. 208–233.

Stewart, F. (1986). Food aid: pitfalls and potential. In *Food aid and the well-being of children in the developing world*. UNICEF, New York, pp. 67–84.

Stewart, F. (1989). Recession, structural adjustment and infant health: the need for a human face. *Transactions of the Royal Society of Tropical Medicine and Hygiene* **83**: 30–31.

Streeter, P. (1981). *First things first*. World Bank/Oxford University Press.

Taylor, C., Jolly, R. (1988). The straw men of primary health care. *Social Science and Medicine* **27**: 971–977.

Tomkins, A. (1987). Improving nutrition in developing countries: can primary health care help? *Tropical Medicine and Parasitology* **38**: 226–232.

Torun, B. (1982). Environmental and educational interventions against diarrhea in Guatemala. In Chen, L. C., Scrimshaw, N. S. (eds) *Diarrhea and malnutrition: interactions, mechanisms and interventions*. Plenum Press, New York, pp. 235–266.

Ulbricht, T. L. V. (1976). Priorities in agricultural research. *Food Policy* **1**: 313–319.

UNICEF (1987). *The state of the world's children*. Oxford University Press.

UNICEF (1990). *The state of the world's children, 1990*. Oxford University Press.

Van Lerberghe, W. (1990). *Kasongo: child mortality and growth in a small African town*. Smith-Gordon, Nishimura, London.

Walsh, J. A., Warren, K. S. (1979). Selective primary health care. *New England Journal of Medicine* **301**: 967–974.

Walt, G., Perera, M., Heggenhougen, K. (1989). Are large scale volunteer community health worker programmes feasible? The case of Sri Lanka. *Social Science and Medicine* **29**: 599–608.

Warren, K. S. (1990). Beyond universal childhood immunization: Bellagio IV. *Lancet* **335**: 651–652.

Waterlow, J. C. (1981). Crisis for nutrition: Boyd Orr Memorial Lecture. *Proceedings of the Nutrition Society* **40**: 195–207.

Waterlow, J. C. (1986). Famine relief in Africa. *Lancet* **1**: 547–548.

Waterlow, J. C. (1989). Diet of the classical period of Greece and Rome. *European Journal of Clinical Nutrition* **43**: Suppl. 2, 3–12.

Wiesner, B. (1988). GOBI versus PHC? Some dangers of selective primary care. *Social Science and Medicine* **27**: 963–969.

World Health Organization (1981). *The role of the health sector in food and nutrition*. Report of a WHO Expert Committee. Technical Report Series No. 667. WHO, Geneva.

World Health Organization (1989). *Strengthening the performance of community health workers in primary health care*. WHO Technical Report Series no. 780. World Health Organization, Geneva.

Zumrawi, F. Y., Vaughan, J. P. *et al.* (1981). Dried skimmed milk, breast-feeding and illness episodes—a controlled trial in young children in Khartoum Province, Sudan. *International Journal of Epidemiology* **10**: 303–308.

Index

Abbreviations used in the index

AIDS	Acquired immuno-deficiency syndrome	IGF-1	Insulin-like growth factor 1
ARP	Adenosine triphosphate	NADP	Nicotinamide-adenine diphosphate
BCG	Bacillus Calmette-Guerin	NADPH	Reduced nicotinamide-adenine diphosphate
BMR	Basal metabolic rate	PDS	Persistent diarrhoea syndrome
CMI	Cell-mediated immunity	PEM	Protein energy malnutrition
DNA	Deoxyribosenucleic acid	PHC	Primary health care
DPT	Dipheria-pertussis-tetanus vaccine	RNA	Ribonucleic acid
EEG	Electroencephalogram	SGA	Small for gestational age
GOBI	Growth monitoring-oral rehydration-breastfeeding-immunization	SmC	Somatomedin-C
IgA	Immunoglobulin-A		

Absorption
amino acids 89
fat 68
fibre 230
iron 271, 310
nitrogen 68, 306
phosphate 49
sugars 67
trace elements 129, 130, 295
vitamins 295
water 302
Achlorhydria 298
Acidosis 32, 169, 301
Acrodermatitis enteropathica 71, 127, 311
Active cell mass 33–4, 85
Activity of children 232, 237–40, 269, 345–6, 356, 377
Acute phase proteins 93, 97, 115, 129–30, 153, 158, 251, 292–3

Adaptation 21–2, 156
amino acid metabolism 90, 95, 98
heart to reduced load 55
hormones 112, 122
low energy intake 239
protein depletion 244
reduced oxygen demand 59–60
stunting 203–4
Adequacy of breast feeding 273 et seq.
see also Breast feeding
Adipose tissue, see fat
Adolescence 200
Adoption of malnourished children 197, 353
Adults
PEM 2
oedema 148 et seq.
Adult height 198–9
Aeromonas sp. 297
Aflatoxins 138, 159

Africa
early descriptions of PEM 2 et seq.
food production 363
institutions 365
intestinal changes 66
mortality 327, 330, 334, 338
population 362
see also Kenya, Nigeria, Sudan, Zaïre
Age
of hospital admission 7
biological 16, 30, 180
critical periods 229, 263
diarrhoea prevalence 296
errors in estimation 214
impact of infection 316–18
mortality 174, 327
relation to risk 338–9
starting supplements 278
weight for height 215

Age-incidence of PEM and
    policy 190
Aid programmes 365–6, 368
AIDS 170, 290, 308
Albumin
    breakdown 97
    congenital deficiency 149
    distribution 97
    intravascular mass 94, 150, 172
    leakage from capillaries 98
    loss from gut 94
    metabolism 97–9
    regeneration during catch-up
        179, 252
    synthesis 93, 97, 155, 293
    see also Enteropathy,
        Hypoalbuminaemia,
        Leakage
Albumin concentration in
        serum/plasma
    and hormones 114–17
    and immune response 295
    in malaria 306
    in schistosomiasis 307
    during treatment 174
Albuminuria 70
Aldosterone 150
Alertness 201
Alkaline phosphatase 5, 47, 67,
    180
Alkalosis 42
Allergens
    entry through gut 275
    as cause of PDS 299
Allergy to milk 149
Alma Ata, Declaration of 361,
    383
Alpha-l-antitrypsin 94, 108,
    293–5
Alpha-l-antichymotrypsin 108
Alpha-2-macroglobulin 108
Amenorrhoea, lactational
    279–80, 380
Amino acids
    absorption 89
    bacterial synthesis 98
    branched chain 96
    in breast milk 267
    and composition of proteins
        243
    deficiencies 108
    endocrine effects 115
    and loss of oedema 150
    metabolism 90–1, 94–8, 158,
        172
    requirements 95, 246
    score 246
    and water absorption 302
    see also Nitrogen, Protein
Amino-acyl t-RNA synthetase 94
Aminogram in PEM 108
Aminopeptidases 67
Amino-sugars in breast milk 267,
    271
Aminotransferases 63, 107
Ammonia production from urea
    95
Ampicillin 170, 303

Amylase 107, 282
Anaemia
    in chronic infections 305
    in copper deficiency 130
    and iron deficiency 310
    and mental development 346
    oxygen uptake 87
    in PEM 58–61
    treatment 171, 173
    in trichuriasis 307
    see also Bone marrow,
        Haemoglobin,
        Haemopoiesis
Analbuminaemia 149
Anorexia
    in AIDS 308
    in ascariasis 307
    in diarrhoea 279, 303, 174
    and growth failure 251
    in infections 292 *et seq.*, 318
    in measles 304, 88
    nervosa 10, 115, 122
    and PEM 9, 10
    in *Trichuris* infection 307
    in zinc deficiency 15, 127, 128
    see also Appetite
Anthropologists 374, 387
Anthropometry
    applications 220–2
    for diagnosis of malnutrition
        16, 187 *et seq.*, 212 *et seq.*
    for growth monitoring 378
    predictive value 291
    and risk of death 336
    and risk of infection 291
    for screening 220–1, 377
    see also Assessment, Risk
Antibiotics
    to preempt infection 170
    in treatment of diarrhoea 303
Antibodies
    in breast milk 270–1
    in immune response 295
    in immunization programmes
        374–5
Antidiuretic hormone 44, 151
Antioxidants 139–40, 172, 282
Apathy 10, 42, 177, 345
    in zinc deficiency 128
Apolipoproteins
    and fatty liver 64, 155, 158
    see also Lipoproteins
Appetite
    during recovery 172–4, 177,
        180–1, 269
    see also Anorexia
Arm circumference 213, 220
    and risk of death 334, 336–8
Arousal
    effect of supplements 346
Arrhythmias, and potassium
    deficiency 43
Ascaris 307
Ascites 35, 149
Ascorbic acid
    deficiency and anaemia 59
    concentration in infection
        294

Asia
    mortality 329, 338–9, 381
    prevalence of stunting *222*
    see also China, India,
        Indonesia, Nepal, Myanmar
Assessment
    of mental function 347 *et seq.*
    of nutritional state 212 *et seq.*
    of risk 336 *et seq.*
    see also Anthropometry
ATP
    and ion pumps 137
    in muscle 87
    see also ATPase
ATPase
    calcium 45, 137
    in gut mucosa 67–8
    in red cell membranes 136
    sodium-potassium 43, 132, 172
    in zinc deficiency 127
    see also Ion pumps
Atrophy
    of basal layer of epidermis 71
    of gut mucosa 66–7, 303, 308
    of lymphoid tissues 295
    of pancreas 65
    of salivary glands 65
    of stomach mucosa 310
    of thymus 127
Atwater factors 230
Avitaminoses 14
    see also individual vitamins

Bacteria
    colonization of upper bowel by
        68, 138, 170
    in Giardiasis 307
    in iron deficiency 310
    contamination of foods by 281
    killing of
        by lymphocytes 295
        by free radicals 138
Balances
    energy 232
    for measurement of absorption
        68
    nitrogen 68, 94, 237 *et seq.*,
        243, 247
    zinc 129
Bangladesh
    arm circumference and risk
        217, 336–7
    breast feeding and mortality 279
    diarrhoea and growth 294, 317
    lactation 268
    malabsorption 68
    measles 334
    mortality 279, 325, 330, 334,
        374
    neonatal tetanus 329
    oral rehydration 302
    stunting 195
    treatment with zinc 128
    water supplies 373
Barbados
    mental development 348, *349*
Barley
    in weaning foods 281

Basal metabolic rate 83 *et seq.*, 172
and energy requirements 231,
232, 237, 240
expression of 17–21
and cardiac output 55
in infections 293
and ion pumps 137
in marasmus 84
in PEM 83–6
prediction of 20
and thyroid function 122
in stunted children 19
Basement membrane
of glomeruli 70
Basic Needs Approach 363
Bayley Development Scales 347,
355
BCG vaccination 375
Behaviour
in malnutrition 345
at school 351
personal-social 355
Bengal, measles in 334
Beri-beri 3
Bifidus factor, *see Lactobacillus*
Bile acids/salts 68
effect of bacterial overgrowth
298
effect of giardiasis 307
Bilirubin 63, 177
Binding proteins 112
sites for trace elements 130
Bioelectric impedance 29, 37
Biological age 16
Biological value of proteins 247,
281
Biopsies
of gut mucosa 67, 299
liver 62
muscle 33, 42, 45, 48, 86, 87
Biotechnology
for food production 363
Birth
interval 279, 333, 380
rate 380
weight, effect of supplements
333
see also Low birth weight,
Fertility
Bladder stones 49
Blindness, *see* Vitamin A,
Measles
Body
composition 28–34, 188
conductivity 29
impedance 29
mass index 268
size as basis of reference 17
potassium 28 *et seq.*
water 28–37, 244
see also Water
Bolivia
plasma renin activity 151
muscle mass 265
Bomb calorimetry 265
Bone
age 16
density 46

growth 46, 115
retardation of 198
marrow
in malaria 306
in PEM 58, 59
minerals 40
Bottle feeding
risks of 272 *et seq.*
see also Formula feeding
Brain
changes in, rats 344
DNA in 74
growth spurt 199
metabolic rate of 27, 85
potassium content 27, 42
weight of 26, 27, 74
Brazil
early surveys 2
studies on
Ascariasis 306
effect of supplements 276
infections and growth 314
lactation 267
mortality 367
Breast feeding
and birth spacing 380
in diarrhoea 303
exclusive, duration of 272 *et
seq.*
in infections 293
partial 275 *et seq.*
and prevention of infection
272, 376
protective factors in 270–1
promotion of 376
and weight of infants 196, 228,
230, 260 *et seq.*
see also Human milk
Breast milk, *see* Human milk;
Lactation
Bromsulphthalein retention 5
Bronchopneumonia 170
after measles 304, 374
Brush border, changes in 67
Buccal lesions
as cause of anorexia 293
in dehydration 300
in measles 304
in PEM 5

Caeruloplasmin 93, 126, 130–1,
139
in infections 294
Calcification
of pancreas 66
Calcium
in foods 45
and height growth 47, 201, 251
in human milk 46
intracellular accumulation of 137
and membrane damage 42
and membrane rigidity 136
changes in PEM 45–7
pump 45
requirement 46
serum concentration in
Ethiopia 180
see also Rickets

Calcutta
PEM in 6, 65, 156
rickets in 47, 180
skin lesions in 71
Campylobacter sp. 297
Candidiasis
in iron deficiency 310
in zinc deficiency 311
Capillaries 146, 153
see also Leakiness, Permeability
Carcass analysis of children 28, 44
Carcinoma of liver 65
Cardiac function 54–5
failure 56, 132, 172
overload 169
Cardiomyopathy 131
Caribbean, position of women 372
Carotene
as antioxidant 140, 159
in infections 294
in leaf protein concentrate 281
Carrier proteins
for retinol 106, 304
for somatomedin-C 118
for trace metals 126 *et seq.*
Cartilage
and somatomedin-C 115, 118
and stunting 202
and sulphur amino acids 251
Casein *see* Cow's milk
Cassava in weaning foods 279,
281, 283
Catabolic losses
in infections 292
in measles 304
Catch-up growth, *see* Growth
Cell-mediated immunity 127,
292, 295 *et seq.*, 305, 309–12
Cell membranes, *see* Membranes
Cellular oxidation 85, 86
Central America 2, 372
see also Guatemala
Central nervous system, changes
in 74–5, 347
Cereals in weaning foods 281–2
Cereal-based rehydration
solutions 302
Chemoprophylaxis of malaria
306, 334
Child mortality 327 *et seq.*
see Mortality
Child survival
and ecology 366
policy for 368, 369 *et seq.*
see Survival
Chile
age of admission of PEM in 7
basal metabolic rate 85
copper deficiency 131
electrolyte changes 41
mortality from PEM 327
rehabilitation 182
China
famine oedema in 97, 148
infant mortality 326
rickets 47,180
selenium deficiency 326
Chloramphenicol 170

Chloroquine 306
Cholecalciferol, *see* Vitamin D
Choline and fatty liver 64
Cholesterol
  in cell membranes 136
  in serum 65
Chromium
  deficiency of 113
  as essential mineral 126
  and glucose tolerance 132
Chronicity
  diagnosis from hair-bulbs 73
  in marasmus 8
  in relation to stunting 8, 189,
    195
  see also Length/height,
    Duration
Circulatory failure 55
Cirrhosis of liver 65
Classification
  of growth deficits 188 *et seq.*
  of severe PEM 5 *et seq.*
Clubbing of fingers, in
  trichuriasis 307
Coconut oil, in recovery diet
  141, 179
Code of practice, for infant
  formulae 378
Coeliac disease 197
Collagen
  content of body 33
  and copper 130
  formation in growth 251
  labile 72
  in skin 72
  synthesis of 91
  in vascular tree 58
Cognitive development 345, 356
Colloid osmotic pressure
  of plasma 146, 150
Colombia
  effects of interventions 367
  effects of supplementary
    feeding 355, 376
  studies on work capacity 202
Colon, absorption from 96
Colonization of upper bowel, *see*
  Bacteria
Colstrum, protective factors in
  270
Commercial weaning foods 281
Community
  assessment of PEM in 2, 5,
    212 *et seq.*
  felt needs of 382
  health workers 374, 383 *et
    seq.*, 384
  participation by 361, 366–9,
    372, 378, 382 *et seq.*
Complement 295, 309
Conduction velocity in nerves 75
Conductivity of whole body 29, 37
Confounding variables in data
  analysis 23, 291, 336, 352
Congo
  electrolyte changes in PEM 41
  growth of pygmies 199
  see also Zaïre

Conjunctival damage
  in measles 304
  in vitamin A deficiency 309
Contamination
  of weaning foods 272, 294,
    298
  of rehydration solutions 304
Copper
  anaemia and deficiency of 59
  classification of deficiency *16*
  as essential mineral 126
  in infections 294
  in PEM 130–1
  in superoxide dismutase 142
  in treatment 172, 180
Corticosteroids
  and albumin metabolism 99
  in PEM 112, 115–16
  relation to kwashiorkor 158
  in infections 293
Cost of PHC 386
Cotrimoxazole
  for treatment of dysentery 303
                       of pneumonia
                       334
Counter, whole-body 28, 41
Covariance analysis
  for age 191
  for weight 19
Cow's milk
  quality of 247
  see also Allergy, Intolerance
C-reactive protein 293
Creamatocrit 266
Creatine 28, 85
Creatinine
  and arm muscle area 214
  excretion of, as measure of
    muscle mass 27, 34, 93
  height index 34, 107
  in relation to urinary nitrogen
    109
Crisis
  of Third World debt 364
  for nutrition 387
Critical periods
  for brain growth 75
  for energy requirements 199
Crohn's disease 197
Crude protein 297
Cryptosporidium 308
Cultural factors
  and beliefs 374
  and growth 318
  and separation from the
    mother 10
  see also Social environment
Curative services 385
Cut-off points 6, 213 *et seq.*, 216
    et seq., 222, 337
Cystic fibrosis 200, 352
Cysteine
  in acute phase proteins 93
  in glutathione 143
Cystine
  in hair 73
  see also Sulphur amino acids
Cytokines 93, 127, 292

Death, *see* Mortality
Debt
  crisis in Third World 226, 325,
    364
Decalcification, *see* Bone
Deficiency
  definition of 14, 16
  see under individual nutrients
Deficits in growth
  and diarrhoea 314 *et seq.*
  see Growth
Dehydration 30, 36–7, 168 *et
    seq.*
  as cause of anorexia 293
  management of 300 *et seq.*
  and mortality 374
  signs of 300
Demand
  and infant intake 244, 269 *et
    seq.*, 273
Demography 379, 380
Dendrites, changes in 75, 347
Density, *see* Energy density
Dependency, effect of aid
  policies 365, 372, 377, 382
Depigmentation
  of hair 73
  of skin 71
  in essential fatty acid
    deficiency 141
Depletion
  concept of 15, *16*
  of trace elements 126
  of potassium 41 *et seq.*
Deprivation, maternal 8, 10
  see also Poverty, Psychosocial
    factors
Dermis 72
Descriptors of prevalence of
  PEM 216–20
  see also Indicators
Desferrioxamine 139
Detoxification 170
Deuterium, *see* Isotopes
Developed countries,
  contributions of 364 *et seq.*
Development
  economic 363
  mental 344 *et seq.*
Developmental quotient 188,
  203, 347 *et seq.*
Diabetes, malnutrition-related
  66
Diagnosis
  biochemical 14
  of kwashiorkor and marasmus
    5, 104, 108
  of potassium deficiency 42
  of magnesium deficiency 48
  of zinc deficiency 128
Diarrhoea
  and absorption of nutrients 69,
    294
  age incidence 279
  and bacterial overgrowth 68
  as cause of
    growth deficit 253, 314 *et
    seq.*

growth faltering 274
marasmus 159
oedema 153
potassium loss 44
chronic *see* persistent
effects of in PEM 296 *et seq.*
and iron deficiency 310
jejunal perfusion in 94
management of 169 *et seq.*,
  300
morbidity from
  effect of hygiene and
    sanitation 373
  protection by breast feeding
    272 *et seq.*
mortality from 272, 329–30
  after measles 375
and mucosal malnutrition 169
onset after start of treatment
  137
and rehydration 301–4
prevalence in relation to
  nutritional state 312 *et seq.*,
  334
persistent
  aetiology 299
  definition 298
  mucosal damage in 69
  treatment with fermented
    milk 283
  and risk of death 337
  and zinc deficiency 127, 130,
    311
Diet
  meaning of 14
  protein deficient 156
Digestibility, of protein 246
Digoxin 173
Dilemma, weanling's 275
Dinka, heights of 199
2-3 Diphosphoglycerate 60
Disaccharidases 67
DNA
  in brain 74
  in hair follicles 73
  in jejunal perfusion 94
  as reference base 15, 129
Doubly labelled water 234,
  239
  see also Isotopes
DPT vaccination 375
Drug metabolism 170
Duration of PEM
  as determining clinical picture
    8
  effects on mental development
    353
Dwarfism
  nutritional 6
  and zinc deficiency 128
Dysentery 171, 303, 304

ECG
  in potassium deficiency 42
  in magnesium deficiency 48
Ecology 366
Economic factors 344, 361 *et
  seq.*, 374

Economy
  of nitrogen 94
  see also Adaptation
Education
  as element of PHC 362
  in health 384
  in hygiene 373
  of mothers 335, 371
  as preventive strategy 367
EEG changes 347
Egypt
  diarrhoeal disease, reduction
    of 304
  rickets in 47
  somatomedin, studies on 119
Elastin 130
Electrolytes 40–5
  absorption during infection
    294
  measurement in treatment 174
Electron microscopy
  of glomeruli 69
  of gut mucosa 67
  of liver 63
Emergencies
  indicators for use in, 221
Endotoxins 293, 294
  see also E. Coli
Energy
  balance in measles 304, 318
  in breast milk 265 *et seq.*
  consumption of 226
  cost of growth 83, 233 *et seq.*
  deficiency of 4, 150
  density in feeds 179, 229, 255,
    279–81
  expenditure
    measurements of 234 *et seq.*
    in infection 293
  intakes
    in infections 314–15
    in kwashiorkor 157
    in marasmus 85
  metabolism 83–8
  requirements 229 *et seq.*
  storage 236 *et seq.*
  see also Requirements
Entamoeba histolytica 303
Enterocytes, turnover 94
  see also Gut mucosa
Enterokinase 67
Enteropathy, protein-losing 94,
  295
Enterotoxins, protective effect of
  breast milk 271
  see also E. Coli
Enthalpy, of protein and fat
  deposited in growth 230
Enzymes
  of amino acid metabolism 96,
    244
  of brush border 67
  oxidative 87, 94
  pancreatic 66–7
  of urea cycle 94
Epidemiology
  of protection by breast milk
    272

of interactions of nutrition and
  infection 290
Epidermis 72–3, 127
Epithelium, *see* Conjunctiva,
  Gut mucosa, Vitamin A
Errors
  in anthropometry 214
Erythrocytes
  glutathione reductase 142
  see Red Blood Cells
Erythropoietin 60
Escherichia coli
  endotoxins in 293–4
  enteroadhesive 298
  enteroinvasive 297, 303
  enterotoxigenic 297, 373
Essential amino acids, *see*
  Amino acids
Essential fatty acids, *see* Fatty acids
Ethiopia
  brain changes 74
  breast feeding 276
  breast milk immunology 270
  growth of children 197
  rickets 180
Ethnic differences in growth
  potential 214, 224
  see also Genetic
Exclusive breast feeding 272 *et seq.*
Excretion
  of acid 70
  of sodium 70
Expanded programme of
  immunization (EPI) 375
Exploratory activity of children
  345
  see also Activity
Export proteins 93, 106, 153
  see also Acute phase proteins,
  Albumin, Transferrin
Extracellular fluid 32 *et seq.*
  during growth 244
  in potassium deficiency 42–4
  during recovery 177
  volume 146, 172

Factorial estimates
  of energy expenditure 232 *et
    seq.*
  of protein requirements 242 *et
    seq.*
Faeces
  IgA, lactoferrin in 270
  losses in diarrhoea 298
  nitrogen in 94
Faltering in growth
  definition of 194
  in breast-fed children 273–4
  in supplemented children 276
  in infections 293
  after measles 304
Family planning 367, 380 *et seq.*
Family as target group 369
Famine
  and infections 290
  and loss of fat 71
  oedema 2, 3, 32, 97, 147–9
  and population growth 382

Fat
  absorption of 68, 294
  area in arm 213
  in breast milk 266 *et seq.*
  deposition during growth 177
    et seq., 233, 251
  maternal stores 269, 333
  measurement of in body 33
  metabolism in infections 293
  oxidation of 83
  transport of 64
  in weaning foods 179, 252, 282
  see also Fatty acids,
    Skin-folds
Fatality rate, *see* Mortality
Fatty acids
  essential fatty acids and skin
    changes 141
  and fatty liver 64
  peroxidation by free radicals
    138, 140, 141
  serum levels of
    effect of growth hormone
      117
    in PEM 114
Fatty liver *1*, *5*, 61–5
  biopsies 62
  in essential fatty acid
    deficiency 141
  and ferritin 151
  free radicals and 159
  histology of 62
  and oedema 61, 155
  and prognosis 177
  sequelae of 65
Feedback control of lactation
  270
Feeding
  in diarrhoea 302
  programmes 376–7
  frequency of 269, 279, 282
  see also Breast feeding,
    Supplementary feeding
Fermentation
  in bowel 68
  of weaning foods 282, 304, 373
Ferritin
  and antidiuretic hormone 151
  serum concentration of 59,
    139–40, 159
Fertility, control of 280, 380
Fever 88, 170, 293
Fibre, dietary 94, 129, 294
Fibrinogen 93, 115, 293
Fibronectin 106, 177
Fibrosis
  of liver 65
  of pancreas 66
Filtration, in glomeruli 70
Fitness, cardio-respiratory
  203
Flour-feeding injury 2
Folic acid
  absorption of 295
  deficiency 9, 59, 171, 180
Food aid 364, 365
  subsidies 367
  contamination 373

Food and Agriculture
    Organization
  early surveys 2
  reports on requirements 157,
    230 *et seq.*
Foods
  calcium in 44
  iron in 60
  magnesium in 49
  patterns in relation to PEM
    157
  phosphorus in 50
  potassium in 44
  production 362, 363, 369
Foot processes, of glomeruli 69
Formula feeding 231, 272 *et seq.*,
  376
France, war oedema in 147
Free radicals, 2, 93, 131, 136 *et*
  seq., 152 *et seq.*, 155, 158,
  172–3
  protection by lactoferrin 271
Frusemide 137

Gain
  in length 181
  in weight 177
    during pregnancy 333
  see also Growth velocity
Gambia
  children, studies on
    activity 240
    bone mineral 46
    diarrhoea prevalence 312
    dietary intakes 248, 293, 303
    endocrine changes 112,
      114–15
    energy expenditure 238
    growth velocity *197*
      effect of infections *316*,
      317
    malabsorption 68, 69
    metabolic rate 88
    mortality 325, 333–5, 375
  breast milk, studies on
    adequacy 273
    composition 129
    immunoglobulins in 270
    volume of 262, 268–9
  malaria in 375
  supplementation of pregnant
    women 278
Gamma-globulins in malaria 306
Gangliosides of brain 267
Gastritis 310
Gastroenteritis
  relation to marasmus 8
  and potassium deficiency 42, 44
  see also Dehydration,
    Diarrhoea
Gastrointestinal function 66–9
Genetics
  application to food production
    363
  effects of
    on body composition 214
    on growth potential 192,
      203, 205, 224

Gentamycin 170
Germination of cereals 282
Giardiasis 170, 303, 307
Glomerular filtration 70, 150
Glucagon 112–13
Glucocorticoids, *see*
  Corticosteroids
Gluconeogenesis 83, 115, 117
Glucose
  in blood 113, 171, 174
  in infusion fluids 169
  oxidation in infection 293
  production 83
  in rehydration fluids 301
  tolerance 113, 114, 132
  and water and salt absorption
    301
  see also Sugar
Glutamine 169
Glutathione 139, 141, 152, 159,
  172
  peroxidase 131, 142
  reductase 142
  S-transferase 142
Glycine
  in bile salts 68
  in collagen 91, 93, 251
  in glutathione 143
  in haemopoiesis 59
Glycogen
  in muscle 32, 87
  stores 83
Glycoproteins 106, 294, 305,
  309, 311
GOBI programme 371 *et seq.*,
  382, 385
Gomez classification 188
Gram negative
  septicaemia 170
  bacilli in weaning foods 283
Griffiths scale of mental
  development 347, 356
Gross National Product *326*
Groundnuts in weaning food 282
Growth 187 *et seq.*
  catch-up
    after faltering 274
    in height 198 *et seq.*
    and infection 314 *et seq.*
    in mental development 353
    requirements for 251 *et seq.*
    in tuberculosis 305
  see also Anthropometry,
    Stunting
  factors, see Growth hormone,
    Somatomedin-C
  failure, as sign of malnutrition
    7, 14
    in infections 313 *et seq.*
    and mineral deficiencies 46,
      50, 61, 128
  monitoring 378
  potential 192 *et seq.*
  rate and BMR 84
    and hormones 112–13
    and physical activity 240
    and protein breakdown 91
  requirements

for energy 83, 233-4
for protein 244-6
for skeletal growth 91,
250-1
and supplementary feeding
377
velocity 188, 194 *et seq.*, 244,
337,-8, 378
Growth hormone, 83, 112,
116-17
deficiency of 10, 200
Growth plate 118
Guatemala
birth weight 333
breast milk immunoglobulins
270
diarrhoea 294, 303, 313, 373
energy expenditure of children
238-40
folic acid deficiency 59
infection and growth 318
mortality 325, 330, 339
plasma and red cell volumes
57, 58
selenium 131
supplementation 355
Gut mucosa 66, 67, 73
in zinc deficiency 127
regeneration of 169
requirement for glutamine 169

Haemoglobin
in fatty liver disease 5
in PEM 58
synthesis of 139
Haemophilus sp. 170, 334, 375
Haemopoiesis 59 *et seq.*
during growth 251
limiting factors 180
in malaria 306
in tuberculosis 305
Hair
changes in PEM 5, 73, 212
in essential fatty acid
deficiency 141
effects of supplementation on
201
zinc content of 129
Half-lives of plasma proteins
106
Halidixic acid, for treatment of
dysentery 303
Haptoglobin 93
Harvard standards 6, 188, 191
Head circumference 74, 213
Health
basic system of 385 *et seq.*
passport to 380
rights to 363
sector, responsibilities of
385-6
technology 363
see also Primary Health Care
Heart
disease and stunting 200
rate 55, 87
see Cardiac, Myocardium
Heat production 84, 88

Height
as basis of reference 18 *et seq.*, 58
calcium and phosphorus and
growth in 46, 49, 201-2
catch-up in 181, 254
growth and infections 317-18
as measure of duration of
malnutrition 7, *8*, 156
and mental development 354
stunting in 189 *et seq.*
see also Catch-up, Growth, Stunting
Hepatomegaly, *see* Fatty liver
Histidine
and anaemia 59
distorted metabolism of 96
History
of kwashiorkor 1, *2*
of paediatrics 1
of supplementary feeding 377
Homoeostasis of energy
metabolism 83
see also Adaptation
Hookworm 307
Hospitals, role of 385
Human capital 363, 366, 369
Human milk
calcium content of 46
intake in diarrhoea 303
iron content of 60
magnesium content of 49
non-protein N in 244
protective factors in *270*-1
requirements of 229 *et seq.*,
241 et seq.
urea in 244
zinc in 129
see also Lactation
Human rights 361, 363
Humoral response, *see* Immune
response
Hungary, studies in
of body composition 26
of fatty liver 61
of pancreatic enzymes 66
of plasma and red cell volumes
57, 58
Hunger oedema, *see* Famine
oedema
Hungry season, effects on
diarrhoea prevalence 312
growth 194, 222
milk output 268
mortality 330
physical activity 240
Hydrogen in breath 68
Hygiene, personal 373
Hyperkeratosis 71
Hyperpigmentation of skin 71
Hypoalbuminaemia
as cause of oedema 146 *et seq.*,
155, 158
in diagnosis of kwashiorkor 15
and fatty liver 64
and growth hormone 117
pathogenesis of 94, 96-9, 105
and serum calcium 46
and zinc absorption 129

Hypocalcaemia 46
Hypoglycaemia 83, 113, 171
Hypokalaemia 43
Hyponatraemia 29, 44-5, 109,
136, 151, 153, 177
Hypopigmentation, of skin and
hair 73
Hypothermia 88, 113, 171
Hypothyroidism
and cardiac function 54, 122
in PEM 121
and stunting 200
Hypotonicity 42, 44
in dehydration 301
Hypovolaemia 55-6, 58, *151*

IgA
in breast milk 270-1
response in PEM 295, 298
in vitamin A deficiency 309
IGF-1, *see* Somatomedin C
Ignorance
as cause of PEM 10
and cultural beliefs 278, 372
see also Education
Immune function
in low birth-weight children 299
in iron deficiency 310-11
in response to infection 295 *et seq.*
and supplementary feeding 275
in zinc deficiency 127, 311
see also cell-mediated immunity
Immunization
in malnourished children 295
programmes 374 *et seq.*, 382
Immunosuppression
in malaria 375
Immunoglobulins
in breast milk 270
response of to infection 295
see also Immune function
Inborn errors of metabolism 996
Income transfer, food as 377
India
brain changes 74
diarrhoea prevalence 312
dietary staple 156
energy consumption 370
famine oedema 149
fatty liver 62
feeding patterns 276
programmes 376
trials 201
folic acid deficiency 59
institutions 366
intervention projects 367
measles 334
mental development 348
mortality 176, 330, 386
oral rehydration solutions 302
persistent diarrhoea 298
PEM 7
plasma volume 57
rickets 47
somatomedin C 119
village health workers 383,
384-5
vitamin A trials 335

Indices, anthropometric 212 *et seq.*
Indicators, definition 212
Indochina, early description of PEM 3
Indonesia
    colonization of bowel 68
    iron deficiency 310
    nutritional rehabilitation 165
    costs of GOBI programmes 386
    interventions, success of 367
    supplementary feeding and lactation 268
    vitamin A trials 335
Industrialized countries, breast milk intakes 262
Industrial development 363
Infant formula 260
Infant mortality, *see* Mortality
Infections
    as cause of
        anaemia 59
        PEM 8, 158
    diagnosis of 88
    and free radicals 138
    and glucocorticoids 115
    and iron 139
    nutritional state, impact on 290, 314 *et seq.*
    and onset of oedema 36
    and requirements
        for energy 229
        for protein 250 *et seq.*
    and stunting 203, 225
    from supplementary feeding 275 *et seq.*
    treatment of 170, 305 *et seq.*
    and zinc deficiency 129
Inflammatory disease
    of gut 94
Inflammation
    and capillary permeability 148, 153
Infrastructure, need for 363
Inhibition of lactation 270
Initiation of cure 172
Injury, metabolic effects of 92, 295
Insulin 99, 112–14, 122, 158
    resistance 114, 293
Intakes
    of breast milk 260 *et seq.*
    of energy 230 *et seq.*
    of protein 241 *et seq.*
Intelligence tests 347
Interleukins 292, 293, 305
Intermediate technology, *see* Village technology
International Water Decade 372
Interstitial space 146
Interventions
    effects on mortality 331
        on mental development 353, 356
    GOBI programmes 371 *et seq.*
    vitamin A trials 335

Intestinal parasites 306 *et seq.*
    see individual parasites
Intestine, *see* Gut
Intolerance
    to cow's milk protein 69, 180
    to lactose 299, 303
Intracellular water 32
Iodine
    essentiality of *16*
    deficiency 121, 122, 126, 131, 347
Iodinase 121
Ion pumps, *see* ATPase
Iran, rickets in 47
Iron
    absorption of 271, 295
    and behaviour 346
    in breast milk 60
    in catch-up growth 251
    deficiency of 59, 60
    excretion of, effect of lactoferrin 271
    and free radicals 138
    and infections 291, 310
    in leaf protein concentrate 281
    in liver 59
    and mental development 61
    overload of 139, 140
    stores of 60
    toxicity of 139
    in treatment 173, 180, 310, 311
Isotopic measurements
    of breast milk intake 261 *et seq.*
    of faecal loss 94
    of fat absorption 67
    with iodine 97
    of nitrogen 90, 95, 96
    of pancreatic enzymes 66
    of potassium 41
    with sulphur 118
    of urea production 244
    of water 29, 235
    of zinc 129
Ivory Coast, biochemical tests 105, 108

Jamaica, PEM in
    age at admission 7
    ascites 149
    BMR 84
    bottle feeding 272
    colonization of bowel 68
    drug treatment 170
    electrolyte changes 41, 43
    fatty liver 61, 62
        and oedema 6
    ferritin 139
    folic acid deficiency 59, 171
    free radicals 160
    glutathione *142*
    growth patterns 197
    high energy diet 180
    insulin 113
    magnesium deficiency 48
    mental development 203, 348 *et seq.*
    mortality 107, 173, 176, 320

muscle mass 27
nitrogen balances 239
oedema 6, 147
plasma and red cell volume 57, 58
social policy 363
somatomedin 119
thyroid activity 121, 122
trace elements 128 *et seq.*
weaning diets 156
weight gains in the community 252
zinc deficiency 127 *et seq.*, 311
Jejunum
    absorptive capacity 67, 94
    damage in measles 304
    in infection 294
    in protein deficiency 298
Jordan
    adequacy of breast feeding 273, 274
    chromium and glucose tolerance 132
    PEM 7, 156

Kanamycin 170
Kasongo study, *see* Zaïre
Kenya
    cereal-based rehydration 302
    feeding patterns 276, 278, 376
    measles and BMR 293
    schistosomiasis 307
    social factors as cause of PEM 10
Kerala, mortality 326
Keratin 73
Keratinization of mucosae 309
Keratomalacia 171
Keshan disease 131, 132
Khartoum
    adequacy of breast feeding 274, 276, 278
    infection and growth 316
    food supplements and growth 377
    see also Sudan
Kidney
    functional changes 70
    glomerular filtration rate 70, 150
    histopathology 69
    plasma flow 70, 150
    Klebsiella sp. 170
Knemometry 188
Korea, mental development of children from 353
Kwashiorkor
    body water 31–2
    cell membranes 137
    description and classification 1–9
    fatty liver 61 *et seq.*
    free radicals 138 *et seq.*
    glutathione 142
    oedema 36, 146 *et seq.*
    pathogenesis 154 *et seq.*
    and stunting 157

Lactase deficiency 67, 299, 307
Lactation 260 *et seq.*
  in Gambian women 133
  supplementation, effect on 355
  see also Breast feeding,
    Human milk
Lactobacillus
  bifidus 271
  bulgaricus 283
Lactoferrin
  in breast milk 270, 271
  in infections 294
  iron-binding by 311
Lactoperoxidase 270
Lactose 67
  intolerance 299, 303
Lactulose 69
  lactulose/mannitol test of
    absorption 299
Latin America
  early descriptions of PEM 2
  infant mortality 329, 334
  prevalence of PEM *223*
  see also Brazil, Chile,
    Guatemala
Latrines 373
  see Sanitation
Leaf protein concentrate 281
Leakiness
  of capillaries 96, 98
  of cell membranes 45, 136–7,
    152–3. 156
  of gut mucosa 69
Lean body mass 33 *et seq.*
  as basis of reference 85
  gains in 231, 233
  loss of 15
  potassium as a measure of 42
  and zinc 127, 180
  see also Body composition
Lebanon
  biochemical tests 105
  PEM in 6
Length, *see* Height
Lesotho
  mortality in hospital *164*
  types of PEM 7
Lethal day 50 328, 331
Leucocytes
  bactericidal activity 296
  electrolyte transport in 41, 45
  lactoferrin in 311
  and membrane damage 137,
    144
  metabolites in 87
  zinc content 180
  and zinc deficiency 127, 129
Leucocytosis 170
Liberia, potassium deficiency in
  43
Life expectancy 326, 363
Life span, of red cells 60, 136
Limiting factor
  concept of 15
  for catch-up growth 251
  energy as 249, 252
  women's time as 283
  zinc as 180

Lipolysis 117
Lipoproteins 64–7, 108
Literacy and child survival 371,
  373
Liver
  in PEM 61 *et seq.*
  protein content 99
  mass, effect of glucocorticoids
    115
  see also Fatty liver
Low birth weight
  determinants of 333
  energy expenditure of LBW
    children 84
  and growth hormone 117
  and maternal malnutrition
    268, 269
  and PDS 299
  and stunting 199
  and supplementation of
    mother 333
  and zinc deficiency 129
Lymphocytes
  in breast milk 271
  production of in PEM 296
Lymphokines 271, 299, 307
Lysozyme
  in breast milk 270
  in vitamin A deficiency 309

Macromolecules, entry through
  gut 69
Macrophages
  in breast milk 271
  and cytokine release 292
Magnesium 48–9
  and catch-up growth 251
  supplements 173, 180
  tetany-like signs of deficiency
    46
  in routine treatment 169
Maintenance requirements
  for energy 232 *et seq.*
  for protein 239, 243 *et seq.*
  during treatment 173
Maize
  adequacy of diets 281, 282
  flour in oral rehydration 302
  as staple of weaning foods
    156
Malabsorption
  in AIDS 308
  in *Cryptosporidium* infection
    308
  in giardiasis 307
  in infections 292 *et seq.*
  of sugars 67, 169
  see also Absorption
Malaria
  and anaemia 59, 306
  control of 382
  diarrhoea in 294
  immunosuppression by 375
  in iron deficiency 310
  and liver fibrosis 65
  metabolic effects 306
  and mortality 165, 330–1, 334,
    375

  and nutritional state 306
  parasitaemia, effect of diet
    292
  and response to rehabilitation
    291
  screening for 170–1, 174
Malaysia
  breastfeeding and mortality
    272, 276
  feeding patterns 278, 376
  Trichuris infection 307
Mali, health systems 385
Maltase 67
Malting of porridges 282
Manganese 126, 142
Mannitol, absorption 69
Mantoux test 305
Marasmus
  BMR 84
  body water 30, 32
  description and definition 1, 4
    et seq., 158 *et seq.*
  fatality rate 176
  gastrointestinal changes 66
  glutathione in 142
  hair changes in 71
  iron overload in 139
  pathogenesis 158
  skin changes in 71
  trace element status 127 *et seq.*
  urinary mercapturic acid
    excretion in *143*
Marasmic kwashiorkor
  age incidence 7
  cortisol levels 115
  cell membranes 136
  definition of 5, 6
  difference from kwashiorkor
    153
  and ferritin 151
  and fatality rate 175
  and glutathione *142*
  growth hormone levels 116,
    117
  hyponatraemia in 44
  mercapturic acid excretion
    143
  oedema, distribution of 36
  prevalence, relative 7
  renin activity 152
  selenium in plasma 131
  severity 160
  and stunting 158
Marginal diets 254, 268, 281
Marketing, code of practice 260
Maternal
  competence 10
  deprivation 10
  height and mortality 203, 370
  nutritional status and lactation
    263 *et seq.*, 267
  weight and birth weight 333
Maturity and metabolic rate
  18
Maturation of skeletal
  development 117, 198, 202,
    250
  see Bone age

Measles
  and albumin loss 94
  and anorexia 304, 318
  and diarrhoea 94
  energy balance in 318
  growth deficit 318
  gut permeability 294
  immunization against 374, 375
  in Kenya 293
  metabolic rate in 88, 293
  and mortality 165, 330, 334,
    339
  and nutritional state 304
  and oedema 94
  and onset of PEM 156, 159
  PDS in 299
  protein losses in 295
  protein metabolism in 92, 293
  response to rehabilitation 291
  weight loss in 290
  and vitamin A deficiency 335
Mebendazole for treatment of
    worms 308
Megaloblastic bone marrow 59,
    171
Melanin 73
Membranes, cell 32, 33, 136 *et
    seq.*, 159
Memory, tests of 347
Menarche 198
Meningitis 330
Mental development 344 *et seq.*
  and anaemia 51
  and hypothyroidism 122, 123
  as outcome 218
  and stunting 203
Mercapturic acids 143, 159
Messenger RNA, for albumin
    97, 98
Metabolism in PEM 83–99
  in infection 293 *et seq.*
  metabolic mass 18, 19
  see also Amino acids, Energy,
    Nitrogen, Protein
Metabolizable energy of food
    230, 265
Metallothionein 93, 126, 130,
    141, 294
Methionine and fatty liver 64
Methicillin 170
3-Methylhistidine excretion 91,
    93, 293
Metranidazole 170, 303, 308
Metrifonate 307
Mexico
  activity of children 240
  breast feeding 376
  causes of PEM 10
  classification of PEM 1, 188
  electrolyte changes 41
  growth deficits 318
  infant feeding patterns 278
  mental development 348, 355,
    356
  mothers' education 371
  plasma and red cell volumes 57
  skin lesions 71
  staple of diet 156

Micelle formation and fat
    absorption 68, 294, 295
  impairment by *Giardia* 307
Microbial proliferation
  effect of iron 311
  host response to 291
  see also Bacteria, Colonization
    of bowel
Micro-environment 352
  see also Socio-cultural factors
Micronutrients
  absorption in infections 292,
    295
  in breast milk 279
  classification of deficiencies *16*
  depletion of 9
  during treatment 18
  see also Trace elements,
    Vitamins
Milk
  allergy 149
  intolerance 180
  supplementary feeding 201
Millet in weaning diets 283
Mineralization of bone 46
Minerals
  classification of deficiencies *16*
  depletion of 9
  in human milk 267
  during treatment 180
  see also Calcium, Iron,
    Magnesium, Phosphorus
Mitochondria
  abnormalities in liver 63
  superoxide dismutase in 142
  swelling of 43
Molybdenum 126
Monosaccharides, absorption 69
Moonface 35
Morbidity
  and breast feeding 272
  and iron deficiency 310
  and nutritional state 311 *et
    seq.*
  and sanitation 373
  and treatment with iron 311
  and vitamin A deficiency 309,
    335
Mortality 9, 58, 325–43
  age of death 327
  and albumin concentration 107
  anthropometric prediction of
    213, 217, 225
  causes 167
  after discharge from hospital
    165
  and fatty liver 63
  and ferritin 140
  in hospital 171–6
  hypothermia and 88
  hypoglycaemia and 113
  immunization and 374
  and maternal height 203
  after measles 165
  and nutritional state 311
  in PDS 298
  prevention of 367
  prognostic factors 175

  and skin lesions 71
  sanitation and *272*, 373
  and transferrin saturation 139
  and treatment with iron 139,
    173, 310
  trends in 364
Motility of gut 68
Mothers, demands on 369
Motor skills 355
Mucosae
  changes in 1, 5, 212
  of gut 66, 67, 89
  in zinc deficiency 311
  see also Conjunctival damage,
    Gut mucosa, Skin
Multiple deficiency states 3, 4, 8,
    9, 155
Muscle
  area in arm 213–14
  biopsies
    distribution of water in 33
    electrolytes 42, 45
    magnesium 48
    metabolites 87
    protein/DNA 28
    respiration 86
  fibre types 122
  mass
    in Bolivian children 214
    in PEM 27–8, 34, 107
    increase in growth 251
  protein
    breakdown 91, 93, 99, 293
    depletion 115
    synthesis 90, 120, 122
Myanmar
  feeding in diarrhoea 303
  health programmes 384
  lactation 269
  mortality 326
Myelin 75, 121
Myocardium
  damage in K deficiency 43
  contractility 56
  see also Cardiac

NADP 159
NADPH 142
National Center for Health
    Statistics 192 *et seq.*, 214
N/E (non-essential/essential
    amino acids) 108
Neonatal deaths 328
Nepal
  growth velocity 195, 197
  vitamin A supplementation
    335
Nephrotic syndrome 70, 298
Net protein utilization (NPU)
    247–8
Neutrophils 138
Nervous system 74–5, 344
Neutron activation analysis 28,
    34
Nicotinic acid
  and fatty liver 64
  and skin lesions 71
  see also Pellagra

Nigeria
  biochemical tests 106, 107
  birth weight 306
  breast feeding 376
  essential fatty acid deficiency 141
  iron supplements 310
  magnesium deficiency 48
  mental development 348
  mortality 176
  schistosomiasis 307
  somatomedin 119
  weaning diets 157
Nitrogen
  balance 89, 91–2, 94, 237 *et
    seq.*, 243, 293
  excretion in urine 109
  extracellular 34
  in faeces 94
  metabolism 89–96
  in whole body 33
Non-essential amino acids 108
  see also Amino acids, Cystine,
    Glycine
Non-protein nitrogen
  in breast milk 244
Noxae 138, 155, 158–9
Nutrients, classification of 15, *16*
Nutritional Rehabilitation
    Centres 165
  see also Rehabilitation

Obesity 177, 254
Obligatory loss of nitrogen 243
Oedema
  amino acids and loss of 150
  causal factors 36–7, 70,
    146–54
  characteristics in PEM 35, 36
  and classification of PEM *1, 2,
    5,* 167
  and copper deficiency 130
  experimental 97
  in famine 3, 32, 97, 147–50
  and glutathione peroxidase
    activity 142
  in hookworm infestation 307
  and hypovolaemia 56, *151*
  and leakiness of membranes 137
  after measles 94
  and mental development 351
  prognostic significance 175,
    334, 337
  pulmonary 169
  and selenium deficiency 131
  and sodium retention 150–2
  in trichuriasis 307
  and vanadium deficiency 132
  and vitamin E deficiency 140
  and zinc deficiency 127
Oral rehydration 168–9, 300 *et
    seq.*, 374
Organs, *see individual organs*
Organ pattern 26, 85
Osmotic
  stress 136
  diarrhoea 169, 299, 302
  see also Colloid osmotic
    pressure

Osteomalacia 47
Osteoporosis and copper
    deficiency 130
Otitis 170, 294, 305
Overcrowding, risk from 334,
    375
Ovulation and breast feeding 279
Oxidation
  of amino acids 94, 98, 117
  of protein 230
Oxidative
  drive 244
  phosphorylation 87
  stress 159
Oxygen uptake
  demand
    and anaemia 171
    and cardiac function 59
  see Energy metabolism

Pakistan, stunting in 202
Pan American Health
    Organization, child
    mortality 330
Pancreas
  in PEM 65–6
  enzymes of 89
  in infection 299
Papua-New Guinea
  Ascariasis 306
  breast milk outputs 262
Parasites, intestinal 306 *et seq.*
  as cause of anaemia 59
Parenteral nutrition 299
Parity, effect on milk output 268
Partial breast feeding, *see* Breast
    feeding
Participation, *see* Community
Paternalism of aid 367
P/E (protein/energy) ratio 158,
    242 *et seq.*
Pellagra
  infantile *2,* 3–5
  skin lesions 71, 160
Penicillin 170
Perinatal deaths 328
Permeability
  of capillaries 98, 148 *et seq.*
  of cell membranes 32, 137, 141
  of gut mucosa 294, 299
  of red cells 136
  see also Leakiness
Peroxidation of lipids 138, 140,
    179
Persistent diarrhoea syndrome
    (PDS) 298–9, 374
  and giardiasis 307
  and measles 304
  sanitation and 373
Pertussis vaccination 305, 374–5
Peru
  copper deficiency 130
  infections and growth 317
  mental development 348
  stunting 201
Phenylalanine metabolism 96
Phosphorus (phosphate) 49–50
  and catch-up growth 251

and rickets 180
and stunting 202
Phospholipids in red cell
    membrane 141
Physical activity, *see* Activity
Phytate 129
Pituitary 115, 116, 151
Placenta, in malaria 306
Planning, family, *see* Family
    planning
Plantains, in diet 156, 209, 279,
    281, 282
Plasma volume 56–8, 150, 172
Plasmodium sp. 306
Play, in treatment of PEM 353
  see also Activity
Pneumococcus sp. 170, 375
Pneumocystis carnii 170
Pneumonia, as cause of death
    329
  see Respiratory infections
Policy, nutrition 155, 203–4
  on breast feeding 273
  stunting and 190, 224
  targeting of 368
Poliomyelitis vaccination 375
Politics and PEM 9, 361–2
Polyamines 75
Polyunsaturated fatty acids 138,
    179, 180
  see also Essential fatty acids
Population increase
  effect on deaths 326, 363
  and fertility control 379, 381
  food production and 362
Post-neonatal deaths 329, 332
Positive
  deviants 11
  discrimination 367
Potassium 41–4
  concentration and capacity 15
  in catch-up growth 251
  depletion 33
  efflux from red cells 136
  and insulin response 113
  and lean body mass 33
  and oedema 150, 153, 155
  in rehydration solution 301
  in treatment 169, 173, 177, 180
  and sodium excretion 70
  in whole body 28
Poverty
  as basis for aid 366
  as cause of PEM 4, *9,* 362
  and stunting 187, 199, 200, 225
Prealbumin 106
Prediction
  of future weight 378
  of long-term outcome 218
  of metabolic rate 20
Predictors, *see* Anthropometry,
    Cut-off points, Growth
    monitoring, Indicators,
    Mortality, Prognosis, Risk
Pregnancy
  and brain growth 344
  supplementation in 355–7, 376
  weight gain in 333

Prematurity
  cost of weight gain 234
  as cause of death 328
  maintenance energy
    requirement in 233
  and protein synthesis 91
Prevalence
  of kwashiorkor 156
  of infection 311 *et seq.*
  method of estimating 218 *et
    seq.*
  and sanitation 312
  of wasting and stunting 195,
    203, 222 *et seq.*
Primary health care 2, 165, 362,
    382 *et seq.*
Prognosis
  and albumin level 107
  in early stage of treatment
    174, 176–7
  and ferritin level 139
  and oedema 36
  and selenium deficiency 132
  and skin lesions 71
  and weight deficit 188
  see also Risk
Programming of growth 198–9
Prolactin 279
Proline 9
Prospective studies
  of growth *200*
  of mortality 336
Protective factors
  in breast milk 270 *et seq.*, 279
  against free radicals 138
Protein
  absorption in infections 294
  breakdown *89*
    in potassium deficiency 43
    in infections 92, 293
  in breast milk 265 *et seq.*
  cellular 34
  deficiency of
    as cause of kwashiorkor 2,
      3–4, 155 *et seq.*
    in hookworm infestation 307
    and SmC levels 121
  tests of 105, 107
  depletion 108
  diurnal rhythm of metabolism
    84
  in foods 244 *et seq.*
  in hair bulbs 73
  metabolism of 89–96
  oxidation of 83
  quality
    in foods 246 *et seq.*
    and stunting 201
  requirements 95, 229 *et seq.*
  reserves 338
  in serum 5
  in skin 72, 73
  structural 34
  synthesis
    energy cost of 233 *et seq.*
    in infection 295
    insulin, effect on 115
    in malaria 306

  in potassium deficiency 43
  see also Albumin, Amino
    acids, Collagen, Muscle,
    Nitrogen
Proteases 43, 108
Proteoglycans
  in kidney 70
  in cartilage 118
Proteus sp. 170
Pseudocholinesterase 107
Pseudomonas 170
Psychomotor stimulation 183
Psychosocial deprivation 9, 117,
    165, 174, 200
  stimulation 356
Puberty 118, 188, 198–200
Public health
  basic system 384–5
  distinction between
    kwashiorkor and marasmus,
    relevance to 5, 160
  improvements in 363
  infections and policy for 313
  role of health sector 386
Pulse rate, *see* Heart rate
Punjab nutrition intervention
    339
Pygmies, SmC in 201
Pyelitis 170
Pyloric stenosis and mental
    development 352
Pyrexia 170, 292, 375

Quality of protein in foods 246 *et
    seq.*

Rash, eczematous 180
  see also Dermatosis, Skin
    changes
Receptors
  of hormones 112, 113, 118,
    121
  of volume 152
  and growth 201
Rectal prolapse, in trichuriasis
    307
Red blood cells
  destruction of 59, 60
  fragility 60, 131
  glutathione reductase in 142
  life-span 60
  membrane transport in 136 *et
    seq.*, 144
  volume 54, 57, 58
  see also Anaemia
Reference
  bases 16–21
    for BMR 85
    for cardiac output 55
    for plasma and red cell
      volumes 56
  pattern of amino acids 246
  standards for anthropometry
    191 *et seq.*, 213 *et seq.*, 231,
    273
    Harvard *6*, 192
    NCHS 192
    velocity 194, 274

Rehabilitation
  centres for 165, 182–3
  from malnutrition 177–81
  and mental development 344
Rehydration
  intravenous *169*
  oral *300*–4, 374
Renal, *see* Kidney
Reproduction rate 363, 379–*81*
Requirements
  for calcium 46
  for energy 157, 229–41, 273
  for magnesium 49
  for phosphorus 50
  for protein 155–7, 241–51
Resources, human 204, 366
Respiratory infections 274,
    305
  as cause of death 329, 334
  and iron deficiency 310
  immunization for 374, 375
  and vitamin A deficiency 309
  treatment 334
Retardation
  of brain growth 74
  of development 26
  of linear growth 189–91, 195 *et
    seq.*
  see also Stunting
Retinol, *see* Vitamin A
Retinol-binding protein
  as marker of PEM 106
  synthesis of 304
Reye's syndrome 62, 159
Rhesus haemolytic disease 140
Riboflavin
  deficiency
    and anaemia 59
    mucosal changes 212
    in PEM 291
    and glutathione reductase 142
    in infections 294
Rice
  diet in PDS 299
  in rehydration solutions 302
  in weaning foods 281, 282
Rickets 9, 47, 180, 251
Risk
  assessment of 336
  of bottle feeding 272, 276
  breast feeding, reduction by
    279
  of early discharge 181
  indicators of 213, 217
  of infections 291
  and oedema 175, 212
  of postneonatal deaths 332
  strategies 367
  in vitamin A deficiency 309
RNA synthesis 127
Rome report on energy and
    protein requirements 230 *et
    seq.*, 267
Rotavirus 271, 294, 297, 373
Rwanda, *Cryptosporidium*
    infection 308

Safe level of intake 239, 245, 248

Sahel
  kwashiorkor in 156
  mortality in 222, 224, 326
  P/E ratio in foods 156, 250
  stunting in 224
Saint Lucia
  rehabilitation of PEM 181
  trichuriasis 307
Salivary glands, atrophy 65
Salmonella sp. 170, 297
Sample size 218
Sampling, of milk 265
Sanitation
  effect on mortality 272, 335,
    372 *et seq.*
  and prevalence of infection
    291, 312, 313
Scavenging, of free radicals 141
  et seq.
Schistosomiasis 307
School achievement 346–8, 354,
  356
Scoring of malnutrition 5, 106
Screening 193, 194, 221, 339, 377
  et seq.
  see also Growth monitoring
Scurvy 130, 141
Secretory IgA, *see* IgA
Secular changes in height 199
Selection of PHC workers 383
Selenium 126, 131–2, 159
  and glutathione peroxidase
    142
  and iodinase 121
  and red cell fragility 60
  in treatment 172, 180
  and type of deficiency *16*
Self-reliance, promotion of 365,
  366
Senecio poisoning 35, 149
Senegal
  birth weight 333
  mortality 325, 334
  thyroid studies 122
Sensitivity
  of anthropometric indicators
    217 *et seq.*, 337, 338
  of biochemical tests 106
  of measures of zinc deficiency
    129
Septicaemia
  and iron therapy 310
  in PEM 170
Serine, in collagen 251
Sesame, as antioxidant 282
SGA infants, risk of death 332
Shigella sp. and diarrhoea 294,
  295, 297, 298, 303, 304, 375
Shock, hypovolaemic 55
Siblings, studies on 348
Sick cell syndrome 45, 136, 137,
  153
Single photon absorptiometry 46
  see also Bone, Calcium
Skeletal growth, *see* Maturation,
  Stunting
Skin
  in copper deficiency 130

and oedema 6, 71
changes in PEM *1, 5*, 155, 159,
  160, 212
and protein loss 28, 34
and supplementary feeding
  201
in zinc deficiency 127, 128
Skinfolds 33, 42, 231, 268
Sleep 83
Small for dates, *see* Low
  birthweight
Social development 363
  research 374
  see also Poverty
Sociocultural environment
  and growth 318
  and infection 290, 313
  and mental development 344,
    347, 352
  and mortality 335
  and type of malnutrition 8
Sodium
  in blood, during treatment
    174
  excretion 70, 151
  influx to red cells 136
  intracellular 137
  load 150, 169, 177
  in muscle biopsies 45
  in oral rehydration solutions
    301
  pump 43, 67, 136
    see also ATPase
  retention 151, 153
  transport 143
  in whole body 44
  see also Hyponatraemia
Somalia, iron deficiency 310
Somatomedin 112, 115, 117–21,
  200, 201
Sorghum, in weaning foods 281,
  283
Souring, in preparation of
  weaning foods 282
South Africa
  magnesium 48
  mental development 348, 349
  nutrition education 372
  potassium 40
  red cell membranes 136
  somatomedin 119
Soya
  allergy to proteins of 299
  milk in lactose intolerance 180
Spacing of births 380
  see also Reproduction rate
Specificity of indicators 217 *et
  seq.*, 337, 338
Spectrum of malnutrition 4, 138
Sri Lanka
  mortality 326
  primary health care 384
  social development 363
Standards, anthropometric 191 *et
  seq.*
  see also Harvard, NCHS,
    Reference standards
Stanford-Binet test 347

Staples 156
  see Maize, Plantain, Rice,
    Wheat
Starch, in weaning foods 281
Starling hypothesis 146, 150
Staphylococcus 170
Starvation 115
  see also Famine
Stimulation
  and nutritional state 10
  and mental development 353
    et seq.
Stomach volume 177, 281
Storage, of energy 233
Strength, of grip 348
Streptococcus sp.
  haemophilus 283
  and otitis 170
  and pneumonia 334
Stress, vulnerability to 345
Strongyloides 308
Stunting
  and diarrhoea 203
  in height 16, 26, 121, 127, 157,
    189 *et seq.*, 222 *et seq.*
  and infections 317
  and mental development 351
  and trichuriasis 307
  see also Growth, Height
Subclinical malnutrition 4, 5, 14,
  105, 248
Subsidies, for food 367
Sucking, and stimulation of
  lactation 270
Suckling's dilemma 275
Sucrase 67
Sudan
  aflatoxins 138
  breast feeding 273
  folic acid deficiency 59
  heights of children 199
  infections and growth 316 *et
    seq.*
  mortality 176
  PEM
    dermatosis 6
    prevalence of different
      forms 7
    supplementary feeding 377
Sugar
  in blood, *see* Glucose
  in oral rehydration solutions
    301, 302
Sulphation, of proteoglycans
  70
Sulphur amino acids
  and cartilage 91
  and stunting 202
Superoxide
  dismutase 131, 141, 142
  free radical 138
Supplementary feeding
  and activity of children 240
  and birth weight 333
  of breast-fed children 263, 275
    et seq.
  and growth in height 199–201
  with iron 346

Supplementary feeding – *cont'd.*
  and mental development 355, 356
  of mothers 268, 269, 356
  and mortality 339
  and prevention of PEM 376
  in primary health care 382
  with vitamin A 335
  with zinc 311
Surface area 17, 18
Survivors of PEM, mental development 344, 348
Survival, policy for 368, 386
Synapses 75
  see also Dendrites

Tachycardia 137
Taiwan nutritional supplementation 355
Tanzania
  feeding patterns 278
  vitamin A supplements 335
Targeting 367 *et seq.*
  of food supplements 376
  of oral rehydration 374
  by village health workers 384
Taurine 68
Technical cooperation 366
Technology, village 281
Teenage mothers 376
Temperature, body 84, 88, 171
  see also Pyrexia
Test weighing 261 *et seq.*
Tetanus, neonatal 377
Tetany, 46, 48
Thailand
  health volunteers 384
  iron dosage in PEM 180
  milk intake 261
  nitrogen balance 239
  phosphate deficiency 49
  plasma volume 57
  red cell membranes 136
  selenium 131
  somatomedin 119
  stunting 199
Therapeutic tests 153
Therapy, *see* Treatment
Thermic effect of food 84, 232, 252
Thiabendazole, for worms 308
Threshold responses 204
Thymulin 296
Thymus, atrophy 127, 296
Thyroid
  hormones 112, 121–3
  releasing hormone 122
  stimulating hormone 122
T-lymphocytes, *see* Lymphocytes
Tolerance tests 67
  see also Glucose
Toxicity of iron 139, 319, 311
Toxins of *E. coli* 297
  see also Aflatoxins
Trace elements 40, 126–32, 141 *et seq.*
  in catch-up growth 251
  in human milk 267

in treatment 173
  see also individual trace elements
Traditional patterns of feeding 276–9, 376
Training programmes
  for community health workers 384
  and technical cooperation 366
Transferrin
  as test for PEM 106, 107
  in malaria 306
  saturation 59
  synthesis 115
Transport proteins, *see* Carrier proteins
Transthyretin 106
  see Retinol-binding protein
Trauma, *see* Injury
Treatment 164–83
  of dehydration *300–4*
  with iron, effects of 310
  of magnesium deficiency 48, 49
  of respiratory tract infections 334
  of worms 308
Trichuriasis
  effects of 307
  and stunting 197
  and zinc deficiency 311
Triglycerides
  lipase 64
  in liver 63
  in serum 64
  synthesis 233
  see also Fat
Tryptophan deficiency 71
Tube wells 373
Tuberculosis 170, 291
  diagnosis 305
  in Expanded Programme of Immunization 375
  and liver fat 62
  and PDS 297
Turkey
  cardiac function 54
  PEM 7
Tyrosine,
  in hair 73
  metabolism 96

Uganda
  activity of children 239
  albumin levels 114, 117, 146, 147, 149
  basal metabolic rate 85
  biochemical tests 105
  brain weights 74
  cardiac failure 56
  diarrhoea, risk from 334
  diet 155
  fatty liver 61
  growth pattern 197, 201
  health services, utilization 383
  hormones 112, 114, 115
  hypothermia 88
  mental development 348

mortality 107, 176
P/E ratio of diet 248
PEM, characteristics 7
prediction of death 337
psychosocial factors 10
red cell membranes 136
weaning foods 283
Ulceration, of skin 71
Ultrasound, and liver size 61
Ultraviolet radiation 160
Unemployment
  in Glasgow 204
  in India 203
UNICEF
  breast-feeding policy 273
  child survival policy 369, 387
  code of practice for marketing 260, 376
  GOBI programme 371
  and oral rehydration 301
  prevalence of PEM 222
  State of the World's Children 362, 385
  targets 387
  village health workers, tasks 384
United Nations
  anthropometry, report on applications 221
  Declaration of Human Rights 363
  mortality statistics 327, 329
  PEM, early surveys 2
  rights of children 205
  Subcommittee on Nutrition 222, 226
  targets 365
  see also UNICEF, UNU, FAO, WHO
United Nations University (UNU)
  report on requirements 230
Urbanization
  and breastfeeding 278, 279, 376
  and education 372
  code of practice of marketing 376
  and feeding patterns 277
  and transmission of infections 375
Urea
  enzymes 94, 244
  excretion 3, 109
  in human milk 244, 267
  production 172
  recycling 95, 244
Urine, estimates of intake from 212
  see also Creatinine, Nitrogen balance
Utilization
  efficiency of 269
  of protein 96, 243, 252
  of urea 244

Vaccines 374, 375
  see also Immunization

Vanadium 132
Variability
  of breast milk
    energy content 260
    fat content 266
    volume 264
  of composition of growth 251
  of energy expenditure 241, 244
  of growth velocity 194, 218
  of intakes 241
  of P/E ratios 242
  of protein requirements 250
Variables, confounding 23, 291,
    336, 352
Vegetable
  oils 179, 282
  proteins
    as allergens 299
    in diet 120, 129, 179
Velocity of growth 194 *et seq.*,
    244, 337, 338, 378
Venezuela, gastrointestinal
    changes 66
Veno-occlusive disease 35, 149
Vertical programmes 385
Village
  health workers 334, 383 *et seq.*
  preparation of weaning foods 281
  weighing of children 378
Villi, of small gut
  atrophy 67 *et seq.*
  damage from infections 307–8
  morphology in diarrhoea
    298–9
Viscosity, of weaning foods
    281–2, 303
Vitamins 3, *16*
  deficiency and anaemia 59
  and fatty liver 64
  see also individual vitamins
Vitamin A
  absorption 295
  as antioxidant 140
  deficiency 9, 291, 292
    early signs 212
    treatment 171
  function 294
  and measles 304
  and morbidity 309
  and mortality
    in the community 335 *et seq.*
    in hospital 177
  and skin lesions 71
Vitamin B complex
  in catch-up growth 251
  in treatment 172
Vitamin B$_{12}$
  absorption 295
  and haemopoiesis 59
Vitamin C
  as antioxidant 140

see also Scurvy
Vitamin D
  in catch-up growth 251
  and rickets 47, 80
  see also Rickets
Vitamin E
  as antioxidant 140, 159, 172
  and mortality 177
  in recovery diet 180
  and red cell fragility 60, 131
VO$_2$ max. 202, 203
Vomiting, treatment 169, 303
Vulnerable periods, *see* Critical
    periods

Wasting 189 *et seq.*
  and mental development 351
  prevalence 222
Water
  absorption in diarrhoea 301
  in body 31
    distribution 32
    expression of 29, 30
    increase with high energy
      feeding 173
    measurement of 29, 37
  doubly labelled 234 *et seq.*
  in lean body mass 33
  supplies of 363, 372 *et seq.*
Weaning
  definition 275
  diets
    contamination 373
    deficiencies 44
    energy density 281–3
    iron in 310
    protein quality 247, 255
    staples 156, *see also* Maize,
      Plantain, Rice, Wheat
    and onset of kwashiorkor 3,
      10–11
  Weanling's dilemma 275
    and diarrhoea 313
Wechsler Intelligence Scale 347
Weight
  as basis of comparisons 18
  of brain 73
  see Assessment, Growth
Wellcome classification 2, 5, 6,
    36, 137
Wheat
  as staple 156
  in weaning foods 281, 282
Work capacity 202, 204
  and iron deficiency 61
Women, special role 368 *et seq.*
World Bank 362, 363, 367, 371
World Food Programme 377
World Health Organization
  anthropometric methods,
    report 213

breast-feeding policy 273
code of practice for marketing
    260, 376
collaborative breast-feeding
    study, report 260, 266
diarrhoea, monograph 313
disease statistics 334
energy and protein
    requirements, report 157,
    230 *et seq.*
health sector, role 386
oral rehydration, promotion of
    301, 302
persistent diarrhoea (PDS),
    report 298
prevalence of PEM, 216, 222
reference data for
    anthropometry 192, 194
risk approach, report 367
surveys of PEM 2
survival, policy 368, 387
Wound infections, susceptibility
    to, 290

Xerophthalmia
  and mortality 335
  and risk of infections 309
  see also Vitamin A
Xerosis of skin 71
Xylose excretion test 68

Yams, in weaning foods 279
Yeast protein 96
Yoghurt 283

Zaïre 3, 7
  albumin levels 107, *176*
  anaemia 59
  cardiac function 54
  gut mucosa 66
  hospital stay 180
  lactation 279
  morbidity and growth 318
  mortality 58, 176, 325, 330,
    338
  oedema 58
  plasma and red cell volumes
    57, 58
  potassium and magnesium 169
  selenium 131
  treatment, dietary 180
Zinc 126–30
  absorption 129, 295
  body content 40
  deficiency of 291
    and fluid loss 298
    and skin lesions 71
  and growth 15, 180, 251
  and infections 294, 311
  protective role of 159, 160
  and sodium pump 137